The Exercise Professional's Guide to Optimizing Health

STRATEGIES FOR PREVENTING AND REDUCING CHRONIC DISEASE

Jeffrey L. Roitman

EdD, FACSM

Chair and Associate Professor
Department of Exercise and Sports Science
Rockhurst University
Kansas City, MO

Tom LaFontaine

PhD, ACSM RCEP, NSCA-CPT, FACSM, FAACVPR

Clinical Exercise Physiologist, PREVENT Consulting Services, LLC
Optimus: The Center for Health
Columbia, MO

. Wolters Kluwer | Lippincott Williams & Wilkins
Health

Philadelphia • Baltimore • New York • London
Buenos Aires • Hong Kong • Sydney • Tokyo

Acquisitions Editor: Emily Lupash
Product Manager: Andrea M. Klingler
Marketing Manager: Allison Powell
Designer: Stephen Druding
Compositor: Aptara, Inc.

First Edition

Library of Congress Cataloging-in-Publication Data

Roitman, Jeffrey L., author.
 The Exercise Professional's Guide to Optimizing Health : Strategies
for Preventing and Reducing Chronic Disease / Jeffrey L. Roitman,
Tom LaFontaine.
    p. ; cm.
 Includes bibliographical references and index.
 ISBN 978-0-7817-7548-9 (pbk. : alkaline paper)
 1. Chronic diseases. 2. Chronic diseases–Psychological aspects.
 3. Chronic diseases–Prevention. 4. Physical fitness. 5. Diet therapy.
I. LaFontaine, Tom, 1946- author. II. Title.
 [DNLM: 1. Chronic Disease. 2. Chronic Disease–prevention & control.
 3. Diet, Reducing. 4. Exercise. 5. Physical Fitness. WT 500]
 RC108.R65 2010
 616′.044–dc22   2010045485

DISCLAIMER

My wife Kay, daughters Lindsay and Shaia, and granddaughters Reilly and Delaney have been the light of my life and my inspiration. My staff and now my students have taught me more than I have ever taught them. I dedicate my efforts on this book to them.
— Jeff Roitman

My wife, Linda, has been my reliable and supportive partner for the past 25 years. My 90-year-old mother has been an inspiration to me throughout my life, particularly during the past 11 years as she has kept her spirit and sense of humor after devastating strokes in the summer of 2000. I dedicate my efforts on this book to them.
— Tom LaFontaine

The etiologies, risk factors, and pathophysiology common to the array of diseases discussed and highlighted in this book are pertinent to exercise professionals and all students of exercise science. The most common and prevalent of the chronic metabolic diseases affecting the population of the United States are discussed in this book. The latest mortality statistics show that almost 36% of all deaths are from the diseases highlighted in *The Exercise Professional's Guide to Optimizing Health: Strategies for Preventing and Reducing Chronic Disease*, and that more than 50% of adults have at least one of these chronic diseases (1). In fact, they are so common that many are risk factors for each other. The direct and indirect costs of identification, diagnosis, and treatment of these diseases and disorders amount to hundreds of billions of dollars annually (1). Health care in the United States is more expensive because of the incidence of these diseases and because of the distinct lack of practicing healthy lifestyles among our general population. The chances that an exercise professional will encounter someone with one or more of these diseases or someone who is at risk for one or more of these diseases are almost 100% during the course of a given year.

The importance of knowing about the diseases and the disease processes, as well as working effectively with people who have them, cannot be understated. *The Exercise Professional's Guide to Optimizing Health: Strategies for Preventing and Reducing Chronic Disease* is designed and written to be of practical value to exercise professionals who work directly with clients who have or who are at risk for these chronic diseases, especially coronary artery disease and other cardiovascular disease, obesity, diabetes, and metabolic disease. Exercise professionals who actively work with clients and patients will encounter people with these diseases every day. This book is meant to provide information and tools that should enable them to promote prevention and to prescribe safe and effective exercise programs for persons with these conditions.

This book is also aimed for undergraduate and some graduate students in Exercise Science courses. We believe (and statistics support) that the frequency of their encounters with this population will increase significantly during the course of the next 10 years; thus, the importance of being able to work with populations effectively becomes progressively more critical. We have attempted to consolidate the scientific information so that it is neither too deep nor too superficial. Some of the physiology and pathophysiology may seem difficult and detailed, but we believe that knowledge of the fundamental basis of the causes of these chronic diseases will help professionals to understand the effects and actions of exercise and diet on the disease process. This, in turn, should enable them to provide better, more effective, and more complete programs and information for their clients and patients.

ORGANIZATION

Chapter 1 is an overview of the epidemiology of chronic disease and of the risk factors for the diseases discussed in this book. It is meant to briefly introduce the science of epidemiology. This chapter presents risk factors in the context of both their influence on the development and progression of the disease and the effects of positively modifying the risk factor. It attempts to present the extent and seriousness of the problem of chronic disease in the United States.

Part I introduces the basic concepts of pathophysiology common to these diseases (Chapter 2) and the preventive effects of exercise and nutrition (Chapters 3 and 4) on the pathophysiology chronic disease.

Part II covers the most prevalent chronic diseases commonly encountered in daily practice by exercise professionals. Atherosclerosis (Chapter 5), obesity (Chapter 6), diabetes and metabolic syndrome (Chapter 7), hypertension (Chapter 8), and dyslipidemia (Chapter 9) are the core chapters of this section. Each chapter is organized by sections on epidemiology and pathophysiology, followed by a comprehensive discussion focused on the efficacy of exercise with respect to modifying the disease process and prevention. After that is a section on specific recommendations for prescribing effective exercise programs for this particular disease entity and the accompanying pathophysiology. The information about exercise prescription is based on the large body of research on exercise and its effects on the pathophysiology of the specific disease process.

The final section of this book, Part III, contains a chapter on behavior change (Chapter 10) and a summary chapter on exercise prescription using information from the pertinent chapter and the appropriate exercise prescription for each of the conditions that we discussed (Chapter 11). The critical importance of effectively intervening in the behavior change process is perhaps the most important piece of this puzzle. Chapter 10 summarizes major theories and research that relate to changing behavior, specifically exercise behavior. We feel that this information is not only important but also crucial to the exercise professionals for their work with people with chronic disease. Chapter 11 brings all of the exercise prescription information that is pertinent to each condition to one place in the book. It is a "digest" of all of those exercise prescriptions specific to each disease.

FEATURES

The Exercise Professional's Guide to Optimizing Health contains many pedagogical features that will help students clarify and apply the material presented to them.

Abbreviations—This list at the beginning of each chapter provides the key terms and their common abbreviation.

Introduction—This section provides the basic "entryway" to the material in each chapter. The Introduction is meant to introduce the importance to and prevalence of the specific disease in the population.

Did You Know Boxes?—These are used throughout the book to highlight and expand upon important information. The intent is to further explain something discussed in the text and/or expand on it in a way that will be informative to those wishing to know more.

Key Points—These boxes highlight important points made in the text using brief, succinct statements.

Optimize—These boxes provide the "optimal" levels, measurements, and lifestyle actions in relation to prevention or reduction of the disease being discussed.

Digging Deeper—Each chapter has a concluding section that expands significantly on the discussion of a topic presented in the chapter with respect to the literature and research as well as the technical and scientific level of the information. This section is meant to pique the interest of readers who would like to know more about these topics.

Significant Research—This box highlights two of what are considered to be seminal or very important articles relating to the information presented in the chapter. Our purpose here is to draw attention to the literature in a way that illustrates the practical nature of sometimes complex and technical articles that are often avoided and unread by exercise professionals. There is much practical and useful information to be gained by perusing research literature in exercise science.

ADDITIONAL RESOURCES

The Exercise Professional's Guide to Optimizing Health includes additional resources for both instructors and students that are available on the book's companion Web site at http://thepoint.lww.com/Roitman.

INSTRUCTORS

Approved adopting instructors will be given access to the following additional resources:

- Full Text Online
- PowerPoint lecture outlines
- Image bank

STUDENTS

Students who have purchased *The Exercise Professional's Guide to Optimizing Health* have access to the Full Text Online. Purchasers of the text can access the searchable Full Text by going to the book's Web site at http://thePoint.lww.com. See the inside front cover of this text for more details, including the passcode you will need to gain access to the Web site.

Jeffrey L. Roitman
Tom LaFontaine

REFERENCE

1. Centers for Disease Control and Prevention. Chronic disease prevention and health promotion. Washington, DC: Centers for Disease Control and Prevention. Available at: www.cdc.gov/chronicdisease/overview/index.htm. Accessed November 11, 2010.

Katherine Allogia, RN
Personal Trainer
Pilates Instructor
Palm Beach Gardens, FL

Lisa Marie Bernardo, PhD, MPH, RN, HFS
Associate Professor
Health and Community Systems
University of Pittsburgh School of Nursing
Pittsburgh, PA

Kathy Carter, MS, RD/LD
Instructor
Athens Technical College
Athens, GA

Randal P. Claytor, PhD
Associate Professor
Miami University
Oxford, OH

J. Larry Durstine, PhD, FACSM
Distinguished Professor
Chair, Department of Exercise Science
Codirector, Preventative Exercise Program
University of South Carolina
Columbia, SC

Faith Faatz, MS
Adjunct Faculty
Health Fitness Specialist
Minnesota School of Business
Plymouth, MN

Neil F. Gordon, MD, PhD, FACSM
Chief Medical and Science Officer
Nationwide Better Health
Savannah, GA

Wayne Jacobs, PhD
Dean, School of Education
Kinesiology
LeTourneau University
Longview, TX

Janene Mae Jaynes, AFAA Certified, LMT Certified
Teacher and Instructor of Fitness and Massage Physical Education
Utah Valley University
Baysport Cooperate Wellness at Novell
Orem, UT

Michael R. Kushnick, PhD, HFS
Associate Professor of Exercise Physiology
Director Exercise Biochemistry and Physiology Laboratory
Applied Health Sciences and Wellness
Ohio University
Athens, OH

Paul E. Luebbers, PhD
Assistant Professor
Emporia State University
Emporia, KS

Lesley Lutes, PhD
Assistant Professor
East Carolina University
Greenville, NC

Michael Massis, MA, CSCS, CPT, CMT, CMTech
Lecturer/Consultant
M2-Training Systems
Chula Vista, CA
Director
Personal Fitness Training Program
Mueller College
San Diego, CA

Richard B. Parr, EdD, FACSM
Professor
Central Michigan University
Mount Pleasant, MI

Janet Rankin, PhD, FACSM
Professor
Virginia Tech
Blacksburg, VA

Gail Sas
Fitness Trainer
Fitness Therapy Certified
Health Quest Unlimited
Buellton, CA

Paul Sorace, MS
Clinical Exercise Physiologist
Hackensack University Medical Center
Hackensack, NJ

Paul S. Visich, PhD, MPH
Professor
Central Michigan University
Mount Pleasant, MI

Acknowledgments

We acknowledge the valuable assistance of Tisha Polsinelli, one of the best, most knowledgeable, and most talented personal trainers that we know, for her review of these chapters in their earliest stages. The assistance of many professionals, including Dr. Richard Parr, Margaret Moore, and Kay N. Grossman, was invaluable in providing ongoing review, revision, and suggestions that improved the manuscript in many ways. Our Product Manager, Andrea Klingler, has been vital and critical to this effort; without her experience, gentle prodding, and professional expertise, the manuscript and the book was unlikely to have become a reality.

Finally, I (JR) acknowledge the 25-year relationship with my coauthor, Tom LaFontaine, who has been a mentor and a constant reminder of what is right with respect to exercise, nutrition, and healthy lifestyle. Tom never had time for this book but always made time.

Jeff Roitman
Tom LaFontaine

Contents

Introduction to the Epidemiology of Chronic Disease and Risk Factor Theory

ABBREVIATIONS

BMI	Body mass index		Detection, Evaluation, and
CAD	Coronary artery disease		Treatment of High Blood
CVD	Cardiovascular disease		Pressure
DASH	Dietary Approaches to Stop	LDL	Low-density lipoprotein
	Hypertension	Lp(a)	Lipoprotein a
HDL	High-density lipoprotein	MetS	Metabolic syndrome
JNC7	The Seventh Report of the Joint	WHR	Waist-to-hip ratio
	National Committee on Prevention,		

Chronic disease is defined as a disease that develops over a long period of time and persists. In some cases, if the disease is aggressively treated, the signs and symptoms of the disease may resolve. In other cases, the disease process is chronically present, and despite treatment and symptom relief, the pathophysiology does not go away. Once the genome for a disease has been "expressed," the potential for pathophysiology is known to be present (15,33,34).

Type 2 diabetes is an example. Type 2 diabetes is treated medically with hypoglycemic agents (medications) that lower blood glucose, for example, metformin (Glucophage) or insulin. Neither treatment makes type 2 diabetes go away, but can help control blood glucose; thus, they also may provide some control over the pathophysiology of type 2 diabetes (33). On the other hand, optimal lifestyle management of type 2 diabetes with appropriate amounts of daily exercise, low fat, high fiber, low processed carbohydrate diet, and weight loss has been shown to be successful in reversing the pathophysiology that is associated with type 2 diabetes, as well as complete resolution of some signs and symptoms (15,33,34). No pharmacological/medical treatment has been shown to be equally effective. In many cases, this is because pharmacological agents are the only treatment utilized. In other cases, it is because any lifestyle change is not truly optimal.

In this chapter we will discuss the risk factors associated with heart disease. We will discuss the impact of exercise on those risk factors (if appropriate) and the optimal level of each of those risk factors for prevention of heart disease. It is important to point out that even in the face of eliminating the pathophysiology that is associated with heart disease, susceptibility to those processes remains present. People, who aggressively and optimally change their lifestyle, may diminish or eliminate the disease process. However, if they stop the optimal lifestyle behavior(s) they will, in all likelihood, once again experience the pathophysiology and have signs and symptoms similar to their previous disease state.

RISK FACTOR THEORY

Risk factors for disease are discovered and clarified by "epidemiological" research. Epidemiology is the study of factors ("risk factors") associated with an increased risk of disease (both chronic and communicable) in a large population. Epidemiology does not directly determine "cause and effect", for example, what causes a disease, but rather is the study of characteristics or "risk factors" associated with a specific disease, condition, or injury. Epidemiological studies observe large groups of people, usually with a common geographic or demographic base to determine factors or characteristics that are associated with specific disease patterns in that population (see Fig. 1.1). For example, epidemiologists study heart disease and cancer to try to elucidate patterns of lifestyle (diet or stress, for example) that are associated with the presence of disease in the group (50).

Although epidemiological studies do not determine cause and effect, they can establish a dose–response relationship between the two variables (e.g., a disease and a risk factor). Epidemiology can also discover "timing" relationships between variables, if the study follows a "prospective" cohort. Prospective means that a cohort of similar demographic characteristics was recruited and then followed forward in time in an ongoing study that occurs over many years or decades (often 10–20 years or more, as in the Framingham study). These prospective studies track the same group or groups continuously across those years. It is difficult for most epidemiological studies to determine the relative power of individual risk factors. For instance, it is difficult to determine from most epidemiological research whether smoking or high cholesterol is the most powerful risk factor for heart disease. Epidemiologists use a variable called population-attributable risk that can be used to determine the relative contribution of a risk factor to the onset and progression of a disease such as atherosclerosis.

Recent developments and progress in epidemiological research design has led to a level of sophistication that allows some assignment of causation to the risk factors that are identified. The ability to say that a particular risk factor can be causative is strengthened by several factors, which are outlined in the

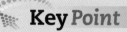

Key Point

Epidemiology is the study of chronic disease in large population groups. Epidemiology generally does not determine cause and effect, but rather association with a particular disease.

DID YOU KNOW?

The Framingham Study

The Framingham study is one of the most well-known and long-term epidemiological projects. For more than 60 years, this study has followed a large group of people (called a "cohort" in epidemiology) in Framingham, Massachusetts. The initial cohort of 5,200 persons was formed in 1948. Since then additional cohorts of offspring have been formed and studied. This study was one of the first to clarify primary and secondary risk factors for heart disease, such as smoking, high cholesterol, and high blood pressure, as well as other modifiable and nonmodifiable risk factors. The Framingham cohort has been followed through as many as three generations of family members who are currently part of the study. The reader is encouraged to review the Web site for the Framingham study (27).

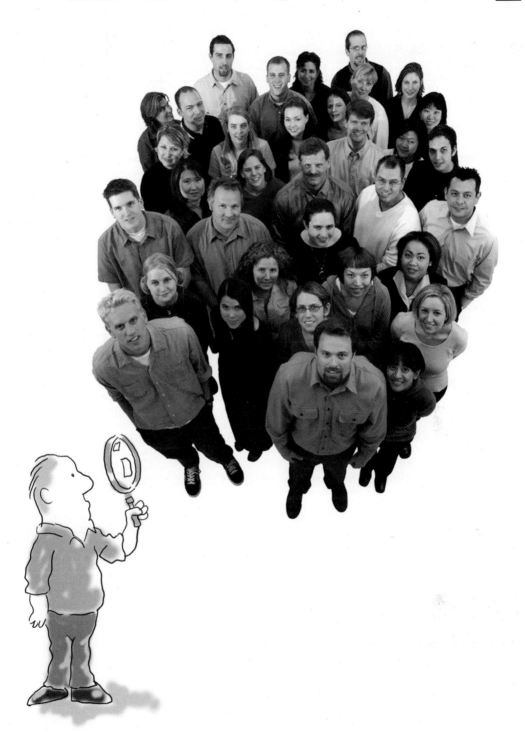

FIGURE 1.1 Epidemiology is the study of large population groups that attempts to clarify risk factors associated with chronic and other disease.

Causality in Epidemiology

Ways to strengthen the ability to show causality in epidemiological research include:

1. **The strength of the association:** In some studies of obesity and risk of type 2 diabetes, people with a BMI >35 had a 9- to 25-fold greater risk of developing type 2 diabetes when compared to those with a BMI of <23 or 25. In this example, the power of a 25-fold increase is much greater than a 2- to 3-fold increase.
2. **Consistency:** Findings that a particular significant relationship occurs consistently in different studies and populations, for example, risk factors that appear in the "7 Countries Study" also appear in other populations.
3. **Specificity:** The finding that a particular risk factor is "specific" for a certain disease. This may be less critical in this case, because most risk factors are not specific to a single chronic disease. Overweight, for example, not only increases risk of type 2 diabetes but also, independently, increases risk for hypertension, high triglycerides, low HDLs, CVD, stroke, and so on.
4. **Temporality:** This is simple and commonsense. If someone's cholesterol level was optimal before a heart attack, it cannot really be a risk factor.
5. **Biological gradient:** This is the concept of dose–response. Clearly many risk factors do occur in a dose–response relationship to a particular disease.
6. **Plausibility:** There must be some biological reason to believe a particular risk factor could "cause" atherosclerosis. For example, sedentary lifestyle is associated with increased systemic inflammation and inflammation may be an underlying cause of both atherosclerosis and type 2 diabetes.
7. **Coherence:** The association should fit with other pieces of the puzzle, other known facts about the history, and pathophysiology of the disease.
8. **Confirming animal or human research:** Such as randomized, controlled trials that demonstrate that controlling specific risk factors decreases the risk for the disease in question.
9. **Analogy:** If similar associations have been shown to be causal then it's more likely the present association is also causal.

box above. Not all epidemiological research is designed to make this case, but epidemiology can identify risk factors for further study and provide clarification to assign causality in different research designs.

The development and importance of epidemiology has mirrored the increased sophistication of the statistical treatment of those data over the years. Thus, for most individuals reading these studies is difficult at best, because of the statistical complexity. We will attempt to translate that literature into useful tools for the exercise professional.

ESTABLISHING THE RISK FACTORS

Risk factors are established by examining the presence of common characteristics among the cohort that is being studied. For example, in the Framingham study the original participants were interviewed and were given thorough physical examinations, their blood samples were obtained, and they completed surveys that assessed lifestyle factors such as smoking, physical activity, and dietary habits. It was not until 1960 in an article published in *Circulation* that the American Heart Association stated that smoking was clearly associated with death from coronary heart disease (18). Other risk factors, such as cholesterol and hypertension, were also identified in the early to late 1950s and 1960s, and physical inactivity became "officially" associated with heart disease in 1967, but not declared a "primary risk factor" until after 1990 (27). Many of these risk factors took longer to identify because these kinds of data are slow to accumulate.

The current list of risk factors (and potential risk factors) for heart disease is long, and there is some support for more than 200 variables that have been shown to be related to coronary artery disease (CAD) and atherosclerosis. Such characteristics range from commonly accepted risk factors like smoking and high cholesterol, thrombogenic risk factors (related to formation of blood clots), disease-related risk factors such as hypertension or diabetes to obscure risk factors such as poverty and a lipid called lipoprotein(a). The list is long, and choosing a single set of factors that work for everyone is difficult. See box below for a list of major, modifiable and nonmodifiable risk factors.

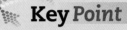

Key Point

Risk factors are characteristics that are related to the presence of disease. They may be lifestyle behaviors, physiological or biochemical values, or even psychological factors that are related to the presence of a specific disease.

American Heart Association lists six clinical and behavioral risk factors for heart disease. These are smoking, abnormal blood lipids, high blood pressure, physical inactivity, obesity, and diabetes mellitus (2). Additionally, The American Heart Association lists three risk factors that cannot be controlled: advancing age, heredity and family history, and sex. The National Heart, Lung, and Blood Institute of the National Institutes of Health studies and informs the interested public about cardiovascular disease and lists the six behavioral risk factors that AHA lists, but adds insulin resistance and metabolic syndrome (MetS) to that list.

There are many additional characteristics that increase risk for heart attack or CAD. It is beyond the scope of this text to discuss all of them. In the following sections, we will

DID YOU KNOW?

CAD Risk Factors (2,65)

Modifiable Risk Factors
- Smoking
- Abnormal blood lipids
- Physical inactivity/sedentary lifestyle
- High blood pressure
- Obesity
- Diabetes
- Abdominal obesity
- Psychosocial factors
- Fruit/vegetable consumption

Risk Factors that Cannot be Modified
- Heredity or family history
- Age
- Sex

Factors That May Contribute
- Stress
- Lack of moderate alcohol intake

discuss the modifiable risk factors listed previously, along with other contributing factors such as nutrition, stress, and various lipid components.

RISK FACTORS FOR HEART DISEASE

Since the initial publication of Framingham data (and other epidemiological studies), many different characteristics have been shown to be associated with heart disease. They are classified in various ways, for example, modifiable and nonmodifiable risk factors and risk factors that have been shown to be "independent" (when controlling statistically for other potential or known risk factors the factor in question remains significantly associated with risk for the disease). Risk factors have also been classified into groups according to whether intervening in a particular risk factor has been shown to reduce risk (5). In this section, we will simply list risk factors as modifiable or nonmodifiable.

MODIFIABLE RISK FACTORS

These risk factors can all be modified. All are associated with lifestyle. They are subject to intervention and research supports that intervention lowers risk for CAD.

Smoking

Smoking is the classic risk factor associated with CAD. It was identified in the Framingham study in 1960 to be strongly associated with the rising prevalence of CAD and increasing death rate over the middle part of the 20th century after World War II (21). Smoking has been biologically linked to the development and progression of atherosclerosis (21,38,47,63). According to the National Institutes of Health, in 2008 23.1% of men and 18.3% of women smoked (12). The percentage of smokers has declined from 24.1% in 1998 to 20.6% in 2008. According to the CDC the rate has been stable for the past 5 years (8).

Two surgeons general reports on the health risks associated with smoking have been published (9,10). Smoking has been shown to be associated with and to facilitate the deleterious effects of other risk factors on such things as the stability of plaque (blockages in arteries), endothelial function (the function of the lining of arteries), and blood clotting (9). It worsens the effects of risk factors such as high blood pressure, sedentary lifestyle, dyslipidemia, diabetes, and blood clotting (42,46). Smoking cessation helps prevent death and reduces morbidity (11). See Figure 1.2 for some of these effects.

Methods for smoking cessation include those that intervene only with lifestyle modification and those that use prescription and/or over-the-counter drugs together with lifestyle change. Lifestyle-change methods, including formal programs using well-known methods for facilitating cessation of tobacco use, have been shown to be successful. However, long-term compliance is a problem. It has been estimated that more than 70% of smokers (or somewhere between 30 and 40 million people) have tried to quit smoking. Likewise, it has been reported that the noncompliance rates at 1 year after many of these programs is more than 90%. That is, more than 90% of those who quit

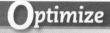

Optimize

Tobacco Use

No tobacco use and avoidance of environmental exposure to tobacco smoke of any kind.

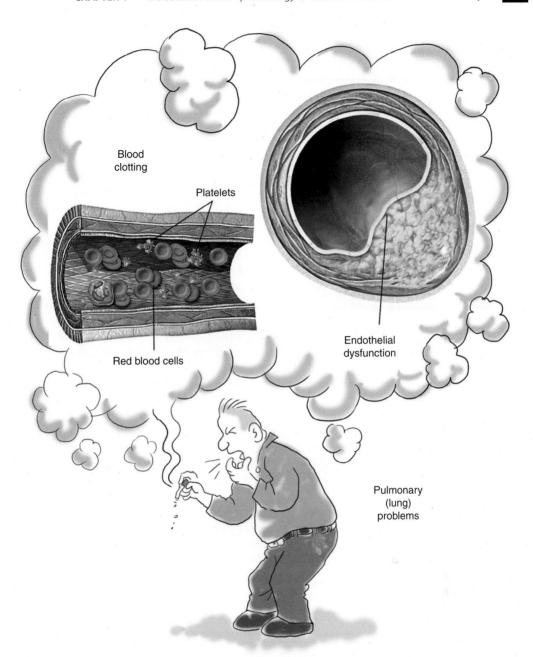

Blood
clotting

Platelets

Red blood cells

Endothelial
dysfunction

Pulmonary
(lung)
problems

FIGURE 1.2 Smoking causes a number of deleterious effects that are directly related to the pathophysiology of chronic diseases.

restart within 1 year (24,58). Compliance may be very difficult because smoking is both chemically and behaviorally addictive.

Blood Lipids

"Lipids" are fats in the blood. Because fats (e.g., cholesterol) are not soluble in blood plasma, they must be transported in the blood attached to lipoprotein molecules. Thus, high-density lipoprotein (HDL) and low-density lipoprotein (LDL) are lipoprotein carriers that facilitate the transport of cholesterol to peripheral sites (muscles, for example) for metabolic use. There are two avenues for cholesterol to enter the blood stream. First, many of the foods we eat contain cholesterol that is absorbed into the blood through the stomach and intestines. Second, our bodies are capable of manufacturing cholesterol. Cholesterol is necessary for many important physiological and anatomical processes, including production of vitamin D, bile acids, sex hormones, and cell membranes (including nervous system). Most cases of abnormal lipids (cholesterol, high LDL, etc.) are the result of consuming too much fat, especially saturated and trans fat.

There are several blood lipids aside from cholesterol, including LDL, HDL, and triglycerides and others. Blood cholesterol has been shown to be a strong risk factor for CAD (24). In addition, all of the lipid components have been shown, in more than one study, to be predictive of CAD and to be independent risk factors (24).

Periodically, a group of expert professionals is assembled by the National Institutes of Health called the "Adult Treatment Panel" (comprised of experts from such organizations as the American Heart Association, American Diabetes Association, American College of Cardiology, etc.). This group issues guidelines recommending lipid levels and also makes recommendations for treatment of abnormal blood lipids. The group last made recommendations in 2001, but additional recommendations were made in 2004 after some studies showed that additional lowering of lipids, especially LDL, was more effective in reducing events (24,29). Those updated recommendations can be seen in the box on the left. The fourth treatment panel has been appointed, and its recommendations are due for publication in 2010. All exercise professionals working with persons with chronic disease should be knowledgeable of these guidelines and alert for updated information.

Key Point

Blood cholesterol is manufactured by the body, but is most commonly increased by foods that contain saturated fat, trans fat, and cholesterol.

Optimize

Levels of Blood Lipids (29)

Cholesterol	<200
LDL	<100
	or <70 in persons with CAD or "CAD equivalent"*
HDL	>60
Triglycerides	<150
Non-HDL Cholesterol	<130

*CAD equivalent: diabetes, other atherosclerotic disease (e.g., PAD) or a 10-year risk equivalent >20% by Framingham score.

Cholesterol

Though total blood cholesterol remains important and is associated with CAD, it is no longer a primary target for optimizing blood lipids (24,29). One reason for this is that LDL is lowered as other lipids are controlled. Therefore, to make it a separate target is not meaningful. Additionally, it has been shown that LDL is an important, independent determinant of risk. Non-HDL cholesterol has become an alternate target for lipid management in some patients (29). Non-HDL cholesterol is HDL cholesterol subtracted from total cholesterol.

LDL Cholesterol

LDL is sometimes called "bad cholesterol" and is a specific form of lipoprotein. LDL is the main target for lowering lipids to prevent heart disease. LDL can become "oxidized" in the blood (i.e., chemically altered). Oxidized LDL has powerful, negative effects on atherosclerosis, endothelial function, and clotting mechanisms, and inflammation and other factors that stimulate the onset and progression of CAD. Lowering LDL reduces risk for fatal and nonfatal cardiac events (heart attack, sudden death), as well as for further development and progression of CAD (24,29). As we stated earlier, LDL is a transporter for lipid in the blood. In this case, perhaps the easiest way to conceptualize it is that LDL transports fat to arteries and other sites where they are deposited. Thus, elevated LDL actually adds to the total burden of plaque (blockages) found in coronary, peripheral, and other arteries where these blockages develop and progress (see Fig. 1.3).

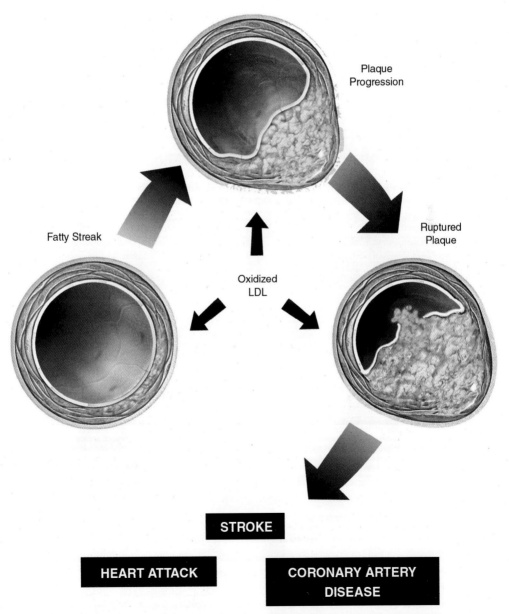

FIGURE 1.3 Oxidized LDL is directly related to plaque development and progression. Occlusive vascular disease is common to heart attacks, stroke, and claudication.

HDL Cholesterol

HDL is often called "good cholesterol" because it is antiatherogenic; that is, it is helpful in preventing the formation and progression of blockages. HDL transports cholesterol from blockages to the liver where it is used to form bile, as a backbone for vitamin D or sex hormones or is eliminated (28). In the research literature this is often referred to as "reverse cholesterol transport" (see Fig. 1.4) (4,23,44).

Raising HDL cholesterol is a major objective of controlling lipids (52). Low HDL is associated with increased risk for developing heart disease, death from heart attack, and stroke even when total cholesterol and LDL are optimal.

Non-HDL Cholesterol

Reducing "non-HDL" cholesterol is another beneficial target for reducing lipids to prevent heart disease (see Fig. 1.5). This can be extremely helpful in people with triglycerides

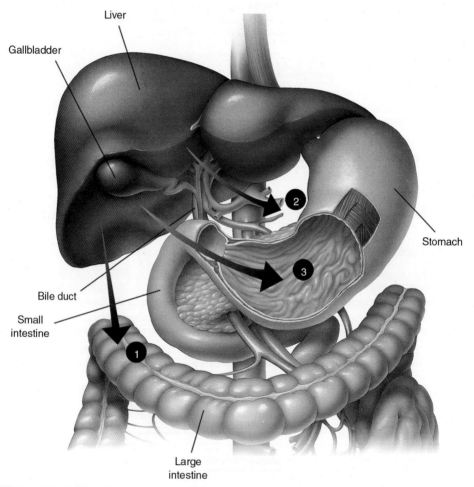

FIGURE 1.4 HDL is called "good cholesterol" because it is responsible for transporting cholesterol away from plaque to the liver for biological functions or elimination.
Key: 1) Some cholesterol is excreted through the intestinal tract, 2) some may be transported through the vascular system to serve critical physiological and anatomical functions and 3) cholesterol is also eliminated through the formation of bile acids in the gall bladder.

>200 mg/dl or in those with MetS or diabetes. (MetS and type 2 diabetes will be discussed later in this chapter and more completely in Chapter 7.) Non-HDL cholesterol is simple to measure (total cholesterol – HDL cholesterol), and the target then becomes the standard LDL target (100) plus 30 (see Optimize box, above, discussing Levels of Blood Lipids) (29).

Triglycerides

The recommendations for triglycerides can be seen in the box above. Triglycerides are another kind of fat found in the blood, muscle, and adipose tissue. They are usually elevated as a result of overweight, sedentary lifestyle, excess intake of dietary fat, excess intake of sugars and refined and processed carbohydrates, and alcohol consumption.

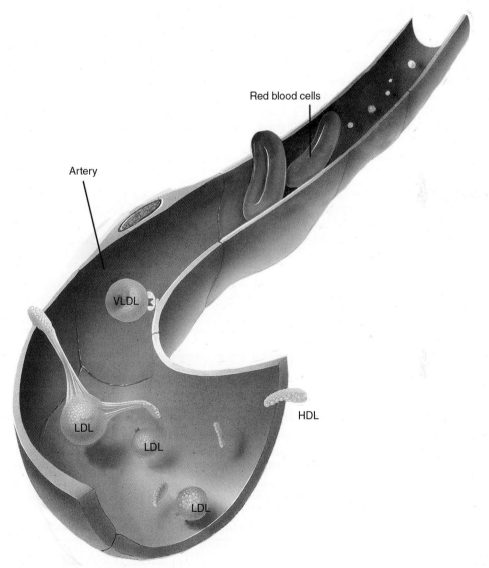

FIGURE 1.5 Non-HDL cholesterol is considered to be atherogenic. It is the sum of LDL, IDL and VLDL cholesterol. All of these have atherogenic components.

Triglycerides can be elevated due to certain medications, such as beta blockers or some diuretics. They are commonly elevated in people with MetS and type 2 diabetes because of the metabolic abnormalities associated with these diseases. Thus, it is recommended that triglycerides should be assessed in all persons with CAD, especially those with MetS or type 2 diabetes (29).

In the updated recommendations, people with diabetes are treated similarly to those with CAD. That is, people with diabetes have the same risk for having a cardiac event as people with diagnosed atherosclerotic disease. High triglycerides are an independent risk factor for CAD (64). Someone with both high triglycerides and LDL (familial combined hyperlipidemia) is at especially high risk, because of the type of LDL that is likely to be present (29,64).

Blood Pressure

In a national report titled "JNC7," hypertension or high blood pressure is defined as resting blood pressure >140 and/or >90 (56). This government report classifies blood pressure into more categories than simply *high* or *normal*. The box below shows the JNC7 blood pressure classifications. Note that "prehypertension" is a new, separate category. The point of this category is that what was formerly called "borderline" hypertension is now known to put a person at greater risk for developing hypertension as well as CAD and CVD. Thus, the recommendation is that those with "prehypertension" should be treated with lifestyle modification (56). Of course, lifestyle modification involves regular (and frequent) exercise as well as sodium restriction and weight loss.

DID YOU KNOW?
Classification of Blood Pressure (56)

Classification	Systolic Blood Pressure	Diastolic Blood Pressure
Normal (optimal)	<120	<80
Prehypertension	120–139	80–89
Stage 1 hypertension	140–159	90–99
Stage 2 hypertension	≥160	>100

High blood pressure has been shown to alter endothelial function by exerting abnormal forces (called "shear forces") on the blood vessels. This chronically increased shear force results in abnormal endothelial function and inflammation, which predisposes arteries to developing atherosclerosis. Changes in lifestyle that promote normal blood pressure improve shear force that allows the vessels to normalize endothelial function. Thus, risk for CAD/CVD and related manifestations (heart attack and stroke) is reduced (35). It has been estimated that reducing blood pressure to "normal" limits will reduce heart attack, stroke, and heart failure by 25% to 50% (35,43,56).

The optimal lifestyle for preventing or lowering high blood pressure includes weight reduction in overweight or obese Individuals. Even small amounts of weight loss have been shown to lower blood pressure. The DASH (Dietary Approaches to Stop Hypertension) diet was originally aimed at hypertension and prehypertension but has been shown to be effective also in controlling other risk factors and reducing overall risk for CAD (51). It is a diet high in potassium and calcium and reduces sodium to <1500 mg/day. Using diet combined with exercise is even more effective than single changes in either one (51,57). The DASH diet will be discussed in more detail in the chapter on nutrition and chronic disease.

> ### Optimize
> **Blood Pressure**
> <120/<80

Obesity

Obesity and overweight are at epidemic proportions in the American population; 67% of adults in the United States are overweight or obese. That percentage has increased every year since 1980. Obesity and overweight in children aged between 6 and 11 years and adolescents aged between 12 and 19 years is also high and increasing; 19% of children and 17% of adolescents are overweight (95% or greater weight for age and sex), and another 14% are at risk of becoming obese (85th to 95th percentile for age and sex) (12).

The definitions of normal weight, overweight, and obesity can be found in Chapter 6. Measuring body mass index (BMI) may not be either the best or the most predictive of those measures used to predict risk of heart disease. Recently, either waist circumference or waist-to-hip ratio (WHR) is often cited as a more powerful tool in predicting risk for chronic disease and mortality (19,20).

Excess adipose tissue is associated with increased systemic inflammation, which establishes a theoretical connection with atherosclerosis and heart disease (7,25,27). Additionally, it has been demonstrated that losing weight results in decreasing the levels of inflammatory markers, including c-reactive protein and interleukin-6 (27,55,66). Finally, it is not certain whether the caloric restriction that is inherent in weight loss programs, or the weight loss itself, is responsible for the reduced inflammation. It is clear that caloric restriction and weight loss are both helpful in protecting persons from type 2 diabetes, hypertension, heart disease, heart attack, and stroke (27,59). Interestingly, a recent study not only confirms this but also demonstrates that although the risk of elevated BMI is decreased with increasing levels of physical activity it is not totally eliminated (60).

Physical Inactivity

For a full discussion of the risk factor, the protective benefits of physical activity and the physiology behind the connection between physical activity, exercise, and heart disease see Chapter 3. Sedentary lifestyle (lack of physical activity) has been shown to be an independent risk factor for heart disease (2). It has also been demonstrated that initiating an exercise or physical activity program is protective from events resulting from heart and vascular disease. Finally, it has also been shown that exercise and physical activity are effective methods for improving other risk factors such as lipids, weight, and blood pressure (31). Again, see Chapter 3 for a full discussion of physical activity, physical fitness, and heart disease.

> ### Optimize
> **Exercise/Activity Levels (49)**
>
> **Exercise**
> *Frequency:* Daily
> *Intensity:* 60% to 85% heart rate reserve or maximal oxygen uptake reserve
> *Duration:* 30 to 60 minutes/day
> *Mode:* Cardiovascular endurance and resistance training for muscular strength and endurance
>
> **Physical Activity**
> 12,000 to 14,000 steps/day
> Both daily exercise and daily physical activity should account for a weekly caloric expenditure of >2000 kCal over basal.

Diabetes Mellitus

Both type 1 and type 2 diabetes mellitus are strong risk factors for CAD and CVD. The following is a limited discussion of type 1 diabetes, its pathophysiology, and risk factor associations (type 2 diabetes will be discussed in detail in Chapter 7).

Type 1 diabetes is an autoimmune disease of the insulin-producing cells (beta cells of the Islet of Langerhans) in the pancreas. The onset of type 1 diabetes is most common in younger people, and the majority of people with newly diagnosed type 1 diabetes are adolescents, though type 1 diabetes can and does have adult onset and diagnosis. Because those with type 1 diabetes ultimately lose the ability to produce insulin, all people with type 1 diabetes must use exogenous insulin (supplied by injection or other means) in most cases, multiple times during the day (13). Best control is always established by regular blood glucose testing, and people with type 1 diabetes may test 3 to 4 or more times per day. It has been shown that close control of blood glucose in type 1 diabetes decreases complications and thus decreases morbidity and mortality (16,48).

Type 2 diabetes is an entirely different disease though with similar signs, symptoms, and complications. Insulin receptors on skeletal muscle (and other) cells become insensitive to circulating insulin; thus, the ability of the body to utilize blood glucose is progressively diminished—this is called "insulin resistance." The ultimate result of the insulin resistance is hyperglycemia (increased circulating blood glucose). This results in increased insulin production by the pancreas, leading to both beta cell and insulin receptor dysfunction and further increases in both circulating insulin (hyperinsulinemia) and blood glucose (hyperglycemia). This cycle is associated with metabolic syndrome (MetS) and the onset of chronic hyperglycemia and type 2 diabetes after some variable amount of time.

The risk factors for MetS are found in the box below. MetS is defined by the presence of three of the five factors listed below. MetS is also accompanied by the general, low-level inflammatory state that we have described associated with both obesity and smoking and will be discussed more completely in other chapters in this book. Both MetS and type 2 diabetes can be prevented with exercise and weight control/loss (24,30,39). If MetS accompanies type 2 diabetes, the risk of complications and morbidity, including heart disease, is much higher (39).

> ### **O**ptimize
> **Blood Glucose Levels**
> Fasting: <100
> Glycated hemoglobin: <5.7

PRACTICING HEALTHY BEHAVIORS

Recently, some interesting and disturbing information about how Americans practice healthy lifestyles has surfaced. Two recent articles are significant. Both studies report data on the number of Americans practicing "healthy lifestyle habits." The risk factors in the

> **DID YOU KNOW?**
> ### Five Healthy Behaviors
>
> 1. 30+ minutes of daily PA
> 2. Normal BMI or WHR
> 3. Healthy diet
> 4. Not smoking
> 5. ½ to 2 alcoholic drinks per day

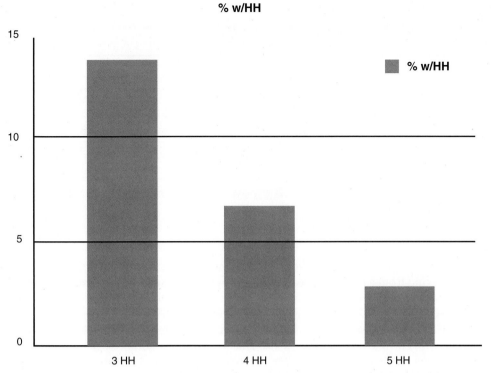

FIGURE 1.6 Percent of Americans practicing 3, 4, or 5 healthy habits, including (1) no smoking; (2) BMI <25.0; (3) exercise ≥30 min/day; (4) moderate alcohol consumption, 5–30 g/day; (5) top 40% of healthy diet scores (14).

three studies (not all were reported in each study) were BMI or abdominal obesity, physical inactivity, smoking, diet, and alcohol use (15,32,36).

King compared the numbers of Americans that actually practice five acknowledged healthy behaviors in 1988 versus 2006. This report states that the percentage of Americans practicing all 5 healthy behaviors decreased from 16% to 8% between 1988 and 2006 (32). Previously, Chiuve (15) reported that less than 4% of the population practiced 5 healthy behaviors. Thus, the prevalence of Americans practicing a healthy lifestyle, as defined by the presence of these health behaviors, is already very small and is diminishing (Fig. 1.6).

Put bluntly, Americans have fewer healthy behaviors than they did 20 years ago, despite the increased knowledge of, research in, and educational efforts about how these healthy behaviors may actually cause chronic disease.

Interestingly (and sadly) the authors also reviewed data for individuals with cardiovascular disease, diabetes, hypertension, and hypercholesterolemia. Individuals diagnosed with these chronic diseases (all of which are discussed in this book) were no more likely to practice these healthy and disease-preventing behaviors than individuals who do not have heart or other chronic disease (32). They speculate many reasons for this startling revelation. Some of those reasons are noted in the box below. It is likely that our tendency to be negligent in practicing these behaviors is multifactorial. Perhaps one overriding reason is that medicine has long been excellent at treating symptoms, but is much less accomplished and effective at treating root causes of chronic disease—lifestyle!

Even more recently, it was reported that men with any 3 "low-risk factors" had almost a 60% lower chance of CAD events and a 77% lower risk of dying from CVD (36). It is

DID YOU KNOW?
Likely Reasons for Not Practicing Healthy Behaviors

1. The societal importance and effectiveness of practicing these behaviors is minimized.
2. Men have been shown to be less willing to accept health advice and counseling from health professionals (doctors, nurses, dietitians, exercise professionals, etc.).
3. Inaccurately low self-assessment of risk for cardiovascular and other chronic disease.
4. Poor medical control and nonadherence to medication of treated risk factors (and chronic diseases), such as hypertension, hyperlipidemia, and obesity/overweight.
5. Reliance of individuals on automobiles and other labor-saving devices, as well as lack of opportunity for increased physical activity exacerbated by urban and suburban neighborhood design, job, and family demands, and so on.

clear that increased healthy habits practiced in daily life equals/lower the risk of having and/or dying from a chronic disease. Interestingly, this last study also examined these data on persons with diagnosed disease who were taking medication. The combined effects of medication and even one healthy behavior further lowered risk of mortality.

Optimally, then, practicing as many healthy behaviors as possible lowers risk even in people with chronic disease. This is also true among older adults—age (according to these numbers) made little difference in the outcome. These same authors also looked at people who added healthy behaviors and found that adding a healthy behavior (one or more) added to the increased protection from disease (36). In summary, it is clearly beneficial to practice as many health behaviors as possible. It is also beneficial to add healthy behaviors to one's list in order to continue to decrease risk.

Table 1.1 shows published statements and guidelines about risk factor modification as well as recommendations for levels of specific risk factors.

DIGGING DEEPER
Genetics of Atherosclerosis

Studies suggest that 50% to 75% of CVD can be explained by traditional risk factors (41). However, it has been shown that having a history of premature heart disease (men older than 55 years of age and/or women older than 65 years of age) in the family (parent or sibling) is a risk factor for heart disease. One large epidemiological study of 15,250 families reported CAD risk levels in the range of 1.7 to 12.9 times among families with a premature history of CAD (45,61,62). Among those with premature CAD in 2 family members the risk increased to almost 13-fold.

On the other hand, the Framingham study has demonstrated that those with a family history of premature CAD with a low-risk profile (low cholesterol, normal blood pressure, nondiabetic, nonsmoker, etc.) have a 10-year risk for CAD similar to persons without a family history (61,62). Another report states that 82% of the heart disease in the Nurses Health Study, a prospective (ongoing) study of health status and risk factors among 84,000 female nurses, can be attributed to risk factors and specifically to lifestyle (54). Thus, it is clear that lifestyle exerts a more significant influence on the risk for having CAD than genetics.

(continued)

TABLE 1.1 Guidelines and Recommendations

Guideline	Smoking	SBP	DBP	Chol	LDL	HDL	Trg	Diet Fat	Diet Sat Fat	Diet Chol	Exercise/ Activity	Blood Gluc	Body wt/ Obesity	Sodium	Alcohol	Other (See Ref for Specifics)
JNC VII (2003)	Complete cessation	<120	<80	NR	NR	NR	NR	NR	Reduce	Reduce	30 min/day most days	NR	BMI = 18.5–24.9	2400 mg/day	<2 drinks/ day or I drink/day if women or low wt.	DASH Eating Plan
AHA Diet and Lifestyle Recommendations: 2006 AHA Diet Guidelines (2000)	Avoid use of and exposure to all tobacco products	<120	<80	NR	Achieve desirable level <100	Achieve desirable level >40-Men >50-Women	Achieve desirable level <150	<30% (but no specific record for CAD)	<7% total cal <1% trans fat	<300 mg/day	≥30 min/ day on all of most days; cal expend of 100–200 kcal/ session	<100	Maintain a healthy body weight; BMI >18.5–24.9	<2300 mg/day	2 drinks/ day for men; 1 drink/day for women	Minimize intake of foods and drinks with added sugar; recommendations for food consumed outside the home is available
NCEP III (2001)	NR	NR	NR	<200	<70	>40	<150	25–35% of total cal	<7% of total cal	<200 mg/day	Increase physical activity	NR	Reduce weight	NR	NR	1. Drug tx
AHA/ACC Guidelines for Sec Prev (2006)	Complete cessation	<140 or <130 (if CHF or CRF) or <130 (if DM)	<90 or <85 (if CHF or CRF) or <80 (if DM)	<200	Primary Goal <100; further reduction to <70 is reasonable	Sec goal >40	Sec goal <150	NR	NR	NR	Min goal: 30–60 min—most or all days of the week Optimal = daily; resistance training 2 days/wk	HbA₁c <7%	BMI = 18.5–24.9	NR	NR	

(continued)

TABLE 1.1   Guidelines and Recommendations (Continued)

Guideline	Smoking	SBP	DBP	Chol	LDL	HDL	Trg	Diet Fat	Diet Sat Fat	Diet Chol	Exercise/Activity	Blood Gluc	Body wt/Obesity	Sodium	Alcohol	Other (See Ref for Specifics)
Fourth Joint Task Force of European Society on Cardiovascular Disease Prevention (2007)	Complete cessation	<120	<80	<190	<115	NR	NR	<30% of total cal; <1/3 of fat intake should be saturated	Reduce through replacing with MUFA	<300 mg/day	30 min of moderately vigorous exercise on most days of the week	HbA1c <6.5 FBG <110	BMI >30.0 should lose weight; 25.0–29.9 should consider losing weight <102 cm in men; <88 cm in women should not gain weight	NR	NR	Numerous additional recommendations based on level of risk, clinical history

ACSM Position Stand on Weight Loss (2009)	NR	NR	NR	NR	NR	NR	NR	NR	NR	NR	NR	NR	150–250 min/week to prevent weight gain (1200–2000 kcal/wk); 250–300 min/week for weight maintenance	NR	NR	NR	lose 5%–10% body weight if obese; change eating and exercise behavior; reduce energy intake by 500–1000 kcal/day; supplement endurance exercise with resistance training
American Diabetes Assoc. Practice Standards (2010)	Complete cessation of use and exposure to all tobacco products	NR	NR	Sat fat <7%; min trans fat	<200 mg/day	w/IGT or IFG, 150 min/week	NR	FBG <100 HbA1c <6.5	BMI <25.0 Indiv w/ IGT or IFG lose 5–10% body weight	NR	NR	NR					

Note: This table includes published statements and guidelines about risk factor modification as well as recommendations for levels of specific risk factors related to the specific topic covered in the statement. All of the recommendations are specific to "secondary prevention" (individuals with clinical evidence of disease); if specific recommendations are made, otherwise, "optimal" levels are selected for goals.

JNC 7, The Seventh Report of the Joint National Committee on Prevention, Detection, Evaluation, and Treatment of High Blood Pressure; NR, no recommendation; DBP, diastolic blood pressure; SBP, systolic blood pressure; chol., cholesterol; LDL, low-density lipoprotein; HDL, high-density lipoprotein; Sat fat, saturated fat; Trg, triglycerides; gluc, glucose; BMI, body mass index; HbA1c, hemoglobin A1C; CAD, coronary artery disease; IFG, impaired fasting glucose; IGT, impaired glucose tolerance; indiv, individual; FBG, fasting blood glucose.

Essentially, hereditary disease can be categorized into two broad areas:

1. Monogenic disorder/diseases: Major single-gene–related diseases such as Huntington's chorea, LDL-receptor deficiency, cystic fibrosis, Duchenne's muscular dystrophy, and so on. These diseases are caused by a gene defect or mutation and can be directly attributed to that gene.
2. Polygenic disorder/diseases: These occur when "polymorphisms" (characteristics or traits from more than one gene) are inherited, predisposing persons to a chronic health problem such as CAD (6).

Phenotype is the interaction of genotype (the DNA, or genetic code, of a person) and the environment, for example, exposure to a risk factor such as tobacco smoke or high-fat diet. The phenotype is determined by this interaction and is responsible for a particular predisposition to have certain nonmonogenic diseases, such as CAD. Polygenic diseases result in people being "susceptible" to the development and progression of specific chronic diseases such as atherosclerosis, particularly when superimposed on an environmental risk factor such as obesity, physical inactivity, high-fat diet, or tobacco use (6). Several phenotypes for CAD risk have been identified (some of these are discussed in the box titled "Polygenic Phenotypes and CAD").

It is estimated that about 5% to 10% of CAD cases may be accounted for by monogenic disorders, but many of them are exacerbated or, in fact, actually realized only in the presence of a high-risk lifestyle, for example, high-fat diet or sedentary living. A striking example of phenotype and risk of CAD was reported by Williams et al. (62). In a family with premature CAD caused by familial hypercholesterolemia, "pioneer" ancestors who had the gene lived into their 80s. Their lifestyle required daily physical activity and a primarily plant-based diet high in fiber, low in saturated fat, and devoid of processed foods (62).

DID YOU KNOW?

Polygenic Phenotypes and CAD (6)

- Plasma lipoprotein (a) or Lp(a) among populations is accounted for by variability in the apoprotein (a) gene.
- Familial hypercholesterolemia (FHC) is caused by mutations in the LDL receptor gene. FHC is a disorder resulting in extremely high cholesterol. This disorder accounts for <2% of CAD cases.
- Familial defective apoliprotein B is caused by a gene mutation.
- Apoliprotein E polymorphisms.
- Approximately 15% of persons with premature CAD have low-HDL syndrome. This may be highly treatable by weight loss, diet, and exercise, particularly if triglycerides are elevated slightly.
- Approximately 15% of persons with premature CAD have high blood homocysteine levels, which is also treatable by folic acid (vitamin B_{12}) supplementation.

The majority of CAD is not monogenic (related to a single gene). Rather most CAD is related to the interaction between the genome and the environment. In the presence of genes that make us susceptible to the pathophysiology of CAD, the influence of environmental factors, such as tobacco use or high LDL, causes the inflammation, endothelial dysfunction, and deposition of plaque in vascular walls, and thus, CAD. So, polygenic conditions, health behaviors (diet, tobacco use, lack of physical activity) imposed on susceptible genes account for the majority of atherosclerosis. Aggressive lifestyle management of risk factors in the primary and secondary prevention of CAD is the answer to resolving the inherent risk in environment–gene interaction.

Significant RESEARCH

Two important studies fit this category for Chapter 1. These two studies highlight the significance of "modifiable" risk factors and, thus, of the importance and effectiveness of treating chronic disease with lifestyle first and foremost.

The Significance of Modifiable Risk Factors

Yusuf S, Hawken S, Ôunpuu S, Dans T, Avezum A, et al., on behalf of the INTER-HEART Study Investigators. Effect of potentially modifiable risk factors associated with myocardial infarction in 52 countries (the INTERHEART study): case–control study. Lancet. 2004;364:937–52.

▪ Summary ▪

INTERHEART is a "case–control" study of heart attack survivors in 52 countries. The participants come from every inhabited continent. Yusuf and his colleagues studied modifiable risk factors in survivors of heart attack. The risk factors included those traditionally associated with CAD, including smoking, hypertension, diabetes, blood lipids, BMI, WHR, abdominal obesity, psychosocial factors, daily fruit/vegetable consumption, regular exercise, and regular alcohol consumption. Additionally, they assessed increased ApoB/ApoA1 ratio. The authors summarize their conclusions quite clearly in the following statement: "Abnormal lipids, smoking, hypertension, diabetes, abdominal obesity, psychosocial factors, consumption of fruits, vegetables, and alcohol, and regular physical activity account for most of the risk of myocardial infarction worldwide in both sexes and at all ages in all regions."

There are several important conclusions within this study.

- Modifiable risk factors account for more than 90% of the risk of heart attack.
- Having multiple risk factors does not simply add to the risk; rather multiple risk factors multiply the risk level exponentially.
- Regular exercise, daily fruit and vegetable consumption, and not smoking would reduce the incidence of heart attack by more than 75% in these populations.

Undeniable evidence of the importance of modifiable risk factors, coupled with evidence of the preventive effect of modifying them makes this study significant. Yusuf and his colleagues in this important piece of research have demonstrated that a healthy lifestyle is associated with significantly decreased rates of myocardial infarction.

(continued)

The Significance of Exercise and Diet

Knowler WC, Barrett-Connor E, Fowler SE, Hamman RF, Lachin JM, Walker E. Reduction in the incidence of type 2 diabetes with lifestyle intervention or metformin. Diabetes Prevention Program Research Group. N Engl J Med. 2002;346(6): 393–403.

■ **Summary** ■

Knowler and his colleagues studied the effects of diet and exercise versus pharmacological (metformin) intervention in a group of nondiabetics with elevated fasting blood glucose. They also randomized a group to placebo treatment; thus, the two treatment groups were compared to a control, placebo group with more than almost 4 years of follow-up. Lifestyle was significantly more effective than metformin (58% vs. 31% compared to placebo) in reducing the incidence of type 2 diabetes in this population.

The lifestyle intervention group was advised to exercise 150 minutes per week at a moderate intensity and to lose 7% of initial bodyweight using a healthy, low-calorie, low-fat diet. At the conclusion of the study, 50% of the lifestyle group had lost the recommended 7% of body weight and 74% had complied with the exercise recommendations. Medication adherence in the placebo and metformin groups exceeded 70%. The lifestyle group initially lost 7 kg of weight over the first year and slowly regained weight at follow-up, resulting in an average weight loss of approximately 4 kg. Neither the placebo nor metformin group lost weight, nor did they significantly change their activity levels. The lifestyle group was significantly different from both groups in activity and weight at the conclusion of the study.

The importance of this study should be obvious. Metformin is a drug that is thought to act on insulin receptors to increase the uptake (and use) of glucose into skeletal muscle. Thus, metformin should also exert control over elevated blood glucose associated with type 2 diabetes. In this study, lifestyle modification, specifically exercise and weight loss associated with diet, was more effective in preventing type 2 diabetes than this drug. Prior to Knowler's important research, no other study has systematically compared lifestyle change to drug therapy for *preventing* chronic disease. Knowler showed the effectiveness of lifestyle in preventing chronic disease conclusively in this research. Its importance lies in the fact that it supports our notion that nothing is quite as effective as lifestyle, especially "optimal" lifestyle in preventing chronic disease.

SUMMARY

Chronic disease develops over a long period of time and persists, sometimes for the lifetime of an individual. Risk factors are determined by epidemiological research using large population groups. Risk factors are associated with, but not necessarily causative of, chronic disease. A common underlying pathophysiology is present in many chronic diseases. There are modifiable and nonmodifiable risk factors for all chronic diseases and modifying health (lifestyle) behaviors is an effective way to prevent chronic disease. Optimal lifestyle changes are most effective for intervening with and managing the pathophysiology of chronic disease as well as for delaying or stopping progression of the disease.

REFERENCES

1. American Heart Association Web site [Internet]. Metabolic Syndrome. Dallas, TX. American Heart Association [Accessed February 14, 2009.] Available at: www.americanheart.org/presenter.jhtml?identifier=4756.

2. American Heart Association Web site [Internet]. Risk Factors. Dallas, TX American Heart Association [Accessed January 12, 2010]. Available from:http://www.americanheart.org/presenter.jhtml?identifier=500.

3. American Heart Association Web site [Internet]. Risk Factors. Dallas, TX: American Heart Association [Accessed January 12, 2010]. Available at:www.americanheart.org/presenter.jhtml?identifier=4726.

4. Barkowski RS, Frishman WH. HDL metabolism and CETP inhibition. Cardiol Rev. 2008;16(3):154–162.

5. 27th Bethesda Conference: Matching the intensity of risk factor Management with the hazard for coronary disease events. J Am Coll Cardiol. 1996;27:957–1047.

6. Brenner S, Miller JH. Encyclopedia of Genetics. San Diego: Academic Press, 2002.

7. Calabro P, Limongelli G, Pacileo G, et al. The role of adiposity as a determinant of an inflammatory milieu. J Cardiovasc Med. 2008; 9(5):450–460.

8. Centers for Disease Control and Prevention Web site [Internet]. Morbidity and Mortality Daily. Washington, DC, [Accessed January 12, 2010]. Available at: http://www.cdc.gov/mmwr/preview/mmwrhtml/mm5844a2.htm.

9. Centers for Disease Control and Prevention website [Internet]. Reducing the Health Consequences of Smoking: 25 years of progress. Report of the Advisory Committee to the Surgeon General of the Public Health Service. Washington, D.C. [Cited, January 15th, 2009]. Available at: http://profiles.nlm.nih.gov/NN/B/B/X/S/_/nnbbxs.pdf.

10. Centers for Disease Control and Prevention and Prevention website [Internet]. Smoking and health. Report of the Advisory Committee to the Surgeon General of the Public Health Service. Washington, D.C. [Accessed January 15, 2009]. Available at: www.dcd.gov/nchs/data/hus/hus07.pdf.

11. Centers for Disease Control and Prevention website [Internet]. The Health Benefits of Smoking Cessation. A report of the Surgeon General. Washington, D.C. [Accessed January 15, 2009]. Available at: http://profiles.nlm.nih.gov/NN/B/B/C/T/_/nnbbct.pdf.

12. Centers for Disease Control and Prevention website [Internet]. National Center for Health Statistics. Washington, DC. [Accessed February 20, 2009] Available at: www.cdc.gov/nccdphp/overview.htm.

13. Centers for Disease Control and Prevention Web site [Internet]. National Center for Health Statis-tics. Washington, DC. [Accessed March 20, 2009] Available at: www.cdc.gov/nchs/nhanes.htm.

14. Chiuve SE. McCullough, ML. Sacks FM, et al. Healthy lifestyle factors in the primary prevention of coronary heart disease among men: Benefits among users and nonusers of lipid-lowering and antihypertensive medications. Circulation. 2006;114(2):160–167.

15. Cris SA, Houmard JA, Kraus WE. Modest exercise prevents the progressive disease associated with physical inactivity. Exerc Sport Sci Rev. 2007;35(1):18–23.

16. Daneman D. Type 1 diabetes. Lancet. 2006;367:847–858.

17. Dawber TR, Kannel WB, Revotskie N, et al. Some factors associated with the development of coronary heart disease: Six years' follow-up experience in the Framingham Study. Am J Public Health. 1959;49:1349–1356.

18. Dawber TR. Summary of recent literature regarding cigarette smoking and coronary heart disease. Circulation. 1960;22:164–166.

19. de Koning L, Merchant AT, Pogue J, et al. Waist circumference and waist-to-hip ratio as predictors of cardiovascular events: Meta-regression analysis of prospective studies. Eur Heart J. 2007;28:850–856.

20. Dobbelsteyn CJ, Joffres MR, MacLean DR, et al. A comparative evaluation of waist circumference, waist-to-hip ratio and body mass index as indicators of cardiovascular risk factors. The Canadian Heart Health Surveys. Int J Obes Relat Metab Disord. 2001;25(5):652–661.

21. Doll R, Hill AB. Lung cancer and other causes of death in relation to smoking. BMJ. 1956;2:1071–1081.

22. Donnelly JE, Blair SN, Jakicic JM, et al. ACSM's position stand on appropriate physical activity intervention strategies for weight loss and prevention of weight regain for adults. Med Sci Sports Exerc. 2009;41(2):459–471.

23. Duffy D, Rader DJ. High-density lipoprotein cholesterol therapies: The next frontier in lipid management. J Cardiopulm Rehabil. 2006;26(1):1–8.

24. Executive Summary of the Third Report of the National Cholesterol Education Program (NCEP). Expert panel on detection, evaluation, and treatment of high blood cholesterol in adults (Adult Treatment Panel III). JAMA. 2001;285:2486–2497.

25. Fantuzzi G, Mazzone T. Adipose tissue and atherosclerosis: Exploring the connection. Arterioscler Thromb Vasc Biol. 2007;27(5):996–1003.

26. Fourth Joint Task Force of the European Society of Cardiology and Other Societies on Cardiovascular Disease Prevention in Clinical Practice. European guidelines on cardiovascular disease prevention in clinical practice. Eur J Cardiovasc Prev Rehabil. 2004;14(Suppl 2):S1–S157.

27. Framingham Heart Study Web site [Internet]. Framingham, MA. Framingham Study [Accessed January 18, 2009]. Available at: http://www.framingham-heartstudy.org/.

28. Fuster V, Topol EJ, Nagel, EG. Atherothrombosis and Coronary Artery Disease. 2nd ed. Baltimore, MD: LWW Publishing, 2004.

29. Grundy SM, Cleeman JI, Merz C, et al. For the Coordinating Committee of the National Cholesterol Education Program implications of recent clinical trials for the National Cholesterol Education Program Adult Treatment Panel III Guidelines. Arterioscler Thromb Vasc Biol. 2004;24(8):e149–e161.

30. Grundy SM. Metabolic syndrome: A multiplex cardiovascular risk factor. J Clin Endocrinol Metab. 2007;92(2):399–404.

31. Haskell WL, Lee IM, Pate RR, et al. Physical activity and public health: Updated recommendation for adults from the American College of Sports Medicine and the American Heart Association. Med Sci Sports Exerc. 2007;39(8):1423–1434.

32. King DE, Mainous AG, Carnemolla M, et al. Adherence to healthy lifestyle habits in U.S. adults, 1988–2006. Am J Med. 2009;122:528–534.

33. Knowler WC, Barrett-Connor E, Fowler SE, et al. Reduction in the incidence of type 2 diabetes with lifestyle intervention or metformin. Diabetes Prevention Program Research Group. N Engl J Med. 2002;346(6):393–403.

34. Kraus WE, Levine BD. Exercise training for diabetes: The "strength" of the evidence. Ann Intern Med. 2007;147(6):423–424.

35. Landmesser U, Drexler H. Endothelial function and hypertension. Curr Opin Cardiol 2007;22(4): 316–320.

36. Lee CD, Sui X, Blair SN. Combined effects of cardiorespiratory fitness, not smoking and normal waist girth on morbidity and mortality in men. Arch Int Med. 2009;169(22):2096–2101.

37. Lee Y-H, Pratley RE. Abdominal obesity and cardiovascular disease risk: The emerging role of the adipocyte. J Cardiopulm Rehabil Prev. 2007;27(1):2–10.

38. Leone A. Smoking, haemostatic factors, and cardiovascular risk. Curr Pharm Design. 2007;13(16): 1661–1667.

39. Libby P, Nathan DM, Abraham K, et al. Report of the National Heart, Lung, and Blood Institute—National Institute of Diabetes and Digestive and Kidney Diseases working group on cardiovascular complications of type 1 diabetes mellitus. Circulation. 2005;111:3489–3493.

40. Lichtenstein AH, Appel LJ, Brands M, et al. Diet and Lifestyle Recommendations Revision 2006: A Scientific statement from the American Heart Association Nutrition Committee. Circulation. 2006; 114;82–96.

41. Magnus P, Beaglehole R. The real contributions of major risk factors to the coronary epidemics. Arch Intern Med. 2001;161:2657–2660.

42. Nakamura K, Barzi F, Huxley R, et al., for the Asia Pacific Cohort Studies Collaboration. Does cigarette smoking exacerbate the effect of total cholesterol and high-density lipoprotein cholesterol on the risk of cardiovascular diseases? Heart. 2009;95: 909–916.

43. Ogden LG, He J, Lydick E, et al. Long-term absolute benefit of lowering blood pressure in hypertensive patients according to the JNC VI risk stratification. Hypertension. 2000;35:539–543.

44. Olchawa B, Kingwell BA, Hoang A, et al. Physical fitness and reverse cholesterol transport. Arterioscler Thromb Vasc Biol. 2004;24:1087–1091.

45. Pereira MA, Schreiner PJ, Pankow JS, et al. The Family Risk Score for coronary heart disease: Associations with lipids, lipoproteins, and body habitus in a middle-aged bi-racial cohort: The ARIC Study. Ann. Epidemiology. 2000;10:239–245.

46. Pyörälä K. Current status and future perspectives in the prevention of coronary heart disease. Cor Vasa. 1991;33(2):91–102.

47. Rahman MM, Laher I. Structural and functional alteration of blood vessels caused by cigarette smoking: An overview of molecular mechanisms. Curr Vasc Pharmacol. 2007;5(4):276–292.

48. Rewers M, Norris J, Dabelea D. Epidemiology of type 1 diabetes mellitus. In: Eisenbarth GS, editor. Immunology of Type 1 Diabetes. 2nd Edition. Wolters-Kluwer Academic/Plenum Publishers, 2004:221–233.

49. Roitman JL, LaFontaine TP. Secondary prevention of coronary artery disease. In Hamm LE, editor. AACVPR Cardiac Rehabilitation Resource Manual Champaign, IL: Human Kinetics Publishers, 2005:27–42.

50. Rothman KJ, Greenland S. Modern epidemiology. 2nd edition. Philadelphia, PA. Lippincott, Williams & Wilkins, Publishers, 1998:24–27.

51. Sacks FM, Svetkey LP, Vollmer WM, et al. Effects on blood pressure of reduced dietary sodium and the Dietary Approaches to Stop Hypertension (DASH) diet. DASH-Sodium Collaborative Research Group. NEJM. 2001;344:3–10.

52. Singh IM, Shishehbor MH, Ansell BJ. High-density lipoprotein as a therapeutic target: A systematic review. JAMA. 2007;298(7):786–798.

53. Smith SC, Allen J, Blair SN, et al. AHA/ACC Guidelines for secondary prevention for patients with coronary and other atherosclerotic vascular disease: 2006 Update: Eendorsed by the National Heart, Lung, and Blood Institute. Circulation. 2006; 113:2363–2372.

54. Stampfer MJ, Hu FB, Manson JE, et al. Primary prevention of coronary heart disease in women through diet and lifestyle. NEJM 2000;343(1):16–22.

55. Tchernof A, Nolan A, Sites CK, et al. Weight loss reduces C-reactive protein levels in obese postmenopausal women. Circulation. 2002;105:564–569.

56. The seventh report of the Joint National Committee on Prevention, Detection, Evaluation and Treatment of High Blood Pressure. (US Department of Health and Human Services: NIH Publication No 03-5233. December 2003) [Internet]. Available at:

http://www.nhlbi.nih.gov/guidelines/hypertension/express.pdf.

57. The Trials of Hypertension Prevention Collaborative Research Group. Effects of weight loss and sodium reduction intervention on blood pressure and hypertension incidence in overweight people with high-normal blood pressure. The Trials of Hypertension Prevention, phase II. Arch Intern Med. 1997;157:657–667.

58. Treating tobacco use and dependence (revised 2000), Washington, DC: NIH Website. [Internet] [Accessed February 15, 2009] Available at: http://www.ncbi.nlm.nih.gov/books/bv.fcgi?rid=hstat2.chapter.

59. Ungvari Z, Parrado-Fernandez C, Csiszar A, et al. Mechanisms underlying caloric restriction and lifespan regulation: Implications for vascular aging. Circ Res. 2008;102(5):519–528.

60. Weinstein AR, Sesso AD, Lee IM, et al. The joint effects of physical activity and body mass index on coronary heart disease risk in women. Arch Intern Med. 2008;168(8):884–890.

61. Williams RR. Genetics of atherosclerosis: Can early familial coronary heart disease be prevented? In: FG Yanowitz, Ed. Coronary Heart Disease Prevention. Marcel Dekker, New York, NY, 1992:45–70.

62. Williams RR, Hasstedt SJ, Wilson DE, et al. Evidence that men with familial hypercholesterolemia can avoid early coronary death: an analysis of 77 gene carriers in four Utah pedigrees. JAMA. 1986;255(2):219–224.

63. Yanbaeva DG, Dentener MA, Creutzberg EC, Wesseling G, Wouters EF. Systemic effects of smoking. Chest. 2007;131(5):1557–1566.

64. Yuan G, Al-Shali KZ, Hegele RA. Hypertriglyceridemia: Its etiology, effects and treatment. CMAJ. 2007;176(8):1113–1120.

65. Yusuf S, Hawken S, Ôunpuu S, et al. On behalf of the Interheart Study Investigators. Effect of potentially modifiable risk factors associated with myocardial infarction in 52 countries (the Interheart Study): A case control study. Lancet. 2004;364: 937–952.

66. Ziccardi P, Nappo F, Giugliano G, et al. Reduction of inflammatory cytokine concentrations and improvement of endothelial functions in obese women after weight loss over one year. Circulation. 2002;105(7):804–809.

CHAPTER 2

Pathophysiology of Chronic Vascular Disease

ABBREVIATIONS

CAD   Coronary artery disease
EPCs   Endothelial progenitor cells
HDL   High-density lipoprotein

LDL   Low-density lipoprotein
PAD   Peripheral artery disease

Chronic diseases such as atherosclerosis and diabetes are considered lifelong or recurrent diseases. They are not temporary, as are communicable diseases (colds or flu), nor are they genetic; that is, they generally are not caused by single gene defects or mutations but rather by the interaction of genes and environmental variables such as sedentary lifestyle, obesity, and overweight; tobacco use; and poor-quality diets. The pathophysiology and symptoms may recur throughout a person's lifetime (see Fig. 2.1), particularly if the person does not adhere to the optimal lifestyle. Most people who undergo typical (medical) treatment programs without adhering to "optimal" lifestyle changes see chronic diseases worsen throughout their lifetime.

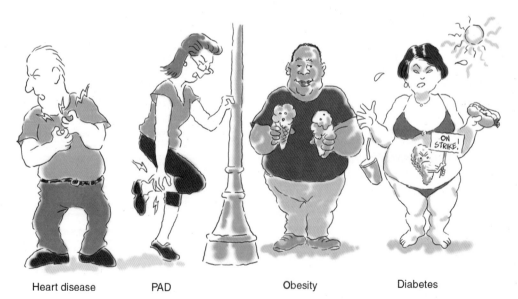

Heart disease   PAD   Obesity   Diabetes

FIGURE 2.1 A low-level, systemic inflammation and endothelial dysfunction are pathophysiologies that are common to the chronic diseases discussed in this book. PAD, peripheral artery disease.

Depending on the level of lifestyle intervention, most chronic diseases respond positively, especially to optimal lifestyle intervention. Optimal lifestyle intervention is often accompanied by long periods of symptom-free states. However, suboptimal lifestyle intervention is frequently accompanied by progression and worsening of the disease. An example of such a negative result is a person with type 2 diabetes, or even prediabetes, who does not lose weight, continues to eat a high-fat diet, and is noncompliant to exercise. This person is insulin resistant and hyperinsulinemic; thus, type 2 diabetes will progress and, at the same time, increase the risk for other chronic diseases (especially heart and peripheral vascular disease) (2).

Although chronic disease is often not diagnosed until later in life when people exhibit signs or symptoms, sometimes well into or after the fifth-to-sixth decade of life. A recent exception is that type 2 diabetes in children is becoming more and more prevalent. Once called "adult-onset diabetes," this is no longer the case.

Almost everyone who gets diagnosed with a chronic disease has "subclinical" disease prior to diagnosis (see Figs. 2.2 and 2.3). For example, this is the basis for the categories of "prehypertension" and "prediabetes." One may not have signs or symptoms, but the pathophysiology associated with the disease is present, often for many years preceding the diagnosis.

Interestingly, 47% of the decrease in deaths from cardiovascular disease is accounted for by improved medical and surgical intervention, rather than health behavior change. Reduction in risk factors is also significant, accounting for 44% of the decreased mortality (11). The decrease in deaths attributed to risk factor reduction comes from decreased incidence of smoking, lowered cholesterol, and lowered blood pressure. These are nearly offset by increased obesity and type 2 diabetes in the United States. Clearly, the death rate from chronic disease (specifically heart disease) is on the decline, but the health of this country is not improving; rather it is also on the decline (1,2).

Optimize

Lifestyle

1. Sixty or more minutes of moderate-to-vigorous exercise per day, including 2 to 3 days of resistance training and stretching (target: >2000 Kcal/week in exercise).
2. No tobacco use.
3. BMI <25.0 or WHR <0.95 (men) or <0.80 (women).
4. Healthy diet (high fiber, whole grains, mostly plant based).
5. One (women) or two (men) alcoholic drinks per day.

DID YOU KNOW?
Vascular Diseases

Atherosclerotic vascular disease: Atherosclerosis is defined by the formation of "plaque" under the lining of the vessel, called the endothelium. Blockages in the artery may limit blood flow to distal tissue.

Coronary artery disease (CAD): CAD is an atherosclerotic disease of the arteries of the heart. It is the primary cause of heart attacks. The medical term for heart attack is "myocardial infarction."

Peripheral artery disease (PAD): PAD is an atherosclerotic disease of the arteries of the arms or legs. PAD is most common in legs and causes "claudication"—discomfort or pain in the muscles with limited blood flow.

Cerebrovascular disease: It is the atherosclerotic disease of the arteries in the head or neck and is most commonly associated with stroke or transient ischemic attack.

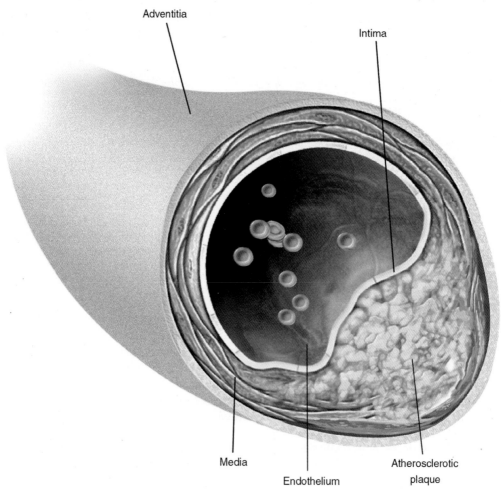

FIGURE 2.2 Atherosclerotic vascular disease is the formation of plaque between the endothelium (the intima) and the middle layer (media) of the artery. Plaque is a collection of cells including lipids, smooth muscle, white blood cells, and other lymphocytes and "cellular debris" that forms in the wall of the artery.

There are some common underlying physiological characteristics (actually "pathology") that occur with many chronic diseases (see Fig. 2.1) (6,34). The pathophysiology of chronic disease is discussed in detail in this chapter and with each disease in this book. These may include low-level systemic inflammation, changes in vascular function, and changes in endocrine function. Early in the disease process (and sometimes even later), these changes

DID YOU KNOW?

Subclinical Disease

Chronic vascular disease does not suddenly develop at the time someone has initial symptoms. The disease process is active for much of the person's life, and symptoms or signs develop when the disease progresses to a "tipping point." The disease, before symptoms are present, is said to be "subclinical." After signs and symptoms are obvious, the diagnosis is usually made.

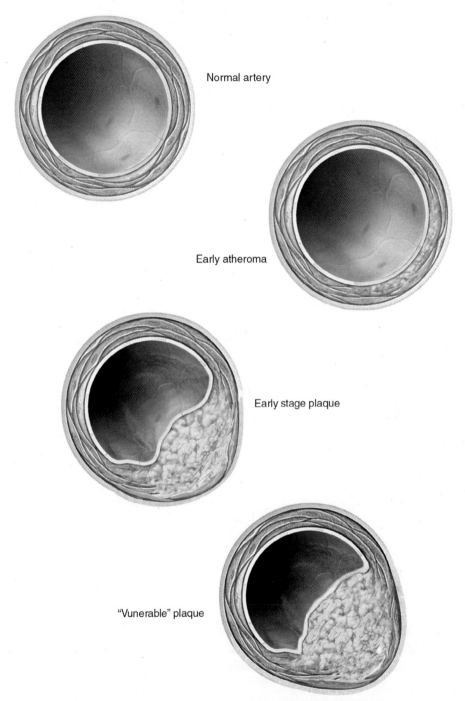

Normal artery

Early atheroma

Early stage plaque

"Vunerable" plaque

FIGURE 2.3 Subclinical atherosclerosis involves blockages that are small enough that they do not cause signs (abnormal exercise tests or electrocardiographic changes) or symptoms (angina or other discomfort related to the blockage) and may not restrict blood flow.

are reversible. Lifestyle intervention, with optimal doses of cardiovascular endurance exercise (and perhaps other types), along with a low-saturated-fat, high-fiber diet not only promotes reversal but has also been shown to prevent these changes (2,8). As the disease progresses, some of the processes probably become permanent physiological (or in some cases, anatomical) alterations, while many remain reversible.

INFLAMMATION AND THE DISEASE PROCESS—WHICH COMES FIRST: THE CHICKEN OR THE EGG?

A low-level systemic (including vascular) inflammation is one hallmark of atherosclerosis as well as other chronic diseases. The question is, where does the inflammation come from? Lifestyle factors that promote low-level systemic inflammation abound in our daily environment. Most Americans are exposed to these lifestyle factors almost every day from infancy throughout life. They are most commonly found in our Western diet and sedentary lifestyle (30).

WHAT CAUSES INFLAMMATION?

Food and many health behaviors (lifestyle) are a prime suspect in this inflammatory condition. Meals high in saturated fat and/or trans fat promote inflammation. High blood triglyceride levels, following high-fat and high "processed" carbohydrate meals promote inflammation. Conversely, consumption of high-fiber diets as well as diets high in polyunsaturated, monounsaturated, and omega-3 fats all suppress or inhibit inflammation. These diets also inhibit the formation of free radicals that, again, are inflammatory. Increased intake of vegetables and fruits is anti-inflammatory and is associated with lower prevalence of diabetes, heart disease, and other chronic diseases (2,8).

High blood triglyceride levels, high low-density lipoprotein (LDL) levels, low high-density lipoprotein (HDL) levels, cigarette smoke, and other inhaled environmental pollutants, overweight and obesity, and stress are associated with vascular inflammation as evidenced by increased inflammatory markers in the blood (3,17,18).

Key Point

Risk factors may be either related to (e.g., blood lipids) or are health behaviors (e.g., sedentary lifestyle). The chronic diseases that we discuss in this book have some common underlying pathophysiology that is directly related to lifestyle.

DID YOU KNOW?
Low-Level Systemic Inflammation

In this case, a "low-level" inflammation is defined as one that is marked by small, nonclinical increases in inflammatory markers, such as high-sensitivity C-reactive protein, interleukin 6, or any other number of inflammatory substances that are found to be elevated. It is not the same as an acute infection (viral or bacterial) that is associated with changes in white blood cells, circulating lymphocytes, or other markers of "frank," infectious inflammatory response. In this case, we term this an "inflammatory syndrome." See the "Digging Deeper" section at the end of this chapter for a more complete and detailed explanation of the inflammatory process.

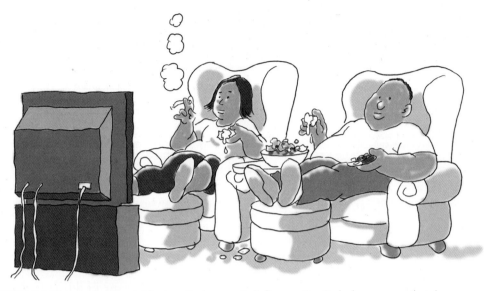

FIGURE 2.4 The environmental factors that promote inflammation include exposure to tobacco smoke, sedentary lifestyle, foods high in saturated and trans fat, and food made from refined grains. There are many other proinflammatory influences in our daily environment that promote chronic disease.

Lack of or very low levels of daily physical activity and low levels of physical fitness are associated with chronic and vascular diseases and are also associated with this inflammatory "syndrome" (Fig. 2.4) (4,29,31).

Moderate exercise has been shown to reduce inflammation and to reduce free radicals in the blood. High-intensity exercise, on the other hand, is known to temporarily increase the inflammatory effect. Therefore, moderation is important in prescribing exercise for most people with chronic disease (11,13,32). (See Fig. 2.5 for factors that are anti-inflammatory.)

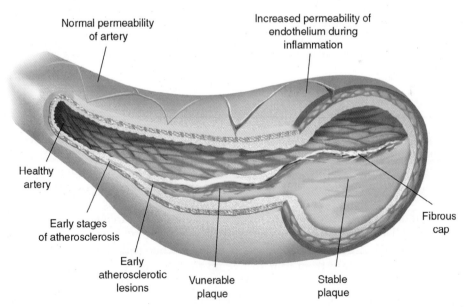

FIGURE 2.5 The inflammatory process is involved in the development, progression, and stability of plaque in arteries.

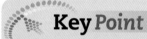

Key Point

Moderate exercise is anti-inflammatory.

In summary, the initial cause of this inflammatory effect is unknown, as is whether it actually precedes or follows the negative lifestyle behaviors associated with the risk factors or the disease state. However, it is apparent that our lifestyle exposes us to inflammatory factors practically from birth throughout life in large part due to the lifestyle choices that we make every day.

VASCULAR FUNCTION

The endothelium is a single cell lining that is found in all arteries and normal endothelial function is essential for healthy arteries. The endothelium plays a critical role in the function of arteries, especially with respect to chronic disease, and has been described as an "organ" in and of itself. Abnormal vascular (endothelial) function is an underlying characteristic of chronic vascular disease as well as other chronic disease (22,23).

NORMAL VASCULAR FUNCTION

Among many functions that the endothelium performs, one is to cause arteries to widen (vasodilation) and constrict (vasoconstriction) when necessary in order to control blood flow to certain areas of the body (see Fig. 2.6). That is, the endothelium is largely responsible for increasing or decreasing blood flow to the heart, brain, muscle tissue, and other organ systems. For example, coronary arteries must dilate in order to increase blood flow to heart muscle during situations of increased metabolic requirements—exercise is one of those times. The heart is critically dependent on this increased blood flow during exercise. During maximal cardiovascular endurance exercise when endothelial function is normal, blood flow can increase from four to five up to 25 times resting. Perhaps the primary control process of normal vascular function is the "nitric oxide system." This is a complex system that results in the production of nitric oxide, which promotes vasodilation under the influence of energy requirements within the cells and other factors, such as pressure on the walls of the artery and chemical factors (22).

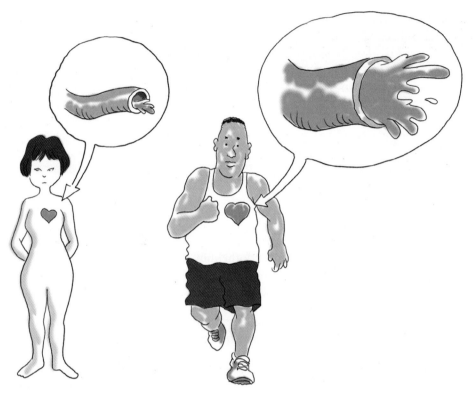

FIGURE 2.6 Exercise normally facilitates vasodilatation in arteries that supply the heart and exercising muscle.

When plaque and endothelial dysfunction are present, coronary arteries may paradoxically constrict in response to increased metabolic demand, rather than expanding. This is called "idiopathic" vasoconstriction. Thus, the vessel is dysfunctional (it constricts) when increased blood flow is most needed (9).

The endothelium is generally in a constant state of repair and regeneration (see the section "Repairing the Endothelium"). It can and does normalize itself, given an appropriate stimulus and the opportunity. For example, after smoking a single cigarette, the

DID YOU KNOW?
Normal Arterial Function

Expansion (vasodilation) and contraction (vasoconstriction) are important functions that must occur for arteries to function normally and for blood flow to accommodate tissue requirements. Vasodilation occurs in situations in which muscle or other organs require increased blood flow. Vasoconstriction, on the other hand, occurs when the amount of blood flowing to a particular area is more than required to meet demand. For example, normal blood flow to the gut is controlled by vasoconstriction when digestion is not occurring; on the other hand, during digestion, blood flow is significantly increased by vasodilation. The endothelium, a biologically active organ, controls much of this process.

Vascular, or endothelial, dysfunction results in an artery (most important, this occurs in coronary arteries) undergoing "paradoxical" vasoconstriction despite the need for increased blood flow to the tissue it serves. In this case, when exercise or other conditions demand increased coronary blood flow, endothelial dysfunction may cause the coronary artery supplying the region to constrict, thus having the opposite effect that is necessary for optimal function. In those with atherosclerotic vascular disease, this may result in symptoms such as angina or other symptoms.

Key Point

The endothelium controls many physiological functions related to arteries, including blood flow and permeability. Endothelial dysfunction is pathophysiology common to the chronic diseases that we discuss in this book.

endothelium begins to function abnormally within minutes (20,36). Subsequently, if there is no exposure to smoke for several hours, the endothelium attempts to normalize its function as much as possible. We have already detailed some of the environmental factors that cause endothelial dysfunction.

The mere presence of fatty streaks and intimal deposits (blockages) within the endothelium also cause endothelial dysfunction. Even so, the vascular system attempts to repair, regenerate, and improve these conditions continuously. In addition, there are other environmental factors such as omega 3 fats, weight loss, lifestyle management of blood pressure, lipids, and diabetes, as well as exercise, that improve vascular and endothelial function (14,16).

ABNORMAL VASCULAR FUNCTION

Vasodilation can occur because of mechanical (increased blood pressure) and neurohormonal factors that directly affect the endothelium, circulating metabolites, and local blood flow. The nitric oxide system is critical to the vasodilation response to exercise (22,27). Normal endothelial function also allows the effects of inflammation to be moderated by chemical factors such as high HDL, low "radical oxygen species," and other anti-inflammatory substances that are present when the endothelium functions normally. Many of these substances are produced and released by the endothelium. When the endothelium functions normally, these inflammatory substances are inhibited (20,22,27). Finally, exercise also promotes improved (or normalizes) vascular function, thus providing beneficial effects with respect to prevention of vascular disease, as well as heart attack (12,22,27).

ENDOTHELIAL PROGENITOR CELLS

Specialized cells (similar to stem cells) produced in bone marrow and called endothelial progenitor cells (EPCs) drive the process of repairing the endothelium. EPCs are primarily responsible for the repair and formation of new endothelial tissue. EPCs are stimulated by many conditions, including regular exercise (41,42). On the other hand, the same environmental factors that promote atherosclerosis also inhibit and depress the functions and formation of EPCs (16).

Exercise exerts many preventive, positive influences on the endothelium. One of the most important of these is the stimulation of the production of EPCs. EPCs promote growth and repair of the endothelium when it is not functioning properly or when it is damaged (42).

There is an entire "cascade" of physiological processes that cause EPCs to be generated. It is likely that there is an appropriate and effective frequency, intensity, and duration of exercise associated with the generation of EPCs, but that is not well defined. It is also likely that increased EPCs is one of the "subacute" changes that occur subsequent to a single exercise session but does not persist without daily exercise. How long this effect lasts is unknown (16,41,42).

CHRONIC VASCULAR DISEASE AND INFLAMMATION

As discussed above, this low-level systemic inflammation underlies atherosclerosis. Various substances within the blood are noted to be "inflammatory markers," but there can be "proinflammatory" as well as anti-inflammatory substances. They are present within the endothelium, especially when inflammation is active. These proinflammatory substances also promote further levels of inflammation, thus making the process self-propagating.

INITIATING VASCULAR INFLAMMATION

One source of the initial inflammation in arteries may be the presence of chemically altered LDLs (e.g., from a high-fat meal, exposure to smoke, obesity, etc.), which attract substances that promote further growth of the plaque. The plaque grows by accumulating fatty materials (LDL, cholesterol), white blood cells, smooth muscle cells, and other substances that cause it to enlarge. There is also evidence that factors such as diet, exposure to smoke (including second-hand smoke), and physical inactivity cause this inflammatory process to be initiated and propagate the process once it is present (23,36).

INFLAMMATION AND THE ENDOTHELIUM

Inflammation is also associated with abnormal endothelial function. It promotes additional cell growth and deposition within the wall of the artery. Blockages can easily grow to occlude from 60% to 90% of the opening of the artery. These kinds of blockages may limit blood flow in high-demand situations (activity or exercise or stress, for example) or even at rest after a large high-fat, high-processed-carbohydrate meal and then cause symptoms. Depending on the location of the blockages, they can also be associated with leg pain or symptoms of transient ischemic attack and stroke. A transient ischemic attack is exactly what it sounds like—a transient or temporary set of symptoms caused by the restriction of blood flow in or to the brain. By definition, the symptoms of a transient ischemic attack are resolved within 24 hours of onset.

INFLAMMATION AND PLAQUE STABILITY

In addition, inflammation at times causes the existing plaque to be unstable, thus making it prone to "rupture." The stability (or more specifically, "instability") of plaque is directly related to the likelihood of rupture. At least 50% and perhaps as much as 70% to 80% of heart attacks and strokes occur through plaque ruptures that occlude less than 50% of the artery. These smaller blockages often have higher lipid content and softer coverings (they have little or no "fibrous cap") and are more prone to rupture (see Fig. 2.7) (37,38).

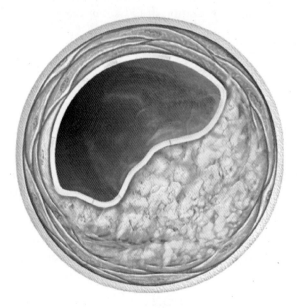

Unstable atherosclerotic plaque

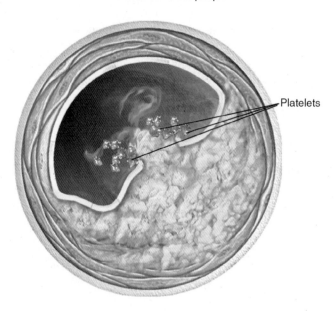

Plaque rupture

FIGURE 2.7 Plaque rupture may result in heart attack or stroke. It is the result of unstable atherosclerotic plaque.

Plaque rupture can result in heart attack (myocardial infarction) or stroke (cerebral vascular accident). During a heart attack, when a plaque ruptures, a large blood clot forms at the site of rupture and it partially or completely occludes blood flow to areas of tissue beyond the blood clot. This occurrence is the most common cause of a heart attack or stroke. What precipitates or initiates this plaque rupture is unknown, but what is known is that the smaller, softer plaques with high lipid content, particularly oxidized LDL, are more prone to rupture. Local inflammation is almost always present when a plaque ruptures and, as was stated earlier, the proinflammatory substances make the plaque more unstable. So, inflammation is certainly a prime culprit in heart attacks and strokes (37,38).

Plaque rupture does not always result in complete occlusion of the artery and heart attack (or stroke). It is likely that there may be times when a plaque ruptures or becomes unstable and it merely incorporates additional material into the plaque, then it restabilizes and subsequently heals. The healing process involves smooth muscle proliferation (smooth muscle cells are contained in most plaques), incorporation of the remains of the blood clot, and a re-formation of the endothelium; thus, the plaque is larger than it was before the rupture (37,38).

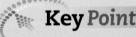 **Key Point**

Inflammation may be the initial and the primary underlying pathophysiology found at the core of many chronic diseases. It can result from many lifestyle behaviors considered to be "unhealthy," including smoking, excess adipose tissue, and low levels of physical activity.

INSULIN RESISTANCE

Another characteristic common to chronic diseases is "insulin resistance." Insulin receptors are found on the membranes of skeletal muscle and other cells. They function to facilitate the entry of glucose into the cell. Insulin has many powerful effects on muscle and fat metabolism, endothelial function, and other hormone function (20,29). Even though this is not a discussion of diabetes (see Chapter 7), it is appropriate to discuss this factor as one that is, perhaps, central to vascular disease. Insulin resistance is associated with many chronic diseases, such as type 2 diabetes, high blood pressure, metabolic syndrome,

DID YOU KNOW?
Insulin

Insulin is a substance that facilitates the entry of glucose into muscles (and other tissue) so that it can be utilized for energy production. There are special receptors on the membrane of muscle cells where insulin attaches in order to promote the entry of glucose into the cell. When these receptors are not readily available or are not working efficiently, "insulin resistance" is the result. Insulin resistance results in restricted entry of glucose into the cells, which then may result in increased glucose in the blood (hyperglycemia). This is a hallmark of diabetes. Long-term insulin resistance ultimately also results in hyperinsulinemia (too much insulin), which leads to even more pathophysiology because of the influence of insulin on so many other physiological processes. Refer to Chapter 7 for a more complete discussion of insulin and insulin resistance.

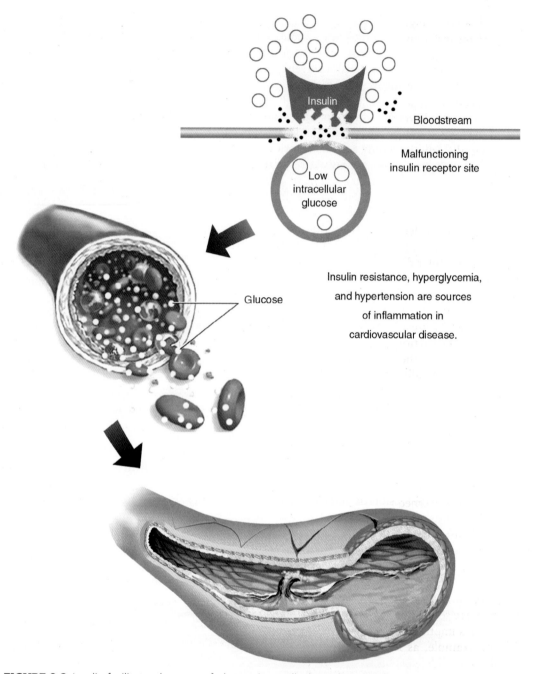

FIGURE 2.8 Insulin facilitates the entry of glucose into cells through an insulin receptor on the cell membrane. The interaction of insulin with the receptor then signals another molecule, glut-4 protein, to transport it through the membrane. Insulin resistance is a result of the receptors being "less sensitive" to the presence of glucose; thus, it does not enter the cells in sufficient amounts, eventually leading to hyperglycemia and hyperinsulinemia.

and obesity (Fig. 2.8). The primary link to vascular disease may be through obesity, or perhaps inflammation (see above), but most likely is both.

Insulin resistance may lead to the inability of circulating insulin to keep blood glucose levels under control. In a fasting state, blood glucose level should be <100 mg/dl. Long-term insulin resistance leads to the overproduction of insulin by the pancreas and a condition called "hyperinsulinemia," or simply too much circulating insulin. Controlling blood glucose is only one of the important effects of insulin. When insulin is present in abnormally high amounts in the blood, many other physiological processes are affected. This is especially true in people with type 2 diabetes or obesity. Insulin stimulates cell growth (essentially production of new cells, for example, growth of the blockages in the arteries), increased lipid metabolism, and decreased synthesis and activation of nitric oxide. All of these conditions are part of the abnormal physiology associated with vascular disease, insulin resistance, and hyperinsulinemia (29).

Insulin accelerates the growth and progression of atherosclerosis by acting on the cells that make up the plaque (blockages). Insulin negatively affects the production of nitric oxide and causes vascular dysfunction. Therefore, it is associated with oxidative stress, endothelial dysfunction, and inflammation. All of these physiological pathways function normally only when insulin is present in normal quantities and when insulin resistance is not present (20,29).

There is a relationship between increased insulin resistance and inflammation, and cardiovascular disease. The connection can be seen in the metabolic influences as well as in the many other actions of insulin. It is safe to say that the insulin resistance associated with inflammation and endothelial dysfunction is a key player in the development of vascular disease, especially in people with obesity and/or type 2 diabetes (8,20,43).

TREATMENT OF CHRONIC DISEASE

Medical treatment of chronic disease is generally aimed at the *signs* and *symptoms* of the disease as well as the physiological and biochemical processes that underlie it. Because this book is concerned with "optimal lifestyle" in the prevention of disease, we will not discuss specific drugs or other medical therapies here.

Unfortunately, drugs are commonly the physician's only answer (as well as the patient's request, in many cases) to prevention and treatment of chronic disease; it is clear that lifestyle management is not only effective but that in most cases it is the *most effective agent* in the prevention toolkit. The key to prevention and management of chronic disease with lifestyle is the word "optimal." Making moderate changes in lifestyle (e.g., 30 minutes of exercise, 3 days per week) or being "moderately overweight" or even being "moderate" in consumption of saturated fat (10% of calories, for example, as recommended by AHA Step 1 dietary guidelines) has not been shown to be particularly effective in either primary or secondary prevention of vascular (or other chronic) disease, and, in fact, it has been shown to be associated with further progression of the disease (32,35,40). The definition of "optimal" is generally known. It is clear, for example, that one cannot use tobacco products "in moderation" or that exercising 3 days per week is not optimal for disease prevention. Daily exercise is preventive. "Optimal" multifactorial lifestyle management is far

> ## Key Point
>
> Pathophysiology (e.g., insulin resistance) can be modified by drugs and lifestyle. However, once the pathophysiology of a chronic disease has been genetically expressed (e.g., insulin resistance), the potential for that pathophysiology remains for life regardless of the effectiveness of treatment.

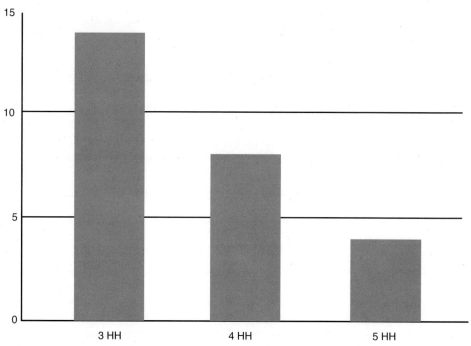

FIGURE 2.9 Percentage of the population practicing three, four, or five healthy habits (HH). 3 HH = no smoking; healthy diet; exercise >30 min/d; 4 HH = no smoking; healthy diet; exercise >30 min/d; BMI <25.0; 5 HH = no smoking; healthy diet; exercise >30 min/d; BMI <25.0; moderate alcohol (5–30 g/d). (Chiuve SE, McCullough ML, Sacks FM, Rimm EB. Healthy lifestyle factors in the primary prevention of coronary heart disease amon men: Benefits among user and nonusers of lipid-lowering and antihypertensive medications. Circulation. 2006;114:160–167.)

more beneficial for improving cardiovascular function than any single pharmacological intervention.

Finally, it is clear that Americans with or without chronic disease do not practice these healthy habits in large numbers (7,21). Figures 2.9 and 2.10 show the percentage of Americans without chronic disease and with cardiovascular disease, respectively, who practice some specific healthy habits. The adoption of these practices would significantly and positively affect their health status.

DID YOU KNOW?

What Are Signs and Symptoms?

- *Signs:* measurable changes in physiology or biochemistry that accompany disease states.
- *Symptoms:* subjective feelings and/or physical changes that are associated with specific physiological changes and disease states.

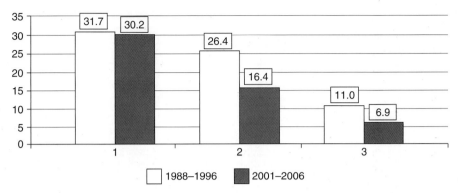

FIGURE 2.10 Percentage of the population with diagnosed cardiovascular disease who practice one, two, or three healthy habits in 1988–1996 vs. 2006. Healthy habits include a body mass index <30.0; physical activity >12 times/mo; no smoking; fruit/vegetable intake >5 servings/d; and moderate alcohol. (King DE, Mainous AG, Carnemolla M, Everett CJ. Adherence to lifestyle habits in US adults, 1988–2006. Am J Med. 2009;122:528–534.)

In later chapters of this book, we will discuss factors that are often thought of as "risk factors" such as lipid (e.g., cholesterol) abnormalities and glucose intolerance that are disease entities by themselves. We will try to point out what is known about "optimal" lifestyle management for preventing chronic disease. The primary goal of this book is to discuss "optimal lifestyle" in the role of chronic disease prevention; thus, we will refrain from discussing medical intervention and medical therapeutics.

DIGGING DEEPER

Inflammation may be the primary underlying pathophysiological process for each of the chronic diseases that we discuss in this book. It may also be the primary, initial pathophysiology expressed in most of these diseases. We have discussed the proinflammatory nature of many of the risk factors and lifestyle behaviors (see Chapter 1) that are associated with many of these chronic diseases. Thus, inflammation is a natural topic for this section.

In this section, a basic explanation of inflammation, including the primary and basic components, will be presented. The reader will be directed to a more complete description in the Significant Research box at the conclusion of this section.

Innate and Adaptive Inflammation

Inflammation has evolved into responses that are classified as *innate* or *adaptive*. The *innate response* protects against infection and "foreign" invaders (antigens). This response occurs quickly, but only to a limited number of invaders or antigens, whereas the *adaptive response* requires that our body be "educated" about the type of invader. Both inflammatory responses are believed to be involved in atherogenesis (24).

The innate response is triggered by receptors that recognize the presence of an invader and "signal" release of cytokines and proinflammatory substances. It is also involved with thrombosis (coagulation), thus directly implicating the innate response in another process that is tied to atherosclerosis. The adaptive response, on the other hand, takes weeks to months to be effective. This additional time is used to "educate" the body about the antigen and to produce specific substances (antibodies) to combat a particular type of antigen.

(continued)

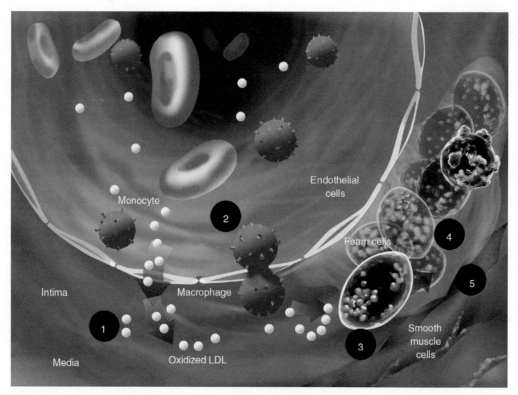

FIGURE 2.11 The development and progression of atherosclerotic plaque is a complex and ongoing process involving the interaction of many cellular and physiological processes. (1) LDL is oxidized and enters the intimal layer through the endothelium. (2) Monocytes are attracted to the area and penetrate the endothelium. (3) Monocytes accumulate fat droplets (LDL) through the process of phagocytosis. (4) The fat-laden cells become "foam cells" containing large amounts of fat, while cytokines signal the initiation of the inflammatory process. (5) Tissue remodeling ensues with the influx of smooth muscle tissue, the formation of scar tissue, calcification, and numerous other inflammation-mediated processes. LDL, low-density lipoprotein.

Inflammation and Atherosclerosis

Excessive amounts of LDL are thought to trigger this process in the endothelium and the intima (the inner layer of blood vessels). LDL, then, is the "invader." Monocytes (a type of white blood cell) function to rid the invader substance. Monocytes are attracted to the endothelium, travel through the endothelial layer to the intima, and engulf LDL (25). Interestingly, though the recruitment of monocytes to the endothelium is one of the first processes to occur, it is not limited to the early stages of atherogenesis, but continues even in long-existing plaque (24).

The monocytes are joined in the intima by another type of lymphocyte (T lymphocyte) that is proinflammatory, and inflammatory processes, already established, are further promoted (see Fig. 2.11). These T lymphocytes are part of the adaptive response and initiate that portion of the immune response. They produce cytokines, other proinflammatory substances, and even trigger the "death by suicide" (apoptosis) of other cells. There are many types of T cells with various functions.

The atherosclerotic process is driven by the monocytes that engulf LDL in the intima and become engorged with fat droplets (so-called foam cells). The T cells and other components of the plaque produce substances that promote cell growth, attracting smooth muscle cells from the middle layer of the artery (the tunica media) and, thus, causing further growth of the plaque. As we have stated, this process becomes "self-promoting"; that is, the presence of the plaque causes the plaque to progress. The foam cells predominate within the intima, forming a fatty core just under the surface of the endothelium.

The final stages of plaque formation occur when smooth muscle cells (and other cell types) are attracted into the area of the fatty core. These smooth muscle cells, along with other matrix components, begin to wall off the fatty core. The barrier is formed between the endothelial layer and the intima, where the lipid core lies. The formation of the matrix within and around these smooth muscle cells includes connective tissue that forms a fibrous cap to the plaque, effectively stabilizing it within the intima (23).

Significant RESEARCH

The first of these articles is a landmark article on atherosclerosis published in *Scientific American* in 2002 that highlighted recent research describing the connection between inflammation and the pathophysiology of CAD and heart attack. The second is also a review of the literature on endothelial function and exercise that outlines the whole of the process and is significant in connecting these primary aspects of health and disease.

Inflammation and Atherosclerosis

Libby P. Atherosclerosis: The new view. Sci Am. 2002;286:47–53.

■ Summary ■

Dr. Peter Libby describes the complex set of physiological relationships involved in the process of inflammation and links them to atherosclerosis. He also brings in some of the "key players" in the atherosclerotic process, LDL, HDL, smoking, diabetes, and other risk factors. He discusses the known relationships (at that time) between the inflammation, coagulation, plaque progression, stability, and rupture. He also introduces the concept that his colleague, Dr. Paul Ridker, has championed—hs-CRP, as an indicator of risk for this inflammatory effect. This article is an excellent way to gather information about the inflammatory process and its relationship to atherosclerosis. Libby recently published another comprehensive review of this research in the *Journal of the American College of Cardiology* that is worth reading: "Inflammation in Atherosclerosis."

Libby's 2002 article is not "research" in the traditional sense but is, in fact, significant in that it draws attention to and summarizes the developing science around the systemic, subclinical inflammation that is, perhaps, the significant underlying pathophysiology for atherosclerosis. Its importance lies in the summary of the material about inflammation and Libby's ability to connect and explain the circumstances of the development and progression of atherosclerosis. Coupled with the more recent 2009 article, it not only introduces important concepts and relationships between inflammation, the disease process, and lifestyle but also connects some of the dots between the risk factors for CAD and the disease process. As outlined in this chapter, health behaviors are intimately involved in the inflammatory process. A high-fat, high-refined, and processed-food diet, sedentary lifestyle, smoking, and other lifestyle choices

(continued)

promote the inflammatory process. These influences most often begin in early childhood and intensify as we age and continue with these habits. Their ongoing effects cause us to be vulnerable to the pathophysiology associated with chronic disease and also cause the expression of genes that cause chronic diseases such as obesity, diabetes, and cardiovascular disease.

Exercise and Endothelial Function

Laughlin HM. Physical activity in prevention and treatment of coronary disease: The battle line is in exercise vascular cell biology. Med Sci Sports Exerc. 2004;36(3);352–362.

■ Summary ■

Dr. Harold Laughlin summarizes the research that highlights the influence of exercise on endothelial function. This is significant because it connects exercise and chronic disease prevention, especially CAD. It is also important because it begins to draw the lines that connect exercise and physical activity to a biological rationale for the preventive effect. No longer does it just seem that the most fit people survive the longest. This was an early and often-used critique of the research showing that the most active people have lower rates of heart disease and die less frequently of the disease.

Dr. Laughlin's laboratory and research group at the University of Missouri is one of the leaders in animal research in endothelial function. In this article he succeeds at outlining the relationships between normal and abnormal endothelial function and exercise. He summarizes the biology of endothelial function. The nitric oxide synthase system is described and related to exercise. The known effects of both "exercise" and "exercise training" are discussed. Dr. Laughlin demonstrates the influence of exercise on endothelial dilation and on gene expression that can either enhance or inhibit normal endothelial function. This is a "seminal" article about exercise and endothelial function that provides the exercise professional with excellent background information to understand this important concept.

REFERENCES

1. American Heart Association Web site. Dallas (TX): American Heart Association. Available at: http://www.americanheart.org/.

2. Bazzano LA, Serdula M, Liu S. Prevention of type 2 diabetes by diet and lifestyle modification. J Am Coll Nutr. 2005;24(5):310–319.

3. Berenson GS, Wattigney WA, Tracy RE, et al. Atherosclerosis of the aorta and coronary arteries and cardiovascular risk factors in persons aged 6 to 30 years and studied at necropsy (The Bogalusa Heart Study). Am J Cardiol. 1992;70:851–858.

4. Blair SN, Kohl HW, Paffenbarger RS, et al. Physical fitness and all-cause mortality: a prospective study of healthy and unhealthy men. JAMA. 1995;273:1093–1098.

5. Centers for Disease Control Web site [Internet] Washington, DC. Centers for Disease Control. Available at: http://www.cdc.gov/nchs/nhanes.htm. Accessed December, 2009.

6. Ceriello A. Motz E. Is oxidative stress the pathogenic mechanism underlying insulin resistance, diabetes, and cardiovascular disease? The Common Soil Hypothesis Revisited. Arterioscler Thromb Vasc Biol. 2004;24(5):816–823.

7. Chiuve SE, McCullough ML, Sacks FM, et al. Healthy lifestyle factors in the primary prevention of coronary heart disease amon men: benefits among user and nonusers of lipid-lowering and antihypertensive medications. Circulation. 2006;114:160–167.

8. Dandona P, Aljada A, Chadhuri A, et al. Metabolic syndrome: a comprehensive perspective based on interactions between obesity, diabetes and inflammation. Circulation. 2005;111:1448–1454.

9. Drexler H, Hornig B. Endothelial dysfunction in human disease. J Mol Cell Cardiol. 1999;31:51–60.

10. Falk E. Pathogenesis of atherosclerosis. JACC. 2006;48(8, Suppl):C7–C12.

11. Ford ES, Umed AA, Croft JB, et. al. Explaining the decrease in U.S. deaths from coronary disease, 1980–2000. NEJM. 2007;356:2388–2398.

12. Green DJ, Maiorana A, O'Driscoll G, et al. Effect of exercise training on endothelium-derived nitric

oxide function in humans. J Physiol. 2004;561 (Pt 1):1–25.

13. Hamer M. Exercise and psychobiological processes: implications for the primary prevention of coronary heart disease. Sports Med. 2006; 36(10):829–838.

14. Haram PM, Adams V, Kemi OJ, et al. Time-course of endothelial adaptation following acute and regular exercise. Eur J Cardiovasc Prev Rehabil. 2006;13(4):585–591.

15. Hill JM, Zalos G, Halcox JP, et al. Circulating endothelial progenitor cells, vascular function, and cardiovascular risk. NEJM. 2003;348:593–600.

16. Jarvisalo MJ, Harmoinen A, Hakanen M, et al. Elevated serum C-reactive protein levels and early arterial changes in healthy children. Arterioscler Thromb Vasc Biol. 2002;22:1323–1328.

17. Kapiotis S, Holzer G, Schaller G, et al. A proinflammatory state is detectable in obese children and is accompanied by functional and morphological vascular changes. Arterioscler Thromb Vasc Biol. 2006;26:2541–2546.

18. Kavey RE, Allada V, Daniels SR, et al. Cardiovascular risk reduction in high-risk pediatric patients: a scientific statement from the American Heart Association. Circulation. 2006 12:114(24):2710–2738.

19. Kim J, Monagnani M, Kwand KK, et al. Reciprocal relationships between insulin resistance and endothelial dysfunction: molecular and pathophysiological mechanisms. Circulation. 2006; 113:1888–1904.

20. King DE, Mainous AG, Carnemolla M, et al. Adherence to lifestyle habits in US adults, 1988–2006. Amer J Med. 2009;122:528–534.

21. Laughlin HM. Physical activity in prevention and treatment of coronary disease: the battle line is in exercise vascular cell biology. Med Sci Sports Exerc. 2004;36(3):352–362.

22. Libby P, Ridker P, Hansson GK. Inflammation in atherosclerosis: from pathophysiology to practice. J Amer Coll Cardiol. 2009;54(23):2129–2138.

23. Libby P. Atherosclerosis: the new view. Sci Am. 2002;286:47–53.

24. Lindstrom J, Louheranta M, Eriksson J, et al. The Finnish Diabetes Prevention Study (DPS): lifestyle intervention and 3-year results on diet and physical activity. Diabetes Care. 2003;26:3230–3236.

25. Linke A, Erbs S, Hambrecht R. Effects of exercise training upon endothelial function in patients with cardiovascular disease. Front Biosc. 2008;13:424–432.

26. Maiorana A, O'Driscoll GO, Taylor R, et al. Exercise and the nitric oxide vasodilator system. Sports Med. 2003;33(4):101.

27. Manson JE, Greenland P, LaCroix AZ, et al. Walking compared with vigorous exercise for the prevention of cardiovascular events in women. N Engl J Med. 2002;347:716–725.

28. Marquezine GF, Bernardo L. Molecular activity of insulin and selective insulin resistance. Endo-crinologist. 2007;17(6):351–356.

29. Miller M, Zhan M, Havas S. High attributable risk of elevated C-reactive protein level to conventional coronary heart disease risk factors: the Third National Health and Nutrition Examination Survey. Arch Intern Med. 2005;165:2063–2068.

30. Myers J, Manish P, Froelicher V, et al. Exercise capacity and mortality among men referred for exercise testing. N Engl J Med. 2002;346(11):793–801.

31. Phillips LS, Branch WT, Cook CB, et al. Clinical inertia. Ann Intern Med. 2001;135:825–834.

32. Plaisance EP, Grandjean PW. Physical activity and high-sensitivity C-reactive protein. Sports Med. 2006;36(5):443–458.

33. Qi L, Hu F. Dietary glycemic load, whole grains, and systemic inflammation in diabetes: the epidemiological evidence. Curr Opin Lipidol. 2007;18(1):3–8.

34. Qureshi AL, Suri FK, Guterman LR, et al. Ineffective secondary prevention in survivors of cardiovascular events in the US population. Arch Intern Med. 2001;161:1621–1628.

35. Rackley CE, Weissman NJ. The Role of Plaque Rupture in Acute Coronary Syndromes. Waltham, MA: Uptodate, 2009. Available at:www.uptodate.com. Accessed March, 2010.

36. Rackley CE. Pathogenesis of Plaque Rupture in Acute Coronary Syndromes. Pathogenesis of Atherosclerosis. Waltham, MA: Uptodate, 2007. Available at: www.uptodate.com. Accessed December, 2009.

37. Rackley CE. Pathogenesis of Plaque Rupture in Acute Coronary Syndromes. Waltham, MA: Uptodate, 2009. Available at: www.uptodate.com. Accessed December, 2009.

38. Schachinger F, Britten MB, Elsner M, et al. A positive family history of premature coronary artery disease is associated with impaired endothelium-dependent coronary blood flow regulation. Circulation. 1999;100:1502–1508.

39. Smith DA, Harnick D, Kilaru R. Comparison of physician-managed lipid-lowering care in patients with coronary heart disease in two time periods (1994 and 1999). Am J Cardiol. 2001;88:1417–1419.

40. Steiner S, Niessner A, Ziegler S, et al. Endurance training increases the number of endothelial progenitor cells in patients with cardiovascular risk and coronary artery disease. Atherosclerosis. 2005;181:305–310.

41. Szmitko PE, Fedak PW, Weisel RD, et al. Endothelial progenitor cells: new hope for a broken heart. Circulation. 2000;107:3093–3100.

42. Thompson, W. (Ed.). ACSM's Guidelines for Exercise Testing and Prescription, 8th ed. Baltimore, MD: Lippincott Williams & Wilkins; 2010.

43. Wang CC, Goalstone ML, Draznin B. Molecular mechanisms of insulin resistance that impact cardiovascular biology. Diabetes. 2004;53:2735–2740.

CHAPTER 3

Exercise and Physical Activity

ABBREVIATIONS

ACSM	American College of Sports Medicine	LDL	Low-density lipoprotein
		LPL	Lipoprotein lipase
AHA	American Heart Association	MET	Metabolic equivalent
BPM	Beats per minute	MetS	Metabolic syndrome
CAD	Coronary artery disease	PA	Physical activity
CRF	Cardiorespiratory fitness	PEH	Postexercise hypotension
EPC	Endothelial progenitor cell	PF	Physical fitness
HDL	High-density lipoprotein	PPL	Postprandial lipemia
HR	Heart rate	RPE	Rating of perceived exertion
HRR	Heart rate reserve	VO$_2$R	Oxygen-uptake reserve

THE CASE FOR EXERCISE: HOW MUCH EXERCISE IS ENOUGH?

The case for exercise as a critical part of a healthy lifestyle for the prevention and management of chronic disease has become well established in recent years. Previously, the American College of Sports Medicine (ACSM) and other organizations (e.g., the American Heart Association [AHA]) suggested that 3 to 4 days, 20 to 30 minutes per day, of vigorous cardiovascular endurance exercise per week was sufficient for healthy people (65). The most recent ACSM/AHA recommendations state that adults should engage in **30 minutes of moderate-to-vigorous exercise on "most or all" days of the week** (25,43,64). Table 3.1 summarizes the ACSM guidelines on providing exercise-prescription recommendations for increasing cardiorespiratory fitness (CRF).

Early recommendations for exercise were based on elegant research conducted by Dr. Michael Pollock more than 35 years ago (18,53–57). Since then a significant body of research has further clarified the question, "How much exercise is enough?" The answer depends on the **goal(s)** of the exercise program that are defined by the needs and health status of each client. Because the topic of **chronic disease prevention** is paramount in this book, the primary question we hope to answer in this chapter is, "What is the optimal amount of exercise required to prevent chronic disease and/or the complications of chronic disease?"

More specifically, we will discuss vascular disease (coronary artery disease [CAD] and other diseases of blood vessels that cause stroke and peripheral vascular disease), diabetes and metabolic syndrome (MetS), and obesity in this book. (See remaining chapters for details on these chronic diseases.) Although the diseases themselves are different, the physiological basis for prevention and for exercise prescription is similar, and, perhaps more than coincidentally, these diseases have a similar underlying pathophysiology (see Chapter 2).

The final piece to the "exercise puzzle" is a discussion of physical activity (PA) and CRF. PA is defined in this book as any type of nonstructured physical movement that results in an increase in energy expenditure. CRF and PA are critical factors in specifying and determining the effects of exercise on chronic disease. In this chapter, we will discuss the importance of

TABLE 3.1	Exercise Prescription for Increasing CRF	
Variable	**Minimum Criteria for Increase**	**Comment**
Frequency	3–5 d/wk Note: for frequencies of 3/wk intensities of 60%–80% HRR or 77%–90% HR Max is required for improvement in CRF	Minimum frequency required to increase fitness. Deconditioned and less-fit individuals may better tolerate increased frequency (including 2 or more 10- to 15-minute sessions per day) and decreased intensity at the initiation of a program.
Intensity	64%–94% Max HR 40%–85% of HRR 40%–85% of VO$_2$R	Lower-intensity cardiovascular endurance training is recommended for less fit individuals. Higher-intensity exercise carries increased risk for orthopedic injury and, perhaps, cardiovascular complications.
Duration	20–60 min/session	Continuous duration is most effective, though intermittent exercise can be used if the rest period is controlled and not excessive. Intermittent bouts of activity and exercise throughout the day (10–15 min, 2–3 times/day) may help novice and less fit exercisers increase CRF until continuous exercise can be tolerated.
Mode	Walking, jogging/running, cycling, swimming, elliptical trainers, stair machines, water aerobics, step aerobics, rowing, other	Weight-bearing exercise may expose deconditioned and overweight/obese individuals to injury and care should be taken when implementing such programs in new exercisers.
Progression	No more than 5%–10% per week for duration and frequency; increase frequency and duration to minimum goal of 1,500 additional calories per week prior to increasing intensity	

CRF, cardiorespiratory endurance fitness; HRR, heart rate reserve; HR, heart rate; VO$_2$R, oxygen-uptake reserve.

With permission from Thompson WR, ed. ACSM's Guidelines for Exercise Testing and Prescription. 8th Ed. Baltimore: Lippincott Williams & Wilkins, 2010.

CRF and PA as well as their influence on prevention and treatment of chronic disease. The "Digging Deeper" section at the end of this chapter discusses this topic in greater detail.

CRF AND PREVENTION OF DISEASE

The scientific literature clearly supports the notion that increased level of CRF is associated with decreased incidence of chronic disease, including hypertension, type 2 diabetes, CAD, and some cancers (63). This is true among populations without a clinical diagnosis (i.e., "primary prevention") as well as for populations with known disease ("secondary prevention").

How Much Exercise?

Exercising for fitness alone is not sufficient for prevention of disease. Daily activity, as well as increased fitness, is important!! The **optimal** amount of exercise to prevent chronic disease includes exercise that improves CRF as well as daily activity/exercise (leisure time physical activity) that may be below the threshold to increase CRF but still provides benefits for prevention of chronic disease.

Each of the primary terms that we will use are defined here:

1. **Exercise:** Exercise (for our purposes) is defined as any activity that is done for the specific purpose of increasing either cardiovascular endurance fitness or muscular strength and endurance. Resistance training is included in this category, if it is intended for either purpose (cardiovascular endurance or muscular strength/endurance).
2. **Physical Activity:** PA is defined as any activity that is not sedentary or quiet sitting. PA can include activities that are very sedentary, such as knitting or even fishing, which can be done in a seated position, to very vigorous activities, such as jogging, cycling, or game and sports activities. PA can be "leisure time physical activity" or job-related activity.
3. **Cardiorespiratory Fitness:** CRF is defined here as the measured value of cardiorespiratory endurance fitness. The "gold standard" is usually VO_2max, but other values can be used. This is always a value that is quantified.

Examples include decrease in mortality from heart attack, incidence of CAD events, and progression and incidence of MetS and type 2 diabetes. Studies show that for each metabolic equivalent (MET) increase in functional capacity there is approximately a 10% decrease in mortality (death) from chronic disease (42). We encourage readers to review some of the "important" studies outlined at the end of the chapter to become familiar with this literature. Your credibility and effectiveness as an exercise professional are enhanced by having scientific information at your disposal.

Because increased CRF is related to prevention and reduced risk for chronic disease, exercise that improves CRF should be included in all exercise programs for treating chronic disease. The principles for increasing the CRF are outlined in Table 3.1. CRF programs must be implemented cautiously and slowly for individuals who are deconditioned, obese, and overweight, have chronic disease, or have little or no experience at maintaining long-term exercise programs (e.g., who have never been able to comply with exercise regularly for longer than 6 months continuously). These clients are the most likely to have difficulty adhering to CRF programs; they are also the most likely to sustain injuries and encounter obstacles that are difficult, sometimes seemingly impossible, to overcome; finally, they are the most likely to perceive (see Fig. 3.1) the discomfort that may accompany higher-intensity exercise as uncomfortable and, therefore, discontinue their program.

Increased Cardiovascular Fitness (4,5)

Even small increases in the CRF level have significant benefits for preventing chronic disease. Part of any client's fitness program should include improvements in CRF. This requires some "vigorous" exercise in the exercise prescription. As defined by ACSM, vigorous is >60% VO_2R.

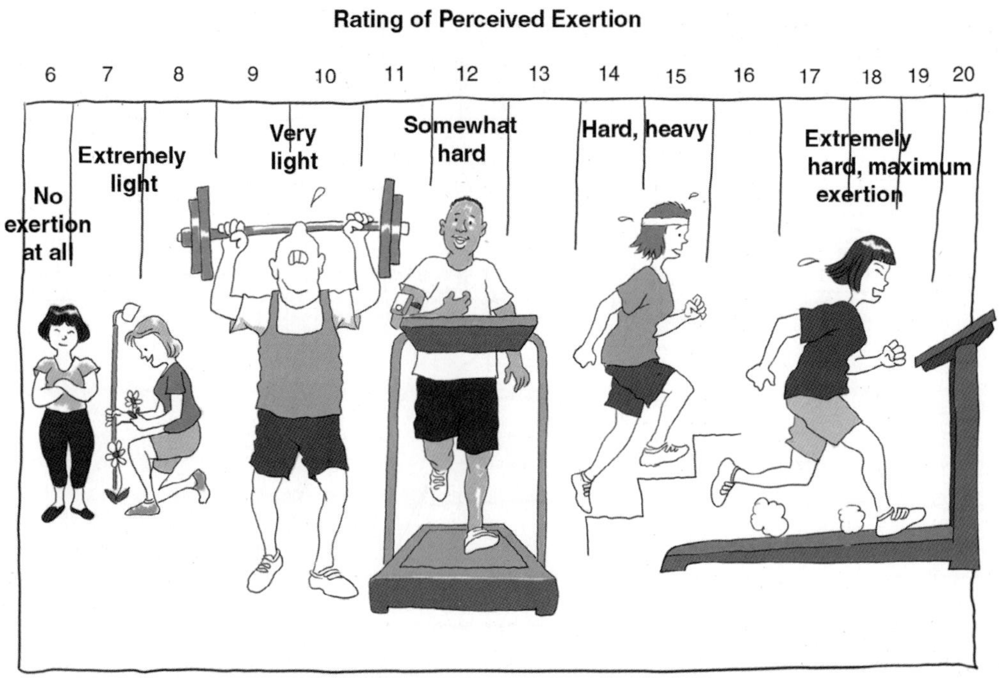

Rating of Perceived Exertion

FIGURE 3.1 One method that is helpful in regulating the intensity of exercise for optimal effects to prevent chronic disease is rating of perceived exertion.

FREQUENCY

Frequency is defined as how often one engages in structured activity each week. It is generally agreed that the minimum frequency required for improving CRF is three nonconsecutive days per week. Exercising every other day (3–4 days/week) is reasonably effective for the development of CRF. Remember, 3 days per week is **not the optimal amount of exercise for preventing disease** or reducing events; it is simply the minimum that should be spent each week on increasing the CRF. (See the box on the next page for optimal frequency guidelines.)

ACSM guidelines state that 30 minutes of physical activity on all or most days of the week is recommended. This means a frequency of at least 4 days per week. We recommend daily exercise and PA for many reasons (see some stated below). Daily exercise is important to obtain and maintain all of the benefits that accrue from both the chronic effects of exercise and the subacute effects that can be extinguished after a few hours to a day (see Fig. 3.2).

Frequency can be manipulated within some limits. For most efficient use of time and best results, it is important that the interval between exercise sessions not exceed 2 days. This allows for flexibility in scheduling around obstacles or events that may interrupt an exercise program. Everyone has interruptions and difficulties. It is important to plan for them as much as possible with people who are new at including exercise into a daily routine.

In addition, shorter, more frequent sessions (even multiple daily sessions) are often useful for *very deconditioned* individuals who may not tolerate longer or more intense exercise sessions. Two to three short exercise sessions per day (e.g., 10–15 minutes each for a total minimum of 30 minutes) may be more easily tolerated than longer, more intense sessions, particularly early in CRF programs. This is also an excellent way to increase overall daily activity levels and to help make activity habitual.

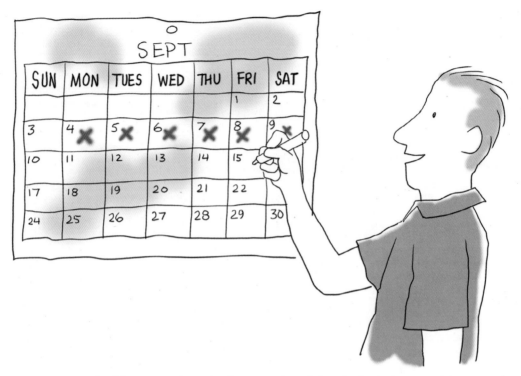

FIGURE 3.2 Optimal frequency of exercise for prevention of chronic disease is 6 to 7 days per week.

An example of using more than one session per day is to attempt 15 to 20 minutes of slow walking either before or after breakfast (a light breakfast is well advised) and another 15- to 20-minute session later in the day. It is best that 3–5 hours separate these two sessions for proper between-bouts recovery. This can be done for three consecutive days with a day off and three (or two) more consecutive days, for a total of 5 or 6 days and a minimum of 150 minutes per week.

These twice-daily sessions may be required for 2 to 4 weeks until the individual is accustomed to continuous exercise for at least 15 to 20 minutes. At that point it is usually possible to progress to once-daily sessions of 30 minutes. Refer to the section on duration for suggestions about balancing intermittent exercise and more frequent exercise.

DID YOU KNOW?

Frequency

- Four to 5 days per week is the minimum for improving CRF.
- Unfit or obese clients may better tolerate more frequent, but shorter exercise sessions (e.g., 2 times/day) at lower intensities (40%–50% VO_2R seems to be the lowest for improving CRF).
- The subacute benefits of exercise, many related to decreasing the risk for chronic disease, appear to require daily exercise, since benefits often accrue from a single exercise session.

Optimally, both *structured exercise* and *lifestyle PA should occur daily.*

INTENSITY

Quantifying intensity during exercise can be challenging. When initiating a new exercise program it may be the most critical part of the prescription for compliance. Excessive intensity may cause musculoskeletal injury and discomfort and is certainly related to noncompliance. High-intensity exercise may be discouraging and uncomfortable, especially for deconditioned individuals. High levels of discomfort during exercise may cause novice exercisers to discontinue a session and, perhaps, an entire program. Heart rate is a commonly used indicator of exercise intensity, but using rating of perceived exertion (RPE or the Borg scale) is also common, and combining both is perhaps the most accurate method of providing an effective exercise prescription, particularly in the absence of a maximal exercise test (59) (see Fig. 3.1).

Formulating an accurate heart-rate prescription based on exercise testing may be difficult because it is rare for most clients or patients with diagnosed disease to have "maximal" graded exercise testing. Therefore, the maximal heart rate, from which the heart rate (HR) for exercise prescription can be derived, is generally not known, and predicting maximum HR is subject to large error ($\pm$20 beats per minute (bpm)). The choice, then, is using estimated maximum HR or a combination of HR and RPE to guide exercise to tolerable and safe limits. However, if submaximal or maximal "metabolic testing" is performed, useful information can be gleaned.

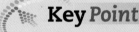

Key Point

Always initiate cardiovascular endurance exercise programs at high levels of comfort, especially in novice or deconditioned exercisers, to prevent injury and to increase the likelihood of compliance. On a 6- to 20-point RPE scale, this would be in the score range of 9 to 11 in initial exercise sessions.

Anaerobic threshold, ventilatory threshold, or respiratory compensation threshold and max VO_2 are all useful measures for quantifying exercise prescription. Knowledgeable exercise professionals can utilize the results of these tests for very accurate and effective exercise prescription.

The use of estimated maximal HR is generally not considered accurate, especially for individuals with stable chronic disease (69). Medications and/or comorbid conditions that affect exercise HR coexist with the chronic disease. In addition, there is a $\pm$20-bpm error in predicting maximum HR, which introduces significant error into the estimation of the appropriate exercise HR range. For example, a 40-year-old person has an estimated maximum HR of 180 bpm ($220 - 40 = 180$). However, even a 10- to 12-bpm error on either side of the 180 figure means that the actual maximum HR may be anywhere between 168 and 192 bpm in almost 70% of clients. The range is even larger (156–204) to be inclusive of 95% of the people. It is not difficult to see that prescribing an exercise HR with the possibility of an error of >24 bpm is not only inaccurate but may also be negligent.

By using a combination of RPE and exercise HR, it is not difficult to determine both the appropriate HR range for most individuals and to allow the individual to control the intensity of exercise for comfort and tolerance. The ACSM recommends an RPE range of 11 to 16 (fairly light to hard) for best CRF results (65). This range corresponds to the ACSM recommendation for HR prescription (60%–90% of maximum HR) and to one metabolic method of prescription (50%–85% of heart rate reserve [HRR] or oxygen-uptake reserve [VO_2R]) (65). (See Table 3.1 for specific ACSM recommendations about prescribing intensity of exercise.)

Gradually progressing exercise intensity from an initial "easy" ("light"; RPE, 11 or 12) workload to a workload closer to the mid- or upper-level recommendation ("somewhat hard" to "hard"; RPE, 13–16) range is advisable, depending on the health and CRF status of the client. Discussing the initial workloads, what to expect, as well as the reason for a slow progression should relieve client misgivings about exercise that is too "easy" or that will not be effective. Using this approach to early progression will allow the exercise professional to implement a program that is tolerable and safe for most clients.

For example, for more fit and physically active clients who have demonstrated compliance to a long-term program or recent exercise training experience as well as many younger clients with stable chronic disease of most kinds (later in this chapter there will be more discussion of precautions), the higher end of the range may be preferred by the client. Higher-intensity exercise has the advantage of eliciting greater physiological change more quickly than lower-intensity exercise (e.g., greater percentage increase in VO_2max). However, it is also more fatiguing, related to a greater risk of overuse and musculoskeletal injury, and is often responsible for new exercisers discontinuing or being noncompliant with exercise training programs. High-intensity training is often required for fit individuals with specific performance goals from a training program, for example, improving 5-km race time. Recent evidence indicates that higher-intensity exercise may be more effective for enhancing certain health benefits (see the "Digging Deeper" section at the end of this chapter).

For novice unfit exercisers, as well as for clients with more significant chronic disease or comorbidities (e.g., coexisting heart disease and diabetes), it is always preferable to begin with light- to moderate-intensity exercise, to progress slowly (5%–10% progression increase in duration per week), and to allow the client to determine the range of comfort and tolerance. Daily and weekly caloric expenditure is, perhaps, most important for prevention efforts. It is probably most important for most clients to be active every day and to accumulate 30 to 60 minutes of daily PA and exercise.

DURATION

The appropriate duration for *increasing* CRF is 20 to 60 minutes per day (3 or more days/week). This may be continuous or intermittent, depending on the initial fitness level and individual preference. Continuous duration is preferable for those who can tolerate it.

If intermittent exercise is required or preferred, both total exercise time and length of rest periods are important to control. Progression toward a minimum of 30 minutes of total exercise time is important, as is decreasing length and number of rest periods. Even in the most deconditioned, the duration of the rest periods should not exceed 5 minutes. Indeed, many new exercisers should be able to tolerate 20 to 30 minutes of continuous exercise at low intensity (40%–50% HRR).

Increasing the length and decreasing the number of rest periods should allow progressing from intermittent to continuous exercise. The ability to perform 15 minutes of continuous exercise shows reasonable ability to progress to 30 minutes of continuous exercise.

DID YOU KNOW?

Duration

- Minimum duration of 20 minutes is required for increasing the CRF.
- Duration is inversely related to intensity. Higher-intensity exercise is generally better tolerated for shorter durations, especially in deconditioned individuals.
- Progressing duration is an excellent method for increasing total caloric expenditure and, at low-to-moderate intensities, is usually well tolerated.

Using total caloric expenditure is an excellent method for progressing individuals toward optimal goals that will provide disease prevention benefits. Approximately 1,500 to 2,000 calories or more of "excess" energy expenditure per week appear to be necessary for optimal disease prevention. Therefore, this is a reasonable goal (15,40,41). In addition, both the long- and short-term benefits of exercise (see the following) are important for disease prevention. Daily or almost daily exercise is required for an optimal prevention program. The goal for an optimal exercise program for disease prevention should be to expend approximately **300 additional calories per day** during exercise and activity.

Shorter durations (e.g., 20 minutes) require somewhat higher intensity (70%–85% VO_2R) for greater improvements in CRF, whereas longer durations (40–50 minutes) allow lower intensity (40%–60% VO_2R) for improved fitness. Generally, duration is inversely related to intensity in exercise prescription. Within ACSM limitations, the greater the intensity, the shorter the duration necessary for fitness improvement, but remember that improvement in CRF is only one factor in the "optimal" exercise prescription. It has, however, been stated that it (CRF) is the most important factor in primary and secondary prevention of cardiovascular disease events (see the section, "Digging Deeper") (4,42).

Progression of duration before intensity is usually better tolerated by new exercisers. This is especially true with less fit clients. Intermittent exercise bouts of 10 to 15 minutes at lower exercise intensities are usually comfortable for everyone, including the least fit individuals.

MODE

The preferred mode, or type, of exercise required to improve CRF uses large muscle groups (legs, arm/legs), is (or can be) continuous movement (walking, jogging, swimming), and has some "rhythmic" qualities (i.e., it is repetitive). Almost any exercise that fits these criteria can be prescribed as part of the program for cardiovascular endurance and, thus, is effective for disease prevention. There may be limitations, however, to the use of some modes of exercise.

Exercise professionals should be aware, however, that it might be more difficult to utilize some activities because of inherent characteristics that may affect the ability to increase intensity. Water aerobics is one example of this. The buoyancy of the water can reduce the intensity of effort. The use of paddles and other devices, as well as the water itself, for increasing resistance increases intensity, but it also requires increased efforts on the part of the exerciser to maintain the intensity. This does not mean that these activities (water aerobics, for example) could not be part of an effective program; it does mean to emphasize that clients need specific instruction with each different modality in order to effectively progress and enhance CRF. In addition, water exercise may not be the best choice for a weight management program because of the lack of weight-bearing and the buoyancy factor. Certainly, using various modes of exercise is both beneficial and useful for obtaining "cross-training" effects.

The use of arm exercise or combined arm–leg exercise may also be considered for CRF programs. Equipment such as arm–leg bicycles,

> ## Key Point
>
> Intensity, duration, frequency, and mode are the essential elements of an exercise prescription. Mixing these three for optimal results in a prevention program aimed at chronic disease is the "art" of exercise prescription. The "science" is prescribing each of these elements at the appropriate level according to the known research literature.

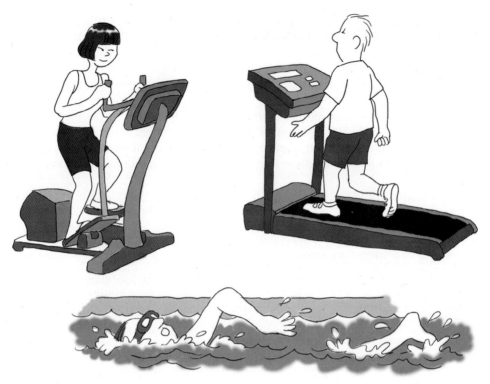

FIGURE 3.3 The mode (type) of exercise should be varied for purposes of cross-training.

arm–leg seated steppers, and elliptical trainers with arm levers and other devices are excellent inclusions (see Fig. 3.3). However, many people are unaccustomed to arm work, and adding large amounts of arm work may increase fatigue and discomfort associated with this mode of exercise. Most individuals are relatively comfortable with 20% to 30% of the "effort" coming from arms with the remainder coming from the legs. Initially, it may be difficult for the new exerciser to judge this correctly.

PROGRESSION OF THE EXERCISE PROGRAM

When the entire exercise prescription is put together, one of the more difficult decisions is how quickly to progress the program. Progression depends on a number of factors, including the initial fitness level, the frequency of training sessions, compliance to the daily exercise prescription, tolerance and response to exercise, and even the ability and willingness of the individual to tolerate discomfort. Fitness goals are another factor that must be included in the decision. Generally speaking, progression (of duration, for example) should not exceed 10% to 15% per week. Duration should be progressed before intensity, and intensity should be progressed gradually to decrease the incidence of overuse injuries and general fatigue from overtraining. Programs should be designed to eventually incorporate activities from light to vigorous in order to optimize outcomes.

Progression to daily exercise from frequencies of 4 to 5 days per week is relatively simple. Adding 1 day, acclimating to that for a period of 1 to 2 weeks, then adding a second day for a total of 7 is relatively straightforward and well tolerated by most individuals. Changing intensity levels from day to day is prudent to prevent injury and undue fatigue.

Once exercise is continuous, increasing the intensity is the next step in progression. This can be accomplished by increasing the pace (e.g., walking speed or steps per minute on the elliptical), resistance, or workload. Using some kind of quantifiable and objective measure of intensity (e.g., HR), coupled with RPE to regulate comfort level, should allow the exercise professional to increase intensity in a gradual, comfortable, and effective manner. HR is one variable that is quantifiable and objective and is relatively easy to measure. As exercise HR decreases at any given workload, physiological tolerance improves and increased intensity is possible.

THE BENEFITS OF EXERCISE

The benefits of exercise have long been assumed to accrue from regular, long-term exercise training (so-called chronic changes). Indeed, there are many benefits from regular exercise training that manifest after a long-term (2–3 months and longer) exercise training program. Classically, these are attributed to maintaining a cardiovascular endurance exercise program (or other fitness-specific program, for example, resistance training) according to appropriate guidelines (see Table 3.1).

Clearly, risk reduction (for chronic disease) is one outcome of a cardiovascular endurance exercise program. Increasing the CRF level (as mentioned earlier) has been shown to be effective in reducing the mortality and morbidity from heart and other chronic diseases. It is also associated with decreased incidence of diabetes and MetS (indeed, it may "cure" MetS) as well as obesity (61).

Engaging in regular, aerobic exercise improves the "gold standard" measure of CRF, **maximal oxygen uptake** (see Fig. 3.4). A cardiovascular endurance exercise program performed according to the criteria mentioned in Table 3.1 can increase VO_2max from 5% to 25% (greater in some studies) in 8 to 16 weeks. As discussed earlier, many studies demonstrate that the incidence of heart disease, stroke, and all-cause mortality decreases with increasing levels or CRF or PA.

In addition, it has been shown that even small increases in CRF improve mortality from heart disease (5,6). The general idea of all this is that increasing both CRF and PA is beneficial for reducing the risk of chronic disease.

It is important to conceptualize the benefits of exercise (especially for clients) into long-term and short-term benefits. The **long-term benefits** develop and accrue over months of

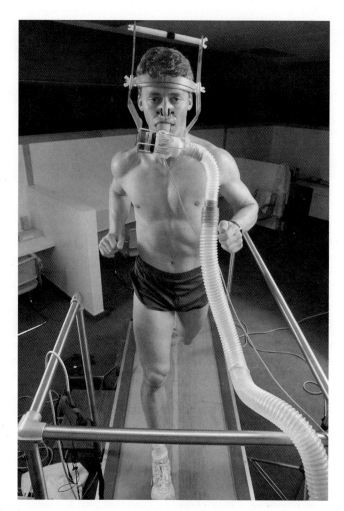

FIGURE 3.4 Maximal oxygen uptake is the "gold standard" for cardiorespiratory fitness.

regular exercise—rather than after days. They accrue in small to negligible amounts with exercise frequencies of 2 days/week or less, or with other levels of exercise that are not consistent with the recommendations described in Table 3.1 (65). Some of the long-term benefits are outlined in Table 3.2 (65).

TABLE 3.2 Long-Term Benefits of Exercise		
Benefit	**Effect**	**Time Course**
Maximum oxygen uptake	↑	8–16 weeks
Cardiovascular endurance fitness	↑	8–16 weeks
Hypertension	↓	4 weeks
Lean body mass	↓	8–16 weeks
Obesity and fat mass	↓	≥6 months

SHORT-TERM (SUBACUTE) BENEFITS

Short-term benefits are those that occur immediately following, and because of, each exercise session. These benefits are also called "subacute" and are, by definition, temporary. They are distinct from the so-called acute effects of exercise such as the changes in HR, blood pressure, lactic acid, and other physiological variables, which occur during exercise (11). In many cases, the time course of the effect is unknown, but preliminary studies confirm that **these benefits occur after each exercise session and last varying amounts of time depending on the intensity and duration of the exercise.** The research that clarifies the principles for obtaining these subacute or short-term benefits is incomplete. Table 3.3 summarizes some of the known subacute benefits of exercise.

TABLE 3.3	The Subacute Benefits of Exercise	
Benefit	**Effect**	**Exercise Prescription**
High-density lipoprotein	↑	Intensity and duration vary; higher intensity may be required
Low-density lipoprotein	↓	
Triglycerides	↓	
Cholesterol	↓	
Postprandial lipemia	↓	Longer duration, lower intensity
Inflammation	↓	Low to moderate intensity
Hemostasis	↑	Low to moderate intensity
Blood pressure	↓	Low to moderate intensity
Endothelial function	↑	Moderate intensity
Glucose metabolism	↑	Longer duration, lower intensity
Insulin sensitivity	↑	Low to moderate intensity

One example, which will be discussed in detail later in this chapter, is insulin resistance and insulin sensitivity. The duration of increased insulin sensitivity after an exercise bout is unknown, but this is a short-term benefit from exercise. The duration of the increased insulin resistance probably depends on some combination of intensity and duration of exercise. Longer, more intense cardiovascular endurance exercise may produce longer-lasting insulin sensitivity, perhaps lasting many hours, whereas shorter duration exercise may be associated with shorter effectiveness.

The same is true for many other subacute benefits. Both the intensity and the duration of the exercise/activity session interact somehow to enhance the particular effect for varying amounts of time after the exercise session. Regardless of the time these changes last, it is likely that they contribute significantly to the preventive effects of exercise. Just as important is the fact that because they are transient, the repetition of exercise and/or activity on a *daily basis* is necessary to sustain and, in fact, to obtain these benefits.

In what follows, several of these effects and what is known about the mode, frequency, intensity, and duration of exercise and PA are discussed. These effects are summarized in Table 3.3.

Key Point

The transient nature of subacute benefits is one reason to exercise on a daily basis. To maintain these important changes, exercise and physical activity must be performed on a continuing and regular basis.

LIPOPROTEINS

Lipoproteins are carriers for lipids (fats) and cholesterol in the blood. The changes in lipoproteins (mainly very low-density lipoprotein, LDL, and high-density lipoprotein, HDL) subsequent to individual exercise bouts are positive with respect to decreasing the risk of chronic diseases. Some of these changes have been clarified, but others are less clear (3,63). HDLs and triglycerides are positively affected; LDL and cholesterol are also affected but are less responsive to exercise (12). There are several factors that seem to affect the amount of change, including the fitness level of the individual and the preexercise lipid levels.

The effects can be summarized as follows:

- HDL is increased. It appears that longer duration, as well as higher intensity, exercise may be more effective. A threshold has not been established.
- Triglycerides are decreased. The decrease is clearly prominent immediately after exercise, but in some cases, this effect has been shown to be present for 18 to 24 hours after exercise and may persist for up to 3 days. LDL is decreased by longer-duration exercise (>90–120 minutes). In particular, it appears that a particular type of LDL (small, dense LDLs) is positively affected by endurance exercise. This type of LDL is very atherogenic (related to increased progression of CAD) and is decreased by exercise, whereas the larger LDL subfractions may actually increase. The effect of this change in the ratio of these two types of LDL is positive with respect to prevention of heart disease (12,30). Finally, LDL "receptors" in the liver may be upregulated by exercise; the harmful effects of the LDL may be decreased. This is also a positive effect with respect to the development of CAD. Total cholesterol is only minimally affected, if at all, by single bouts of exercise.

There may be other effects on various types of HDL and intermediate density lipoprotein (IDL). It is not clear what they are, what the extent of change is and how much exercise is required. However, it is clear that there is benefit to be accrued from each exercise session. Other categories of change in lipid-related variables include those discussed in the following.

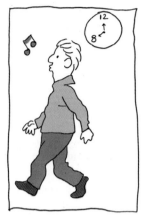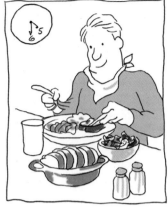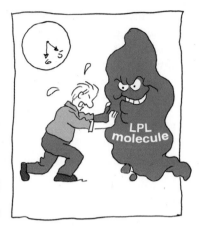

FIGURE 3.5 Exercise moderates postprandial lipemia. The most effective time to exercise is 12 to 24 hours prior to a meal.

Lipoprotein Lipase

Lipoprotein lipase is an enzyme involved in the metabolism of cholesterol and other blood lipids. It has been shown to help mobilize triglycerides from muscle tissue for energy metabolism. Lower-intensity exercise, the type that utilizes more fatty acids for energy metabolism, would seem to be most effective in increasing this enzyme's activity. However, one study found that moderate-intensity exercise, repeated over several days, increased levels of the enzyme (3,30).

Postprandial Lipemia

Postprandial lipemia (PPL) is the surge in lipoproteins (particularly LDL) that is present after a meal. This surge is dependent on the amount of fat ingested during the meal, and high-fat meals produce an especially large surge. The relative degree of this surge is related to the incidence of myocardial infarction; thus, decreasing the PPL surge effectively reduces the risk of cardiovascular event (3).

Abnormal PPL increases coagulability (formation of blood clots), thus further contributing to potential heart attack and stroke. Single bouts of exercise blunt or moderate PPL. Total caloric expenditure, increased postexercise oxygen consumption, and both continuous and intermittent exercise contribute to improving PPL (see Fig. 3.5 above). Some researchers believe that the attenuation of PPL is related to total energy expenditure of the exercise, rather than intensity or duration alone (3). The positive effects of both acute and chronic exercise training on PPL are clear. Both decrease the extent and amount of PPL from a meal (relative to the amount of fat ingested).

GLUCOSE METABOLISM

Enhanced uptake and use of glucose occurs after exercise and PA. Increased energy metabolism within skeletal muscle increases the demand for glucose (and other energy sources), stimulating increased glucose uptake even in the absence of insulin (9,31).

It appears that the increased metabolic demand and nutrient uptake (glucose in this case) by active muscle tissue is facilitated by increased insulin sensitivity (see the following) as well as by glycogen use within the muscles. Various other mechanisms, including adaptation of metabolic enzymes and mitochondria within skeletal muscle and enhanced fat metabolism, contribute to the effect (9,27,40). Regardless of the mechanism, increased metabolic activity stimulates removal of circulating blood glucose, which stimulates increased glucose production in the liver. Therefore, in normal, nondiabetic individuals, blood glucose is maintained in a very tight range during conditions of both exercise and rest.

In people with type 2 diabetes or MetS, blood glucose level can become elevated. Endothelial dysfunction follows, caused by a host of metabolic abnormalities, including oversecretion of insulin (hyperinsulinemia), the presence of metabolic oxidants (oxidized LDL) in the endothelial layer, and inflammation (27,33). Exercise can increase the removal of glucose from the blood in these instances and, thus, provide protection from some of the harmful effects of chronically high levels of blood glucose (see Chapter 7 for a more detailed discussion) (31,40,58). In short, although persons with type 2 diabetes have abnormal glucose metabolism and insulin sensitivity, the outcome of exercise is the same as in those with normal glucose metabolism—increased glucose uptake and increased insulin sensitivity at rest and during exercise.

INSULIN RECEPTORS

People with prediabetes and type 2 diabetes usually have some combination of hypo- or hyperinsulinemia, insulin resistance, and hyperglycemia. The causes of these conditions vary, but generally are a result of sedentary lifestyle and diet (especially insufficient intake of fiber and high intake of trans fat and saturated fat). The end results include obesity and chronic low-grade inflammation. All of these factors are interrelated.

Insulin receptors are found on the membranes of skeletal muscle and in other tissue, including adipose tissue (see Fig. 3.6). They facilitate the uptake of glucose into the cell from blood. The sensitivity of these receptors is usually impaired in people with type 2 diabetes or MetS. This can cause hyperglycemia and, ultimately, hyperinsulinemia. These conditions, in turn, are responsible for other metabolic, coagulation, and

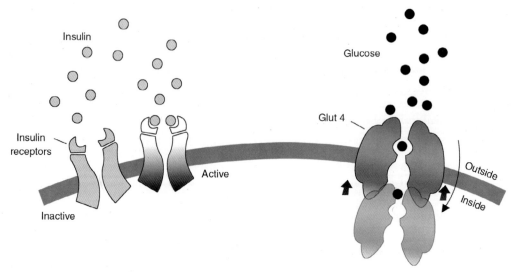

FIGURE 3.6 Exercise enhances insulin receptor sensitivity.

vascular abnormalities that increase the risk of atherogenesis, as well as for cardiac event.

Exercise increases insulin sensitivity. Both single exercise sessions and chronic exercise training are associated with the increase. Single exercise sessions cause temporary changes in insulin sensitivity that are related to the total energy expenditure of the exercise, rather than intensity. There is controversy about the contribution of intensity, duration, or volume of exercise necessary for changes in insulin sensitivity (19). For example, 30 minutes of brisk walking probably causes an increase in insulin sensitivity similar to that achieved in three 10-minute walks separated by rest (28).

In addition, it is known that individuals with higher cardiovascular fitness have greater insulin sensitivity after a single session of exercise than do less fit individuals (9,19,27). Therefore, persons who exercise on a regular basis obtain the beneficial subacute effects of increased insulin sensitivity. This means that there is benefit to both single sessions of activity (being active and exercising on a daily basis) and increasing the fitness level through regular exercise.

Finally, there are connections between the systems of insulin and glucose metabolism and immune function that further support the notion that exercise can improve skeletal-muscle insulin sensitivity and glucose metabolism (31). Immune system "markers" such as tumor necrosis factor and interleukin-6 as well as other immune-related and inflammation modulators are positively affected by acute and chronic exercise. These, in turn, positively influence glucose metabolism, insulin sensitivity, and a host of other factors related to heart disease and contributing to the preventive effects of exercise.

INFLAMMATION

Inflammation is directly related to atherosclerosis as well as to a number of other chronic diseases (23,35). Whether inflammation is a cause or a byproduct of these conditions is not well understood, but it appears that it precedes the vascular dysfunction and may well be the precursor to much of the related pathophysiology (34). The presence of inflammation and influx of inflammatory substances, as reflected by several markers of inflammation (e.g., high-sensitivity c-reactive protein or cytokines), is important in the progression of CAD, acute coronary syndromes, stroke, obesity, chronic heart failure, and diabetes. Many of these inflammatory substances promote atherosclerosis (23,34).

The presence of inflammatory substances may be involved in the deposition of atherosclerotic plaque and probably plays a central role in plaque instability and rupture (thus, heart attack and stroke). This same level of chronic, low-level inflammation has been shown to be associated with increased blood clotting and endothelial and immune system dysfunction, as well as abnormal glucose metabolism (16,23,34).

Epidemiological studies demonstrate that exercise and PA as well as increased CRF correlate with decreased levels of inflammatory markers. Chronic exercise training has been demonstrated to increase substances in the immune system that inhibit the progress of atherosclerosis and to decrease substances that promote progression—the net effect of this is to reduce the development and progression of CAD (16,17,48,51,52). Note that these markers and the response of the immune system to exercise are very closely related to intensity of exercise. High-intensity exercise seems to temporarily increase rather than decrease inflammation. However, that increase does not seem to be either long-lasting or damaging. In fact, some researchers note important differences between that type of inflammatory response and the longer-term response described previously that relates to pathophysiology (16,51). It has been shown that c-reactive protein and

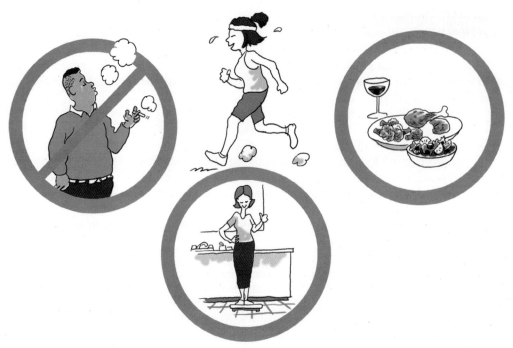

FIGURE 3.7 Moderate exercise and other healthy lifestyle habits are anti-inflammatory.

some other inflammatory markers decrease with exercise training, regardless of changes in other risk factors known to be associated with elevated c-reactive protein (such as diabetes or obesity) (20,22,51).

A relationship between the intensity and/or duration of exercise (i.e., a "dose–response" relationship) and the production of these substances is unclear. **Hard or high-intensity exercise** causes proinflammatory changes in muscle and other tissue that are associated with muscle damage and acute muscle soreness (16). **Moderate-intensity exercise** is associated with improved immune function and enhanced antiatherogenic substances produced by the immune system (52). So far, research seems to indicate that even though short-term, high-intensity exercise increases inflammation, there are no long-term, deleterious inflammatory effects with moderate, regular exercise (16,51). In fact, high-intensity training has recently been shown to have significant beneficial, disease-preventing effects (29).

Clearly, a substantial case can be made for the place of exercise in decreasing inflammatory reactions and in improved immune function (see Fig. 3.7). Moderate-intensity exercise causes subacute and chronic improvement in these physiological functions. Hard or high-intensity exercise causes increases in inflammatory markers and an immune response that are transient and do not appear to be harmful.

HEMOSTASIS

Hemostasis, in this context, is defined as the maintenance of blood volume and normal coagulation. Hemostasis and the coagulability of blood are controlled by extremely complex systems that interact in many different ways with exercise, diet, and other risk factors for heart disease. It has been established that when coagulability is increased, heart attack, angina, stroke, and sudden death are more likely to occur since all are related to the formation of blood clots in arteries. Reducing blood clotting is part of the secondary prevention guidelines for those with cardiovascular disease, including a history of heart attack, stroke, or angina, angioplasty/stent, and coronary artery bypass graft, or as primary prevention in those with risk factors (1).

Diabetes, for example, is associated with a "hypercoagulable" state (increased blood clotting), meaning that people with diabetes (including those with impaired fasting glucose and glucose intolerance [prediabetes as defined by the American Diabetes Association] and MetS) are more prone to forming blood clots than those without these conditions. The reasons are complex and beyond the scope of this discussion. The interested reader is directed to some excellent and detailed reviews in Chapter 7 (14).

The effects of both acute and chronic exercise have been studied extensively in an attempt to understand the relationship between coagulation state and exercise. Positive changes could help explain part of the overall benefit of exercise in reducing mortality from heart disease. The terms *increased coagulability* and *decreased coagulability* will be used to describe changes in the state of blood clotting. They are intended to be broad descriptors of the state of hemostasis and, because of the complexity of the system, they are not intended to be related to any single clotting factor.

A significant problem in interpreting this research is the extreme complexity of the systems. There are many markers and factors inherent to the coagulation process; thus, it is difficult to know which to study and, perhaps more important, whether isolated changes in these factors actually translate to broad changes in coagulability. Finally, any decrease in plasma volume that accompanies acute exercise is a confounding factor. Increased viscosity (thickness of the blood) secondary to this fluid shift can cause increased coagulability, even in the absence of other factors. To date, there is no definitive answer about effects of acute exercise on coagulation, but there are some generalizations that can be made.

Coagulability, depending upon the parameter studied, is generally thought to increase with acute exercise, especially prolonged, high-intensity exercise. However, moderate- and low-intensity exercise may decrease it. In addition, there may be a paradoxical effect in patients with CAD in that exercise may temporarily increase coagulability (2,70). This effect seems to be short-lived (a few hours at most). It is not clear that this is a function of exercise in patients with CAD (or peripheral artery disease) or, perhaps, related to fitness or other variables, which cloud this picture (57,71).

Furthermore, "moderate" exercise training and increased CRF seem to decrease coagulability over the long term. Several epidemiological studies have shown that the most fit and the most active individuals have the lowest levels of coagulability. This is also true in patients with cardiovascular disease, diabetes, and MetS (71).

If, in fact, there is a short-term increased coagulability that is associated with acute exercise, it seems to be counteracted by the long-term changes that enhance fibrinolysis and decrease coagulability (10,14). Thus, the advantages of exercise clearly outweigh the disadvantages.

In summary, though the subacute effects of exercise on coagulation may seem to be in conflict with prevention, viewed in a broader context, they may be part of a bigger picture of enhanced fibrinolysis (dissolving clots) and decreased coagulability. Both have been demonstrated to accompany training in patients with chronic disease and with metabolic derangements as well as in apparently healthy individuals. Regardless of these data, it is certain that high-intensity exercise should be implemented cautiously in patients with CAD and diabetes as well as in those with MetS and hypertension, and, perhaps, in other higher-risk patients (71).

In low-CRF individuals as well as in patients with chronic disease or MetS, with or without hypercoagulable state, exercise is not contraindicated. Because of the known changes in coagulability that accompany higher-intensity exercise, it is best to begin with lower intensity: <40% to 60% VO_2R or HRR, or RPE 11 to 13 or lower. Progression should emphasize duration until 15 minutes of continuous exercise is reached. Then increasing intensity as the cardiovascular response to exercise is enhanced is the best course for progression. The guidelines offered for progression at the beginning of this chapter are applicable to this population. As conditioning progresses, caution is indicated with intensities >70% to 75% VO_2R/HRR, >85% maxHR, or RPE >14.

BLOOD PRESSURE

Hypertension is a widespread cardiovascular disease. More than 30% of all Americans (almost 60 million people) have hypertension, and prevalence is especially high among the elderly people, reaching more than 80% in those older than 75 years of age. Persons older than 55 years of age have a 90% lifetime risk of developing hypertension (36). Approximately 30 million people have prehypertension. Of those with hypertension, only 34% know they have it and keep it under control. The remainder are unaware of their condition; are taking medication, but the condition is not under control; or are not taking medication. (See Chapter 8 for a more in-depth discussion of hypertension.)

The positive effects of exercise on blood pressure are well documented (50). There is evidence that higher levels of PA or increased CRF are associated with reduced incidence of hypertension. What is more clear is that chronic exercise training can lower blood pressure in those with prehypertension and hypertension (50,68). The overall effect of chronic training has been shown to be a decrease of 5- to 7-mm Hg for both systolic and diastolic blood pressure among those with hypertension. Similar decreases have been documented for postexercise hypotension (PEH) in both those with and without hypertension that may last as long as 6 to 12 hours after exercise (49,50). For a more detailed discussion of PEH, please see the section, "Digging Deeper," in Chapter 8.

Resistance training (according to ACSM guidelines) has been shown to reduce blood pressure in both normotensive and hypertensive adults (3). This seems to be a long-term effect, not a subacute or short-term benefit of resistance training. The changes are modest but statistically significant (50). Their clinical significance is not clear, but these changes have been demonstrated to correspond to a 10% decrease in the risk of cardiac event and stroke.

Recommendations for exercise prescription for control of hypertension are based on ACSM guidelines, and the evidence for any particular combination of intensity, duration, frequency, and mode is not well established (50). The effects of PEH are beneficial; therefore, exercising on most, if not all, days is advisable. Moderate intensity (40%–70% VO_2R or HRR) is recommended. Very light (<20%–30% HRR) or very high-intensity (>85%–90% HRR) exercise may not be effective. Again, the most effective duration of exercise is not clear, but it seems that 30 minutes or more of cardiovascular (aerobic) endurance exercise is most effective. Resistance exercise may also be effective if performed according to ACSM guidelines (65).

The potential mechanisms for this effect on hypertension are varied and, again, unclear despite the volume of research. Neurohormonal adaptations are among the most plausible. Effects on sympathetic nervous system activity, including global reductions in sympathetic activity, decreased norepinephrine release, and effects on insulin sensitivity and insulin release (both related to blood pressure and hypertension), are among the possibilities. Changes in the renin angiotensin system are possible but remain unconfirmed (50).

Changes in vascular and smooth muscle function may contribute to the effect. As discussed previously, endothelial function is improved both subacutely and chronically with exercise. Conversely, uncontrolled hypertension impairs endothelial function. Improved endothelial function may be related to the beneficial effect of exercise on hypertension.

Both structural vascular changes and changes in gene expression secondary to the effects of environmental influences (such as diet or exercise) may also provide some clue about how exercise improves blood pressure. These changes include vascular remodeling, increased vessel diameter, and the generation of new blood vessels. Genomic influences on blood pressure and PEH have been observed in humans and that component, though small, probably contributes (50,68).

Because blood pressure is lowered subacutely by cardiovascular endurance exercise, daily exercise is recommended. Aerobic, cardiovascular endurance exercise is most effective for decreasing blood pressure; however, as mentioned earlier, it has been demonstrated that resistance exercise, according to ACSM guidelines, results in decreased blood pressure in adults with hypertension. Intensities of $<70\%$ VO_2R, $<60\%$ maxHR or HRR, or RPE <12 to 13 may be most effective (50,68).

ENDOTHELIAL FUNCTION

The preservation, enhancement, and/or restoration of endothelial function may be one of the most important preventive benefits of regular exercise. Exercise has been shown to be effective in normalizing endothelial dysfunction (33).

Normal endothelial function allows appropriate vasodilation of arteries (most important, coronary arteries) in response to increased metabolic requirements (see Fig. 3.8). Vasodilation can occur because of a number of factors, including mechanical (pressure) and neurohormonal factors on the endothelium itself, circulating metabolites, and local blood flow. The nitric oxide system is critical in the vasodilatory response to exercise (38). Normal endothelial function also allows the atherogenic effects of inflammation to be attenuated, by substances produced in and released by the endothelium. Finally, exercise also promotes improved (or normalizes) function of the underlying vascular smooth muscle, thus also providing beneficial effects with respect to disease and prevention of events (33,35).

Exercise stimulates increased nitric oxide synthase, which improves endothelial function (37). These changes appear to occur particularly in those with abnormal endothelial function, and they may occur as quickly as within 24 to 96 hours after initiating an exercise program (see Fig. 3.8) (24). The aging process is accompanied by some degree of impaired endothelial function, and there is evidence that both acute bouts of exercise and longer-term exercise training can lead to the reversal of this dysfunction even in elderly men (33). The benefits also accrue locally within the coronary and other major arteries and may help explain the decreased incidence and severity of myocardial ischemia associated with exercise training.

The amount of exercise required to enhance this system is not clear. The research seems to indicate that moderate-intensity exercise (40%–60% VO_2max) may be sufficient. More frequent exercise is obviously required, since this benefit of exercise appears to be subacute in nature (22,35).

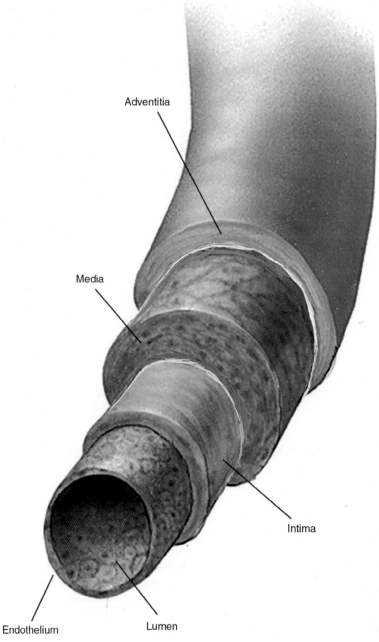

Adventitia

Media

Intima

Endothelium

Lumen

FIGURE 3.8 Normal vascular function is controlled by the endothelium, which facilitates vasodilatation in arteries that supply the heart and exercising muscle.

ENDOTHELIAL PROGENITOR CELLS

Endothelial progenitor cells (EPCs) are produced in bone marrow and are similar to stem cells. They are essential for the formation and maintenance of endothelial tissue. The stimulation of EPC generation by regular exercise is well established, as is their inhibition by many of the health behaviors that are associated with chronic disease, including smoking, insulin resistance, and other risk factors (26,32,60).

It is likely that some mix of frequency, intensity, and duration of exercise is most effective in stimulating the production of EPCs; however, at this time, the most effective combination is unknown. EPC production is probably a subacute change that does not persist without daily exercise. The duration of this effect is unknown (32,60,68).

PUTTING IT ALL TOGETHER

The effectiveness of exercise for primary and secondary prevention is well established (4–8,63). Populations with and without chronic disease who are more active or fit have fewer chronic diseases and related events and have decreased mortality rates. Improving the CRF or PA level in populations with and without chronic disease decreases mortality and events (7,8). Simply put, exercise is a big player in both primary and secondary prevention of cardiovascular and other chronic disease.

The optimal exercise prescription for prevention is also relatively simple. It is likely that both long-term and short-term or subacute effects of exercise are preventive, but the benefits are cumulative, meaning that long-term, regular exercise is optimal for prevention. Therefore, implementing an exercise program that improves the CRF according to ACSM guidelines (see Table 3.1) is one step in prevention. The second and equally important step is increasing levels of daily PA.

Daily exercise and activity levels of sufficient intensity to stimulate some of the changes described earlier are important. This means that the standard exercise prescription of cardiovascular endurance exercise, 3 to 4 days per week, is inadequate. The use of step counters or other devices (accelerometers) to assess daily movement and PA and to assist people to do enough activity is very useful. Using the 10,000-steps-per-day criterion is appropriate for PA. However, if someone's work-related activity is already fairly high (>6,000 to 7,000 steps per day) another 5,000 to 6,000 steps should be added to the baseline. If weight loss is a goal, it may be helpful to exceed 15,000 steps per day. See Table 3.4 for activity classification according to steps per day (66).

It may be just as easy for some individuals to "exercise" 30 to 45 minutes per day, 4 or more days per week. This will ensure the kind of daily PA necessary to obtain most of the benefits discussed previously as well as increased fitness level that is also beneficial.

The prevention of chronic disease is viable and reasonable as an outcome goal for an exercise program. Participants, clients, and patients should be encouraged and, in fact, should be urged to exercise every day for optimal results. The inclusion of short-term benefits into the preventive puzzle makes daily PA and exercise critical in providing the ongoing benefits that contribute to the remarkable preventive effects. The exercise professional should be familiar with and knowledgeable about these benefits and the exercise prescription that provides them.

TABLE 3.4	Categories of Activity in Steps per Day (66)
Highly active	>12,500
Active	10,000–12,499
Somewhat active	7,500–9,999
Low active	5,000–7,499
Sedentary	<5,000

DIGGING DEEPER

The Physical Fitness/Physical Activity Debate

Although it might seem that the debate regarding whether PA or PF is most important in reducing the risk for chronic diseases is academic, it is instructive because exercise professionals should encourage increases in both. Which should take more precedence is the question. There is good, though not conclusive, information that can help provide some answers. The difference is more than semantic because PF indicates an overall level of cardiovascular endurance fitness as well as muscular strength and endurance.

First, we should clarify the difference between PF and PA. In this literature, PF is determined solely by CRF. The "gold standard" in exercise physiology for measuring the CRF is maximal oxygen uptake. Because of the technological difficulty, the expense, the time, and the discomfort to participants, this method is rarely used in large population studies. In fact, neither Williams (72) nor Blair (4) cites a single study using directly measured VO_2max as the independent variable in population studies. CRF has primarily been assessed by treadmill test time in most large-population, epidemiological studies. PA, on the other hand, is frequently used because of the simplicity of the assessment. Self-assessment of PA by questionnaire is a frequently used method. There are many types of survey instrument available, and most research uses a self-formulated and validated survey, as is the case with the Aerobics Center studies, as well as with Dr. Paffenbarger's research (4,7,45,46). The primary criticism of this type of assessment is the self-reporting element of these PA surveys and the errors inherent to self-report of PA.

The early studies (by both Morris et al. [41] and Paffenbarger et al. [47]) used only PA assessed by questionnaire and, in some cases, job analysis. In some studies, PA is expressed as steps per day, MET-minutes per week, weekly caloric expenditure, and so on. Morris et al. and Paffenbarger et al. published most of these early studies, which clearly show that men (all of the early studies used only male participants) with higher levels of PA had lower death rates from heart disease. Morris et al. (41) used "London busmen" who were occupationally divided into men who were inactive (drivers) or active (conductors). Paffenbarger et al. (47) used longshoremen and similarly divided participants into active and sedentary men by job task. The results were similar in that both found about a 20% reduction in cardiovascular disease mortality in the active versus the sedentary group. In addition, in comparing the most active with the least active group, there was a 50% decrease in mortality in the most active longshoremen (47).

Studies that utilize PA as the key measure comprise the largest cohort of participants in the literature. Williams (71,72), in his 2001 meta-analysis used epidemiological studies with 317,908 person-years of data for CRF and approximately 2.29 million person-years of data for PA. He reached three major conclusions:

1. The risk of either cardiovascular disease or coronary heart disease decreases linearly with increasing PA.
2. The greatest decrease occurs between the lowest and the 25th percentile of PF.
3. There is a significant difference between PA and PF, with increased PF being more protective than increased PA.

Perhaps the most interesting conclusion here is that when these data are combined, the lowest-fitness group gains the most from increasing CRF to the next level (72).

Blair (6), in a similar meta-analysis, addressed questions of dose–response effect between PA and CRF and health and which is more powerful. Blair states, "because of the large amount of data and the varied outcomes and methods of assessment of PA, it is impossible to determine a dose-response effect." However, in the next sentence Blair states that there are a few studies (the "exceptions") that demonstrate "a general inverse dose-response gradient across PA categories for most health outcomes" (4).

For the question of CRF and dose–response effect, he found that there was a persistent and significant dose–response effect across all fitness groups. Blair's Aerobics Center studies comprise much of these data; however, other research has confirmed this effect (5–7). The conclusions reiterate what was stated earlier, but perhaps more emphatically. The greatest reduction in risk was seen in men who moved from the lowest quintile of PF to the next lowest (44% decrease in mortality from heart disease). Men who moved from quintile 2/3 to 4/5 decreased death rate by 28% (6). In addition, it is clear that the decrease in mortality between the highest and the lowest CRF groups is at least 50% and, perhaps, up to threefold to fourfold. Thus, Blair confirms Williams' findings that improvements in both PA and CRF are protective. Blair concludes that the effects of CRF are more powerful than those of PA in protection from chronic disease. He also concluded from these data that even though it appears that CRF is more powerful, the reason may lie in how CRF is measured and, more important, in the self-reported measures of PA that may lead to misclassification (6).

Other studies have confirmed these conclusions. Mark states, "The clear implication of the St. James Women Take Heart study and other similar studies is that improving exercise capacity will improve prognosis" (21,38). The St. James study is a large, prospective study of women and PF. Thus, the conclusion that improvement in PF reduced risk was expanded to women. In addition, since these are prospective data, this study allows an additional conclusion relative to prognosis; that is, PF is an indicator of prognosis, not simply a variable that "tracks" mortality. Therefore, low fitness means increased death rates from chronic disease (21).

Myers et al. (42) assessed both PF and PA in a single cohort of men ($n = 6,213$). They used exercise capacity from treadmill tests along with a detailed PA survey (both past and current activity). They found that the best predictors of *mortality* were, in order, (1) peak exercise capacity, (2) recreational energy expenditure during adulthood, (3) recreational energy expenditure during the past year, and (4) energy expenditure from flights of stairs and blocks walked in the past year. The best predictors of *survival* were exercise capacity and energy expenditure from recreational activity in adulthood. In addition, they found that approximately 1,000 kCal/week in energy expenditure was "worth" about 1 MET in PF and that increasing either (PA or PF) yields about a 20% decrease in mortality. They also state that PF is a stronger predictor of mortality than "recent" PA. Myers et al. (42) also found that increased PF yields the largest benefit with regards to mortality, again confirming earlier conclusions by both Williams and Blair.

Finally, in a series of articles Booth and his colleagues (8) have made an interesting and compelling case for the evolutionary and genetic aspects of the "inactivity"–chronic disease connection. They argue that human genomes, especially those interconnected with metabolic pathways, are inextricably linked with PA. Furthermore, that inactivity causes biologically maladaptive physiological and biochemical responses that lead to obesity, diabetes, heart, and other

Key Point

Both physical activity and physical fitness (cardiorespiratory endurance fitness) are related to decreased mortality from various chronic diseases, including heart disease and type 2 diabetes. It is important to increase both for preventing chronic disease.

(continued)

chronic disease. Thus, inactivity, and not decreased PF, is the real perpetrator in increased risk of and death from chronic disease. Booth et al. conclude that humans are genetically built to be active and that prolonged inactivity (sedentary living) promotes chronic-disease pathophysiology. They make an excellent case and, in fact, have begun to provide scientific evidence of these theories (8).

Thus, the essence of the debate is really technical, but, for exercise professionals, the take-home points are as follows:

1. Clients should do a minimum amount of weekly vigorous exercise to meet ACSM's fitness guidelines.
2. Clients should increase physical activity levels so that they get at least 10,000 steps per day (11,000–15,000 for weight loss or maintenance of weight loss).
3. Increased CRF and PA are both protective from chronic disease, especially heart disease, and both should be emphasized by exercise professionals.

Significant RESEARCH

These articles (the first by Dr. Frank Booth) are relatively new and comprehensive (actually an update to a 2000 review by Dr. Booth) on physical inactivity and chronic disease. The second is one of the set of "classic" and landmark articles by Dr. Michael Pollock and colleagues that have defined the principles of exercise prescription for almost 40 years. Although they are very different in scope and content and also very different in complexity, both are worth reading for exercise professionals.

Inactivity and Chronic Disease

Booth FW, Chakravarthy MV, Gordon SE, et al. Waging war on physical inactivity: using modern molecular ammunition against an ancient enemy. J Appl Physiol. 2002;93:3–30.

■ Summary ■

This is an "invited review" in the *Journal of Applied Physiology*, one of the premier scientific journals in the world. Dr. Booth and his colleagues review the evidence and draw out physiological, biochemical, and genetic connections that support the theory that humans are genetically programmed to be active and that to be inactive (sedentary) causes pathophysiologic changes that are at the core of many chronic diseases. Booth has been a crusader for both exercise and PA for many years and this article is both very technical and very informative. He covers these connections for 20 of the most common chronic diseases, including several types of occlusive vascular disease, metabolic disease, pulmonary disease, several types of cancer, musculoskeletal disease, immune system disorders, and even neurological and cognitive disease. This review is too complex to abstract completely here, but it is important and comprehensive and should be read and reread.

The gist of the information in this article is that PA is the "normal" state for humans and that inactivity and sedentariness are abnormal states. Booth addresses this topic by first outlining how the human genome is "programmed" for activity and discusses how inactivity may be behind the "molecular mechanisms of disease." Each chronic disease is then discussed individually in a very organized fashion. The epidemiology of the disease is presented with documentation providing evidence that it is related to inactivity. The intermediate processes (cellular and genetic) by which inactivity provokes the specific disease are then elucidated, and finally, the cellular mechanisms of the disease are described. They state that they intend to "overrun disbelievers" by the weight of the evidence that physical inactivity is abnormal and causes the conditions that precede and accompany chronic disease. This article comes very close to presenting an overwhelming mass of evidence to prove this point.

Exercise and PF

Pollock ML, Ward A, Ayres JJ. Cardiorespiratory fitness: response to differing intensities and durations of training. Arch Phys Med Rehabil. 1977;58(11):467–473.

■ Summary ■

Michael Pollock, PhD, was one of the pioneers of the research that delineates the principles and practices of exercise prescription for cardiovascular endurance fitness. The study that we have chosen is only one from a series of studies that Dr. Pollock carried out to determine the most effective intensity, duration, and frequency for the enhancement of cardiovascular endurance fitness. This particular study focused on intensity, but the others in the series focused individually on frequency, duration, and mode of exercise, as well as the incidence of injury with differing intensities and durations. This is seminal, landmark research that exercise professionals should read.

SUMMARY

Optimal levels of exercise, specifically CRF, and PA, are effective in preventing and reversing several chronic diseases, including heart disease, diabetes, and obesity. The benefits of exercise develop from chronic exercise training and result from both chronic and subacute effects of exercise. Although there is controversy about whether CRF or PA is most important in the preventive effect, it is clear that the optimal program includes both regular exercise for CRF and high levels of daily PA.

REFERENCES

1. ACC/AHA 2005 guideline update for the diagnosis and management of chronic heart failure in the adult: a report of the American College of Cardiology/American Heart Association Task Force on Practice (Writing Committee to update the 2001 guidelines for the evaluation and management of heart failure). J Am Coll Cardiol. 2005;46:1–82.
2. Acil T, Atalar E, Sahiner L, et al. Effects of acute exercise on fibrinolysis and coagulation in patients with coronary artery disease. Int Heart J. 2007;48(3):277–285.
3. Altena TA, Michaelson JL, Ball SD, et al. Single sessions of intermittent and continuous exercise and postprandial lipemia. Med Sci Sports Exerc. 2004;36(8):1364–1371.
4. Blair SN, Cheng Y, Holder JS. Is physical activity or physical fitness more important in defining health benefits? Med Sci Sports Exerc. 2001;33 (6, Suppl):379–399.
5. Blair SN, Kampert JB, Kohl HW, et al. Influences of cardiorespiratory fitness and other precursors on cardiovascular disease and all-cause mortality in men and women. JAMA. 1996;276:205–210.
6. Blair SN, Kohl HW, Barlow RS, et al. Changes in physical fitness and all-cause mortality: a prospective study of healthy and unhealthy men. JAMA. 1995;273:1093–1098.
7. Blair SN, LaMonte MJ. How much and what type of physical activity is enough? What physicians should tell their patients? Arch Int Med. 2005;165(20):2324–2325.
8. Booth FW, Chakravarthy MV, Gordon SE, et al. Waging war on physical inactivity: using modern molecular ammunition against an ancient enemy. J Appl Physiol. 2002;93:3–30.

9. Borghouts LB, Keizer HA. Exercise and insulin sensitivity: a review. Int J Sports Med. 2000;21:1–12.

10. Brun JF, Khaled S, Raunaud E, et al. The triphasic effects of exercise on blood rheology: which relevance to physiology and pathophysiology? Clin Hemorheol Microcirc. 1998;19(2):89–104.

11. da Nobrega L, Claudio A. The subacute effects of exercise: concept, characteristics and clinical implications. Exerc Sports Sci Rev. 2005;33(2):84–87.

12. Durstine JL, Haskell WL. Effects of exercise training on plasma lipids and lipoproteins. Exerc Sports Sci Rev. 1994;22:477–521.

13. El-Sayed MS, El-Sayed Ali Z, Ahmadizad A. Exercise and training effects on blood haemostasis in health and disease: an update. Sports Med. 2004;34(3):181–200.

14. Erbs S, Linke A, Hambrecht R. Effects of exercise training on mortality in patients with coronary heart disease. Coron Artery Dis. 2006;17(3):219–225.

15. Fehrenbach E, Schneider ME. Trauma-induced systemic inflammatory response versus exercise-induced immunomodulatory effects. Sports Med. 2006;36(5):373–384.

16. Ford ES. Does exercise reduce inflammation? Physical activity and C-reactive protein among U.S. adults. Minerva Endocrinol. 2002;27(3):209–214.

17. Gettman LR, Pollock ML, Durstine JL. et al. Physiological responses of men to 1, 3, and 5 day per week training programs. Res Quart. 1976;47(4):638–646.

18. Gill JMR. Physical activity, cardiorespiratory fitness and insulin resistance: a short update. Curr Opin Lipidol. 2007;18:47–52.

19. Gleeson M. Immune function in sport and exercise. JAP. 2007;103(2):693–699.

20. Gulati M, Pandey DK, Amsdorf MF, et al. Exercise capacity and the risk of death in women: The St. James Women Take Heart project. Circulation. 2003;108:1554.

21. Hamer M. Exercise and psychobiological processes: implications for the primary prevention of coronary heart disease. Sports Med. 2006;36(10):829–838.

22. Hansson GK. Inflammation, atherosclerosis and coronary artery disease. N Engl J Med. 2005;352:1685–1695.

23. Haram PM, Adams V, Kemi OJ, et al. Time-course of endothelial adaptations following acute and regular exercise. Eur J Cardiovasc Prev Rehabil. 2006;13:585–591.

24. Haskell WL, Lee IM, Pate RR, et al. Physical activity and public health: updated recommendation for adults from the American College of Sports Medicine and the American Heart Association. Med Sci Sports Exerc. 2007;39(8):1423–1434.

25. Hill JM, Zalos G, Halcox JP, et al. Circulating endothelial progenitor cells, vascular function, and cardiovascular risk. N Engl J Med. 2003;348:593–600.

26. Horowitz JR. Exercise-induced alterations in muscle lipid metabolism improve insulin sensitivity. Exerc Sports Sci Rev. 2007;35(4):192–196.

27. Houmard JA, Tanner CJ, Slentz CA, et al. Effect of the volume and intensity of exercise training on insulin sensitivity. JAP. 2004;96(1):101–106.

28. Kemi OJ, Wisloff U. High-intensity aerobic exercise training improves the heart in health and disease. J Cardiopulm Rehabil Prev. 2010;30(1):1–63.

29. Kraus WE, Houmard JA, Duscha BD, et al. Effects of the amount and intensity of exercise on plasma lipoproteins. N Engl J Med. 2002;347(19):1483–1492.

30. LaMonte MJ, Blair SN, Church TS. Physical activity and diabetes prevention. JAP. 2005;99:1205–1213.

31. Laufs U, Werner N, Link A, et al. Physical training increases endothelial progenitor cells, inhibits neointima formation, and enhances angiogenesis. Circulation. 2004;109:220–226.

32. Laughlin HM. Physical activity in prevention and treatment of coronary disease: the battle line is in exercise vascular cell biology. Med Sci Sports Exerc. 2004;36(3):352–362.

33. Libby P, Ridker PM, Hansson GK. Inflammation in atherosclerosis: from pathophysiology to practice. J Am Coll Cardiol. 2009;54(23):2129–2138.

34. Linke A, Erbs S, Hambrecht R. Effects of exercise training upon endothelial function in patients with cardiovascular disease. Front Biosci. 2008;13:424–432.

35. Lloyd-Jones D, Adams RJ, Brown TM, et al. American Heart Association heart disease and stroke statistics—2010 update: a report from the American Heart Association. Circulation. 2010;121:46–215.

36. Maiorana A, O'Driscoll GO, Taylor R, et al. Exercise and the nitric oxide vasodilator system. Sports Med. 2003;33(4):1011–1035.

37. Mark DB, Lauer NS. Exercise capacity: the prognostic variable that doesn't get enough respect. Circulation. 2003;108:1534–1536.

38. McGavock JM, Eves ND, Mandic S, et al. The role of exercise in the treatment of cardiovascular disease associated with type 2 diabetes mellitus. Sports Med. 2004;34(1):27–48.

39. Morris JN, Clayton DG, Everitt MG, et al. Exercise in leisure time: coronary attack and death rates. Br Heart J. 1990;63:325–334.

40. Morris JN, Kagan A, Pattison DC, et al. Incidence and prediction of ischaemic heart disease in London busmen. Lancet. 1966;2:553–559.

41. Myers J, Kaykha A, George S, et al. Fitness versus physical activity patterns in predicting mortality in men. Am J Med. 2004;117:912–918.

42. Nelson ME, Rejeski WJ, Blair SN, et al. Physical activity and public health in older adults: recom-

mendation from the American College of Sports Medicine and the American Heart Association. Med Sci Sports Exerc. 2007;39(8):1435–1445.

43. Niebauer J, Hambrecht R, Velich T, et al. Attenuated progression of coronary artery disease after 6 years of multifactorial risk intervention: role of physical exercise. Circulation. 1997;96(8):2534–2541.

44. Paffenbarger RSJ, Laughlin ME, Gima AS, et al. Work activity of longshoremen as related to death from coronary heart disease and stroke. N Engl J Med. 1970;282:1109–1114.

45. Paffenbarger RS Jr, Lee IM. A natural history of athleticism, health and longevity. J Sports Sci. 1998;16(suppl.):32–45.

46. Paffenbarger RS Jr, Wing AL, Hyde RT. Physical activity as an index of heart attack risk in college alumni. Am J Epidemiol. 1978;252:161–175.

47. Panagiotakos DB, Kokkinos P, Manios Y, et al. Physical activity and markers of inflammation and thrombosis related to coronary heart disease. Atherosclerosis. 2004;176(2):303–310.

48. Pescatello LS, Franklin BA, Fagard R, et al. ACSM position stand: exercise and hypertension. Med Sci Sports Exerc. 2004;36(3):533–553.

49. Pescatello LS, Kulikowich JM. The aftereffects of dynamic exercise on ambulatory blood pressure. Med Sci Sports Exerc. 2001;33:1855–1861.

50. Plaisance EP, Grandjean PW. Physical activity and high-sensitivity c-reactive protein. Sports Med. 2006;36(5):443–458.

51. Plaisance EP, Taylor JK, Alhassan S, et al. Cardiovascular fitness and vascular inflammatory markers after acute aerobic exercise. Intern J Sport Nutrit Exerc Metab. 2007;17(2):152–162.

52. Pollock ML, Dimmick J, Miller HS Jr, et al. Effects of mode of training on cardiovascular function and body composition of adult men. Med Sci Sports. 1975;7(2):139–145.

53. Pollock ML, Gettman LR, Milesis CA, et al. Effects of frequency and duration of training on attrition and incidence of injury. Med Sci Sports. 1977;9(1):31–36.

54. Pollock ML, Miller HS, Linnerud AC, et al. Frequency of training as a determinant for improvement in cardiovascular function and body composition of middle-aged men. Arch Phys Med Rehabil. 1975;56(4):141–145.

55. Pollock ML, Ward A, Ayres JJ. Cardiorespiratory fitness: response to differing intensities and durations of training. Arch Phys Med Rehabil. 1977;58(11):467–473.

56. Rauramaa R, Gang L, Vaisanen SB. Dose-response and coagulation and hemostatic factors. Med Sci Sports Exerc. 2000;33(6, Suppl):516–520.

57. Rennie KL, McCarthy N, Yazdgerdi S, et al. Association of the metabolic syndrome with both vigorous and moderate physical activity. Int J Epidemiol. 2003;32:600–606.

58. Robertson RJ, Noble BJ. Perception of physical exertion: methods, mediators, and applications. Exerc Sport Sci Rev. 1997;25:407–452.

59. Steiner S, Niessner A, Ziegler S, et al. Endurance training increases the number of endothelial progenitor cells in patients with cardiovascular risk and coronary artery disease. Atherosclerosis. 2005;181:305–310.

60. Thomas DE, Elliott EJ, Naughton GA. Exercise for type 2 diabetes mellitus. Cochrane Database Syst Rev. 2007;2:1–47.

61. Thomas TR, LaFontaine TP. Exercise, nutritional strategies and lipoproteins. In: Roitman JL, et al., eds. ACSM's Resource Manual for Guidelines for Exercise Testing and Prescription. 4th Ed. Baltimore, MD: Lippincott Williams & Wilkins, 2004, pp. 308–316.

62. Thompson PD, Buchner D, Pina IL, et al. Exercise and physical activity in the prevention and treatment of atherosclerotic cardiovascular disease: a statement from the Council on Clinical Cardiology, American Heart Association. Circulation. 2003;107:3109–3116.

63. Thompson PD, Crouse F, Goodpaster B, et al. The acute versus the chronic response to exercise. Med Sci Sports Exerc. 2001;33(6, Suppl):438–445.

64. Tudor-Locke C, Hatano Y, Pangrazi RP, et al. Revisiting "how many steps are enough?" Med Sci Sports Exerc. 2008;40(7, Suppl):537–543.

65. Wahl P, Bloch W, Schmidt A. Exercise has a positive effect on endothelial progenitor cells, which could be necessary for vascular adaptation processes. Int J Sports Med. 2007;28(5):374–380.

66. Wallace JP. Exercise in hypertension: a clinical review. Sports Med. 2003;33(8):585–598.

67. Wallace JP. Principles of cardiorespiratory endurance programming. In: Kaminski LA, ed. ACSM's Resource Manual for Exercise Testing and Prescription. 5th Ed. Baltimore, MD: Lippincott Williams & Wilkins, 2006, pp. 336–349.

68. Wang JS. Exercise prescription and thrombogenesis. J Biomed Sci. 2006;13(6):753–761.

69. Williams PT. Physical fitness and activity as separate heart disease risk factors a meta-analysis. Med Sci Sports Exerc. 2001;33(5):754–761.

70. Williams PT. The illusion of improved physical fitness and reduced mortality. Med Sci Sports Exerc. 2003;35(5):736–740.

71. Womack CJ, Nagelkirk PR, Coughlin AM. Exercise-induced changes in coagulation and fibrinolysis in health populations and patients with cardiovascular disease. Sports Med. 2003;33(11):795–807.

Nutrition and the Prevention of Chronic Metabolic Diseases

ABBREVIATIONS

AHA	American Heart Association	FDA	Food and Drug Administration
AICR	American Institute of Cancer Research	GI	Glycemic index
		GL	Glycemic load
APO	Apolipoprotein	HDL	High-density lipoprotein
BMI	Body mass index	LDL	Low-density lipoprotein
CAD	Coronary artery disease	PD	Portfolio diet
CSI	Cholesterol/saturated fat index	USDA	U.S. Department of Agriculture
CVD	Cardiovascular disease		
DASH	Dietary Approaches to Stop Hypertension	WCRF	World Cancer Research Fund

Nutrition is inextricably linked to chronic disease as well as to good health. This has been confirmed in epidemiological as well as in basic and applied research (1). It has been consistently demonstrated that single micronutrients (i.e., vitamins or minerals) are rarely the cause of a disease process or the determinant of the health of a particular diet. Dietary patterns have become the focus of research in nutritional epidemiology (4,29,61). Dietary patterns account for the overall quality and quantity of foods from various food groups and their interactions in the whole diet. Macronutrients such as saturated fat, trans fat, cholesterol, simple sugars, carbohydrates, and processed meats, and their relative proportional intakes as part of the whole diet, are clearly implicated in chronic disease risk (4,9,22,26,27,29,70).

The Seven Countries Study was initiated in the 1950s and was conducted in the United States and across several diverse European and Asian countries (34) (See Fig. 4.1). This study was designed to investigate the relationships between dietary parameters such as dietary cholesterol and saturated fat and blood cholesterol and cardiovascular disease (CVD) morbidity and mortality. Together with the Framingham Heart Study (see Chapter 1), this large, prospective, cross-cultural epidemiologic study was among the earliest and most important projects designed to study the connection between diet, lifestyle, and chronic diseases (10,14,20,34). Later, the Multiple Risk Factor Intervention Trial (MRFIT) also helped to clarify these relationships (59,60).

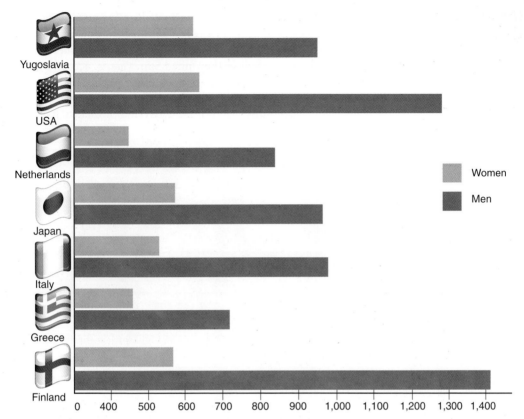

FIGURE 4.1 Sample sizes of participants in the Seven Countries Study.

DIETARY PATTERNS AND CHRONIC DISEASES

About 15 years ago, Drs. Walter Willett and Frank Hu and others identified two primary patterns at opposite ends of the spectrum with respect to chronic disease (22,26,27). Two major dietary patterns were proposed that were intimately related to health and disease: the "prudent" dietary pattern and the "Western" dietary pattern (27). Dr. Hu and his colleagues at Harvard clarified these two patterns using participants in one of their large group prospective studies—The Nurses Health Study (27). The "prudent" dietary pattern is healthy and preventive, whereas the "Western" dietary pattern is not healthy and is associated with increased risk for several chronic diseases (9,22,26,27). The primary dietary pattern in the United States is the Western diet. It is a very different nutritional pattern than was consumed in this country even as few as 50 to 75 years ago (22,26,39,70).

Dietary patterns were first studied as an alternative to studying specific nutrients and their link to health and disease. The argument is that it is not specific nutrients (or the lack thereof) that increase the risk for chronic diseases, but rather the whole diet and the integrated action of the foods and nutrients within the overall "dietary pattern." The Western diet has been demonstrated to be associated with heart disease, diabetes, some types of cancer, and obesity. The prudent diet, conversely, is associated with lower prevalence and death rates from these same diseases and with death from all causes.

The preponderance of foods that compose the Western dietary pattern diet have high caloric density and limited nutrient value. They often are high in fat and sweetened with sugar, high fructose corn syrup, or artificial sweeteners. In addition, the meat is commonly high in saturated fat and may also be "processed." Processed meats may contain trans fats, saturated fats, large amounts of sodium and sugar, as well as other "chemical" flavorings and preservatives.

This introduction is not intended to be a "health-nut" food lecture, but rather simply to state the fact that what the majority of persons in the United States eat is, according to one popular author, not really food but rather factory-raised, color-enhanced, and artificially flavored "food-like" substances (49). Interested readers are referred to the references for more information. See Figure 4.2 for an illustration of these two major dietary patterns.

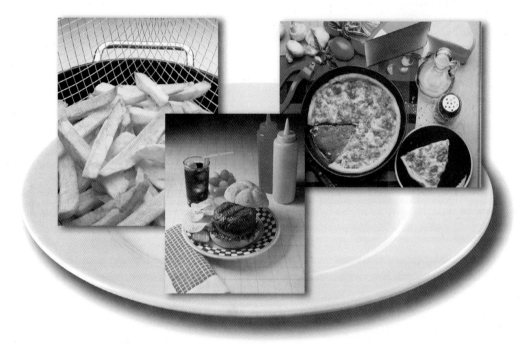

Western diet

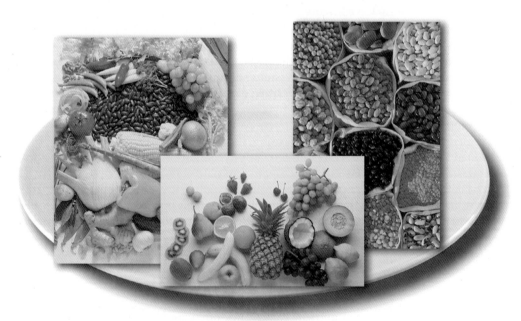

Prudent diet

FIGURE 4.2 The plates illustrate foods typically found in the "Western" and "Prudent" dietary patterns.

TABLE 4.1 Characteristics of the "Prudent" and the "Western Diet"	
Western	**Prudent**
High intake of simple carbohydrates (simple sugar sweetened products)	High intake of complex carbohydrates Few sweetened products
High intake of refined grains Few whole grains, nuts, and legumes Low fiber	Few refined and processed grains, mostly whole grains, nuts, and legumes
Few fruits and vegetables High sodium and fat	High intake of fruits and vegetables High fiber, low fat, lower sodium
High intake of red meat Frequent intake of processed meats Frequent intake of fast foods High or moderate fat dairy	Limited intake of red meats Good fats (unsaturated plant sources) Few meats Infrequent consumption of fast foods Low-fat dairy
Limited intake of fish high in omega-3 fatty acids	Omega-3 fatty acids from fish

It has been conclusively demonstrated that the "prudent" dietary pattern as part of an overall healthy lifestyle is associated with lower risks for hypertension, CVD, coronary artery disease (CAD), type 2 diabetes, abnormal blood lipids, and several cancers (1,7,27,31,40,43,52,67–71). The Harvard Nurses and Health Professionals prospective studies compared the effects of the "prudent" dietary pattern with the typical "Western" dietary pattern in men and women and confirmed the relationship (4,5,67). Recently, more than 72,000 women from the Nurses Health Study were analyzed with respect to dietary pattern. The "prudent" dietary pattern was associated with a 28% lower risk of death from CVD and a 17% lower risk of all-cause mortality (26). Table 4.1 shows common characteristics of the Western dietary pattern and the prudent dietary pattern.

Recently, one or more of nine risk factors were found to be present in 94% of all cases of myocardial infarction in a 52-country study called "INTERHEART" (2,74). Six of the nine risk factors are diet related: apolipoprotein (APO) B:A ratio (see the following box), hypertension, abdominal obesity, diabetes, no alcohol intake, and high-risk diet.

These and other studies have also confirmed the critical role of health behaviors for preventing chronic disease, including dietary patterns, not smoking or use of other tobacco products, maintaining a normal body weight, and engaging in regular physical activity. Van Dam et al. (68,70) recently identified five lifestyle behaviors (see the following box) that are associated with a very low risk for mortality from chronic diseases such as CVD and CAD. Three of the five are related to dietary pattern. Figure 4.3 illustrates the risk factors studied by the INTERHEART study (74).

It is important to remember that the INTERHEART study identified risk factors that are *present* in a large percentage of those who have a heart attack. Van Dam and his colleagues, on the other hand, identified five behaviors that are *preventive* (69). In fact, diet and exercise are at the center of an "optimal lifestyle (35,36)." However, the reality in the United States is that only 3% to 8% of adults can be classified as low risk (1,19,53,70). Figure 4.4 illustrates the important diet-related risk factors identified in the INTERHEART study.

Lipoproteins and Apolipoprotein A and Apolipoprotein B

Apolipoprotein A and ApoB are specific types of lipoproteins. Fat and cholesterol are not soluble in blood plasma. Therefore, lipids (triglycerides etc.) and cholesterol must be attached to protein molecules to be transported through the blood. Protein molecules in combination with the lipid are called "lipoproteins." Thus, all fats are transported through the blood by lipoproteins. There are many forms of lipoprotein, including low-density lipoprotein (LDL), high-density lipoprotein (HDL), and others.

LDL transports cholesterol to tissues for physiological uses as well as depositing it into the walls of arteries, forming atherosclerotic plaque. HDL takes fat to the liver for breakdown and elimination. LDL is often called "bad cholesterol" and HDL, which transports LDL from arterial deposit sites to the liver (reverse cholesterol transport), is called "good cholesterol." Prevention of CAD is associated with lower values of LDL (optimal <100 in persons without CAD or an equivalent such as peripheral artery disease or type 2 diabetes) and higher values of HDL (optimal >60). The ratio of LDL to HDL is often used to assess risk. The optimal LDL/HDL ratio is <2.5.

The two proteins discussed here were studied in the INTERHEART data and are designated as "risk factors." ApoB is the primary protein that carries LDL and ApoA1 is the primary protein associated with HDL. They respond to (and are largely controlled by) diet, exercise, and genes. INTERHEART found that this ApoA/ApoB ratio was important in predicting the risk for death from CAD.

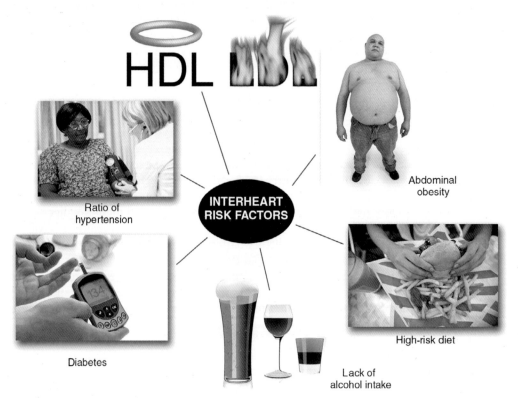

FIGURE 4.3 INTERHEART investigated six important diet-related risk factors associated with heart disease. HDL, high-density lipoprotein.

DID YOU KNOW?

Health Behaviors in a Low-Risk Lifestyle (5)

A "Low-risk lifestyle" is defined by the following behaviors:

- Does not use tobacco
- Body mass index (BMI) <25.0 kg/m^2
- >30 minutes of moderate to vigorous physical activity, 5 or more days/week
- Healthy diet (low in saturated and trans fats and cholesterol, high in fiber, whole grains and legumes, polyunsaturated to saturated fat ratio, low glycemic load (GL), high fish intake, and high intake of fruits and vegetables)
- Moderate alcohol intake (no more than 1 drink per day for women and 1 or 2 for men).

The American Institute for Cancer Research (AICR) in collaboration with the World Cancer Research Fund (WCRF) published a document titled "Food, Nutrition, and the Prevention of Cancer: A World Perspective" (73). They reported that 30% to 40% of all cancers could be prevented by healthier nutrition choices, increased physical activity, and avoidance of overweight and obesity. The box titled "Recommendations for Cancer Prevention from the WCRF/AICR Report" summarizes the recommendations of the WCRF and AICR report.

Of particular importance in this report are the dietary recommendations to consume mostly plant-based foods, no more than 18 oz of red meat per week and no processed

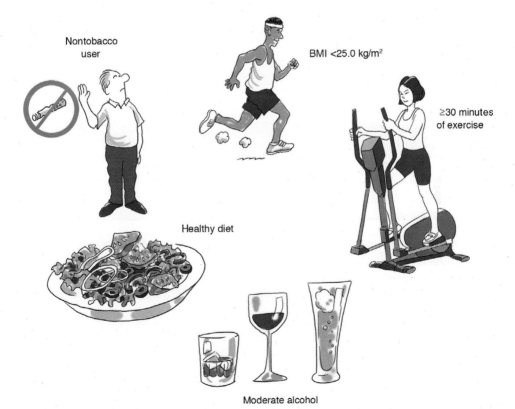

FIGURE 4.4 INTERHEART, Harvard, and other studies have identified five important lifestyle factors associated with low risk for heart disease. BMI, body mass index.

DID YOU KNOW?

Recommendations for Cancer Prevention from the WCRF/AICR Report (73)

1. Be as lean as possible without being underweight.
2. Be physically active for at least 30 minutes every day.
3. Avoid sugary drinks. Limit consumption of energy-dense foods (particularly processed foods high in added sugar, low in fiber, or high in fat).
4. Eat mostly foods of plant origin (i.e., a variety of vegetables, fruits, whole grains, and legumes such as beans).
5. Limit consumption of red meats (such as beef, pork, and lamb) and avoid processed meats (meat preserved by smoking, curing, salting, or by adding chemical preservatives).
6. If you drink alcohol, limit your intake to 2 drinks per day for men and 1 drink per day for women.
7. Limit consumption of salty foods and foods processed with salt (sodium).
8. Do not use supplements to protect against cancer.
9. Mothers should breastfeed infants.
10. Cancer survivors should follow the recommendations for cancer prevention.

meats. In addition, a minimum of 30 minutes of physical activity per day and maintenance of BMI <25.0 are recommended.

In 2006, the American Heart Association (AHA) revised its diet and lifestyle recommendations (39). Key goals of this document are for the U.S. adult and youth populations to consume an overall healthy diet; achieve a healthy body weight; achieve recommended levels for lipoproteins, triglycerides, blood glucose, and blood pressure; and become and remain physically active at recommended levels. Specific recommendations are summarized in the following box. The authors of this statement conclude that by following these

DID YOU KNOW?

Specific Targets of the 2006 AHA Diet and Lifestyle Recommendations (39)

1. Balance caloric intake and physical activity to achieve and maintain a healthy body weight
2. Consume a diet rich in fruits and vegetables
3. Choose whole-grain, fiber-rich foods
4. Consume fish, especially oily fish, twice per week
5. Limit intake of saturated fats to <7% of energy
6. Limit intake of trans fats to <1% of energy
7. Limit cholesterol intake to <300 mg/day by choosing lean meats and vegetable alternatives
8. Consume only fat-free (skim) or low-fat (1% or less) dairy products
9. Minimize intake of partially hydrogenated fats
10. Minimize intake of beverages and foods with added sugars
11. Choose and prepare foods with little or no added salt
12. If you drink alcohol do so in moderation (<1 drink/day for women, not >2 for men)
13. When you eat foods outside the home follow these recommendations as closely as possible

recommendations, U.S. citizens can substantially reduce their risk of developing CVD that remains the leading cause of mortality and morbidity in the United States.

In emphasizing dietary patterns it is important to recognize the significance of two key concepts as follows: (1) macronutrient content of the dietary pattern and (2) the glycemic index (GI) and/or GL of the dietary patterns. These two concepts are discussed below. Table 4.2 presents a brief listing of foods and their GI values.

MACRONUTRIENT CLASSIFICATION

Macronutrients are individual components of dietary patterns that provide energy or biological structure. They are found in the form of carbohydrates, fats, water, and proteins. Each of the macronutrients can be further classified into different subtypes. For example, protein can be complete (contains all essential amino acids) or incomplete (one or more essential amino acids are missing) and can come from either plant or animal sources. Fats can be broadly classified into two types: saturated and unsaturated. Unsaturated fats can be further divided into monounsaturated or polyunsaturated fats. In addition, processing techniques to make vegetable oils more solid results in the formation of trans-fats (there are very limited amounts of trans-fat in nonprocessed foods). Finally, carbohydrates can be classified into two types: simple carbohydrates or complex carbohydrates. Recently, carbohydrates have been classified according to their GI and/or GL (23).

GLYCEMIC INDEX AND GLYCEMIC LOAD

GI measures how rapidly a food breaks down into glucose in the blood. The GI of glucose, e.g., white sugar is 100; thus, this is the "reference" food. Foods with a GI of <60 are better choices because they do not break down as quickly and usually contain greater amounts of fiber and complex carbohydrates and/or lean protein.

GL is similar to GI, but it attempts to add the extent to which a particular food affects blood glucose. GL takes into account the GI, the type, and the serving size of the food. The following Web sites are excellent resources for information on GI and GL: http://www.mendosa.com/gilists.htm and http://www.glycemicindex.com/.

SPECIFIC DIETS AND CHRONIC DISEASE

In this section we will discuss the effectiveness of evidence-based specific whole food, mostly plant-based dietary patterns for the prevention of chronic disease. A summary of the optimal dietary pattern for the prevention and management of chronic disease will be presented. Finally, we will provide recommendations for exercise professionals to assist clients in adopting a low-risk, healthy-eating dietary pattern.

Whole-food prudent dietary patterns that are composed of low saturated and moderately high unsaturated fat, low cholesterol, moderate protein, and high fiber have been studied and confirmed as effective for preventing and managing chronic disease (7,9,22,26,27, 29,40,41,47,52). These whole-food–based diets include the New American Diet, the Dietary Approaches to Stop Hypertension (DASH) Diet, the Portfolio Diet (PD), the OmniHeart Diet, the Ornish Diet, Pritikin Diet, and the Indo-Mediterranean Diet (13,42,47,50,54,55,58). It is clear that some specific food groups and macronutrients have been identified as key to health and disease prevention. Some of these foods include fish (salmon, mackerel, trout, etc.), legumes, nuts, fruits, vegetables, soy products, and whole grains.

TABLE 4.2	Glycemic Index and Glycemic Load of Common Foods	
Food	**Glycemic Index**	**Glycemic Load**
Potatoes, baked	98	High
Carrots	85	Low
Corn	70	Low
Potatoes, red boiled	58	Medium
Green peas	51	Low
Sweet potatoes	50	Medium
Tomatoes	38	Low
Black beans	30	Low
Kidney beans	29	Low
Lentils	29	Low
Cantaloupe	65	Low
Banana	60	Medium
Kiwi	52	Low
Grapes	50	Low
Pears	45	Low
Orange	40	Low
Apple	40	Low
Strawberries	32	Low
Peaches	30	Low
Prunes	29	Low
Grapefruit	26	Low
Cherries	23	Low
Instant rice	87	High
Corn tortilla	72	Low
White rice	70	High
Corn meal	68	Low
Taco shells	68	Low
Refined pasta	65	High
Couscous	61	High
Brown rice	55	Medium
Air-popped popcorn	55	Low
Whole-wheat pasta	45	Medium

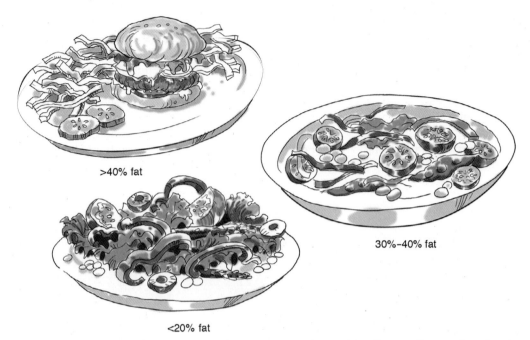

>40% fat

30%–40% fat

<20% fat

FIGURE 4.5 High (>40%), moderate (30%–40%), and low (<20%) fat diets are illustrated on the plates above.

Adherence to low-to-moderate fat, high-fiber dietary patterns has been shown to reduce the risk for numerous chronic diseases, including type 2 diabetes, hypertension, and CVD (3–5,26,27,29). One issue with interpreting the research on the optimal dietary pattern is the lack of an accepted definition of "low" versus "high" fat. Several studies claim to test the difference between low- and high-fat diets when, in fact, the diets were not low fat (28,57). See the following box for definitions of very low- to very high-fat diets. Figure 4.5 illustrates high-, moderate-, and low-fat plates (15,32,46,47,54).

The New American Diet

One of the first and perhaps most practical approaches to a healthy whole-food dietary pattern was the New American Diet that is research based and was developed by the Connors (12). This dietary pattern was based on the concept that a food's hypercholesterolemic

DID YOU KNOW?
Percentage of Calories from Fat in Very Low- to Very High-Fat Diets

Diet Type	Calories From Fat (%)
Very high fat	≥40
High fat	30–39.9
Moderate fat	20–29.9
Low fat	10–19.9
Very low fat	<10

(cholesterol-raising) and atherogenic potential is determined by its cholesterol and saturated fat content (13). As a result of research conducted in metabolic wards designed to improve lipids, the Connors and colleagues developed "the cholesterol/saturated-fat index" (CSI) (13). A low CSI identifies a food that is low in saturated fat and usually cholesterol. The authors calculated the CSI of hundreds of commonly consumed foods and created a diet in which 60% of the calories came from complex carbohydrates, 20% each from fat and lean protein, and 5% from saturated fat. Subsequently, several studies demonstrated the health benefits of the diet that they called "The New American Diet" (12). Table 4.3 provides the cholesterol, saturated fat, and CSI of the 60/20/20 2,000-calorie dietary pattern as well as the CSI of selected commonly eaten foods.

TABLE 4.3	The Cholesterol-Saturated Fat Index (CSI) of Commonly Eaten Foods
Food	**CSI***
Whitefish (snapper, cod, halibut)	4
Salmon	5
Shellfish (shrimp, crab)	6
Ground sirloin beef	9
20% fat ground chuck	13
Pork and lamb chops	18
2% fat cottage cheese	16
25%–30% fat cheeses	19
Whole eggs	29
Egg whites	0
Peanut butter	5
Most vegetable oils	8
Butter	37
Coconut, palm oil	47
Sherbet	2
Rich ice cream, 16% fat	18
Skimmed milk	<1
2% milk	4
Whole milk	7
Sour cream	37

The lower the CSI, the healthier the food.

Modified from Connor et al. (12,13).

*Target CSI = 10–23.

Dietary Approaches to Stop Hypertension Diet

The Dietary Approaches to Stop Hypertension (DASH) project was designed to test the effects of a carbohydrate-rich diet emphasizing fruits and vegetables, low-fat dairy products, low sodium, and whole grains for prevention of hypertension (42,55). The DASH diet is particularly low in saturated fat and dietary cholesterol and moderately low in total fat. It is also designed to be rich in fiber and key micronutrients such as calcium, magnesium, and potassium and low in sodium (a target of 2,300 mg/day in the original version). Table 4.4 summarizes the composition of the DASH diet, and Table 4.5 shows some of the key outcomes of the DASH trial. The results of a subsequent DASH trial studied the effects on blood pressure in participants with prehypertension and hypertension. The sodium content of the diet was lowered from 2,300 mg/day to 1,600 mg/day. These results are summarized in Table 4.6 (55).

In summary, the DASH diet has been demonstrated to effectively lower blood pressure in those with hypertension and prehypertension, especially if sodium intake is limited to

TABLE 4.4 Content of the DASH Diet	
Macronutrient	**DASH (% calories)**
Fat	27
Saturated fat	6
Polyunsaturated fat	8
Monounsaturated fat	13
Protein	18
Protein from vegetable sources	55
Carbohydrates	55
Fiber (g/1,000 cal)	15
Dietary cholesterol (mg)	71

DASH, dietary approaches to stop hypertension.

TABLE 4.5 Outcomes of the DASH Trial (42)		
	SBP (mm Hg)	**DBP (mm Hg)**
All participants	−5.5	−3.0
HTN	−11.6	−5.3
Normotensive	−3.5	−2.2
Total cholesterol (mg/dl) −13.7		
LDL cholesterol (mg/dl) −10.0		

DASH diet also lowered CRP and homocysteine

DASH, dietary approaches to stop hypertension; SBP, systolic blood pressure; DBP, diastolic blood pressure; HTN, hypertension; LDL, low-density lipoprotein; CRP, c-reactive protein.

TABLE 4.6	Selected Outcomes in the DASH-Sodium Trial (55)		
	Sodium Intake		
	High (3,266 mg/d)	**Moderate (2,461 mg/d)**	**Low (1,500 mg/d)**
SBP change (mm Hg)	−5.0	−10.9	−12.1
DBP change (mm Hg)	22.9	25.4	26.4

DASH, dietary approaches to stop hypertension; SBP, systolic blood pressure; DBP, diastolic blood pressure.

1,600 mg/day or less. Of equal importance is that the DASH diet has also been demonstrated to be effective for improving blood lipids and blood glucose and, thus, is also preventive for chronic diseases other than hypertension (3,4).

The OmniHeart Diet

The OmniHeart trial was a randomized clinical trial that compared three diets: the original DASH plan, a second dietary pattern that was similar to the DASH plan in most respects (except that carbohydrate calories were decreased and replaced with increased protein), and a third dietary pattern that also was similar to the DASH plan (except that carbohydrate calories were decreased and replaced with increased unsaturated fat) (4,16,42). The objective of this study was to determine which dietary plan would be most effective for reducing the risk factors for CVD.

Participants had either prehypertension or stage 1 hypertension (see Chapter 8 for definitions). The results demonstrated that all diets were effective for modifying blood pressure, lipids, and risk for heart disease (4,16,42). Table 4.7 presents an example of a daily menu for each dietary pattern, and Table 4.8 presents some selected outcomes from the OmniHeart study.

The Portfolio Diet

PD is based on the origin and evolution of the human genome and dietary consumption (32). The ancestral human diet was high in vegetable protein, dietary fiber, plant starch, sterols and stanols, and nuts. These classes of foods have been approved by the Federal Food and Drug Administration (FDA) for health claims that they may reduce the risk for heart disease (32,65).

The FDA approval encouraged the development and implementation of research into the effects of the PD. Table 4.9 summarizes the typical concentrations of these "functional" foods in the PD. The definition of a functional food is provided in the following box. The PD is low in fat (<27% of calories), saturated fat (<7% of calories), and dietary cholesterol (<200 mg/day). Table 4.10 illustrates a typical PD menu.

The PD including some or all of the foods in the previous box has been tested in several controlled trials with excellent results (32). The specific results of studies where all four of the PD foods were included in the diet reported LDL reductions of 29% to 35% (32). In addition to positive changes in lipids, improvements in other established or potential atherogenic risk factors such as reduced c-reactive protein, homocysteine, insulin resistance, and glycated hemoglobin have all been reported in studies of the PD (32). The PD, including the "functional" foods that comprise the PD, is not only beneficial with respect to promoting

TABLE 4.7	Typical Daily Menu Plan for Each Diet in the OmniHeart Study	
Higher Carbohydrate	**Higher Protein**	**Higher Unsaturated Fat**
Breakfast		
1 cup OJ	½ cup OJ	⅔ cup OJ with calcium
1 slice whole-grain bread	1 slice light bread	1 slice whole-grain bread
1 tablespoon (tbsp) jelly	1.5 tbsp peanut butter	1 tbsp diet jelly
1 large banana	½ cup egg substitute	1 small banana
2 tbsps margarine	3 links vegetable sausage	2 tbsp margarine
1 cup low-fat milk	1 tbsp margarine	1 cup low-fat milk
	1 cup low-fat milk	
Lunch		
½ cup tofu chili*	⅔ cup tofu chili	½ cup tofu chili*
1 & ½ tbsp safflower	¾ oz light cheddar	
	5 tbsp canola oil	
1 & ½ tbsp canola oil	1 oz cheddar cheese	½ oz light cheddar cheese
		12 medium ripe olives
1 & ½ oz tortilla chips	¾ oz tortilla chips	1 oz tortilla chips
¾ cup bulgur wheat salad*	¾ cup bulgur salad*	½ cup bulgur salad*
2 Fig newtons	2 Fig newtons	1 oz unsalted peanuts
½ cup pears in own juice	½ cup pears in own juice	½ cup pears in juice
1 cup low-fat milk	1 cup fat-free milk	½ cup apple juice
Dinner		
6 oz baked cod	6 oz baked cod	6 oz baked cod
1 tbsp olive oil	1 tbsp olive oil	1 tbsp olive oil
1 tbsp plain bread crumbs	Same	Same
1 tsp lemon juice	Same	Same
⅓ cup steamed spinach	¾ cup carrots	⅔ cup steamed spinach
½ cup carrots	2 tsp margarine	⅔ cup carrots
3 tsp margarine	1 slice bread	4 tsp margarine
1 small dinner roll		
1 small peppermint	1 small peppermint	
	2 small peppermint patties	
Snack		
½ cup apple juice	½ cup apple juice	1 medium banana
Trail mix (20 unsalted & 1.5 tbsp raisins)	28 unsalted peanuts	½ cup fat-free yogurt
	½ cup chocolate pudding and 1.5 tbsp raisins	½ cup chocolate pudding

TABLE 4.8 Outcomes in the OmniHeart Study (4,42)			
Diet	CHO	PRO	Unsaturated Fat
PARAMETER			
Blood Pressure			
SBP (mm Hg)			
Stage 1	−12.9	−16.1	−15.8
Pre-HTN	−7.0	−8.0	−7.7
DBP (mm Hg)			
Stage 1	−6.3	−8.6	−8.2
Pre-HTN	−3.6	−4.4	−3.9
LDL (mg/dl)			
>130	−19.8	−23.6	−21.9
<131	−4.4	−6.1	−5.4
HDL (mg/dl)	−1.4	−2.6	−0.3
Triglycerides (mg/dl)	+0.1	−16.4	−9.3
Estimated CHD risk reduction (%)			
Men	−13.8	−18.7	−17.2
Women	−21.2	−30.0	−31.3

CHO, carbohydrate; PRO, protein; SBP, systolic blood pressure; HTN, hypertension; DBP, diastolic blood pressure; LDL, low-density lipoprotein; HDL, high-density lipoprotein; CHD, coronary heart disease.

health, but it also clearly helps to prevent chronic diseases. Figure 4.6 illustrates some functional foods.

The Pritikin Longevity Center Diet and Exercise Program

The Pritikin Longevity Center was established in the 1960s by Nathan Pritikin (51). Dr. James Barnard and his colleagues at the University of California, Los Angeles (54), have studied the metabolic effects of this program extensively. Pritikin participants

TABLE 4.9 Key Ingredients of Portfolio Diet	
Nutrient	Amount (g/d)
Fiber	10–20
Stanols/sterols	1.5–4.0
Soy protein	8–45
Almonds	16.6–46

TABLE 4.10	Typical Menu in the Portfolio Diet	
Breakfast	**Lunch**	**Dinner**
Hot oat-bran cereal	Lentil soup	Tofu ratatouille pasta
Soy beverage	Soy deli slices	Eggplant
Blueberries	Oat-bran bread	Onions
Sugar and psyllium	Stanol/sterol margarine	Sweet peppers
Stanol/sterol margarine	Lettuce	Pearled barley
Double fruit jam	Tomato and cucumber	Steamed vegetables
AM snack	Afternoon snack	Evening snack
Almonds	Almonds	Apple
Soy beverage	Soy beverage	Soy beverage
Fresh fruit	Psyllium	Psyllium

Modified from Jenkins et al. (31).

undergo a complete medical evaluation and history before starting a comprehensive 26-day residential diet and exercise program. Meals are served buffet style, and participants are allowed unrestricted eating except fish or fowl (3.5 oz each per week). The diet contains 10% to 15% of calories from fat, 15% to 20% from protein, and 65% to 75% from carbohydrates as well as <100 mg of cholesterol per day. Carbohydrates are predominantly in the form of high-fiber low-GI/GL whole grains ($\geq$5 servings per day), legumes (several servings per week), vegetables ($\geq$4 servings per day), and fruits ($\geq$3 servings per day). Protein is primarily from plant sources with two servings of nonfat dairy per day and two 3.5 oz servings of chicken or fish per week. All participants engage in 45 to 60 minutes of daily walking or other aerobic exercise at 70% to 85% of the maximal heart rate (55%–75% of VO$_2$ max). Participants also participate in regular flexibility and resistance exercise (51,54).

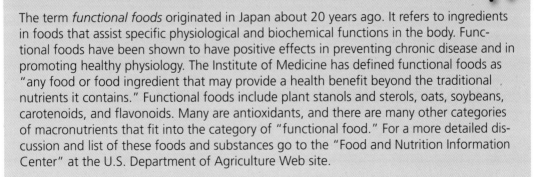

DID YOU KNOW?
Definition of Functional Foods (64)

The term *functional foods* originated in Japan about 20 years ago. It refers to ingredients in foods that assist specific physiological and biochemical functions in the body. Functional foods have been shown to have positive effects in preventing chronic disease and in promoting healthy physiology. The Institute of Medicine has defined functional foods as "any food or food ingredient that may provide a health benefit beyond the traditional nutrients it contains." Functional foods include plant stanols and sterols, oats, soybeans, carotenoids, and flavonoids. Many are antioxidants, and there are many other categories of macronutrients that fit into the category of "functional food." For a more detailed discussion and list of these foods and substances go to the "Food and Nutrition Information Center" at the U.S. Department of Agriculture Web site.

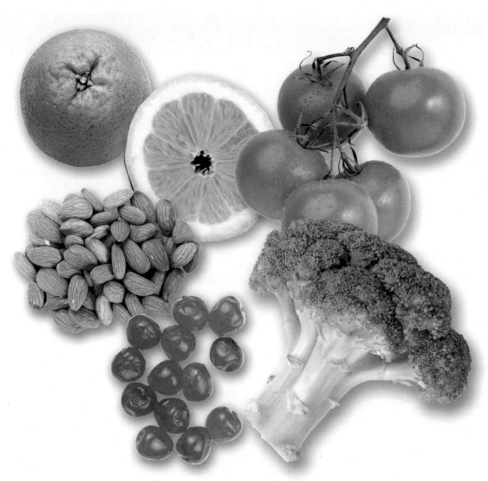

FIGURE 4.6 Functional foods have micronutrients that serve a "functional" purpose in the body. The figure above illustrates some functional foods.

Roberts et al. analyzed the effects of this 26-day program in 4,587 men and women who were followed for 5 years (54). LDL was lowered by 23%, the total cholesterol/ HDL by 11%, and triglycerides by 33%. Body weight was reduced by 5.5% in men and 4.4% in women. The Pritikin program has also been shown to improve blood pressure, blood glucose metabolism and insulin resistance, coronary blood flow reserve, oxidative stress, and inflammatory markers (54). Although most of these studies were single-group nonrandomized designs, it is particularly important to note the short time period (26 days) that yielded these significant improvements in metabolic health of the participants.

The Ornish Diet and Lifestyle Modification Program

The Dean Ornish Lifestyle Modification Program is a comprehensive approach to disease prevention designed to address the underlying causes of chronic diseases (47,50). This program is offered on a residential basis similar to the Pritikin program. The diet is <10% fat and entirely plant based. It is high in fruits, vegetables, legumes, and whole grains. Table 4.11 provides detailed nutritional information about the content of the Ornish diet.

TABLE 4.11	**Nutritional Guidelines of the Dean Ornish Diet**
Fat	10% of calories are from fat. This is achieved by not adding any fats, oils, seeds, nuts, avocados, coconut, and olives to a mostly plant-based diet. The 10% of calories from fat come from natural grains, vegetables, fruits, beans, and soy foods.
Cholesterol	No more than 10 mg of cholesterol per day. To meet this goal, nonfat dairy products are limited to 2 servings per day. Nonfat dairy products are optional. Soy products can be used instead of dairy products because they are cholesterol free.
Animal products	Meat, poultry, fish, and products made from these foods are eliminated. Egg whites are included.
Calories	Unrestricted unless weight loss is desired. Small frequent meals spread throughout the day help avoid hunger and keep energy levels constant. Portion control will assist in reaching and maintaining a healthy body weight and controlling blood sugar.
Sugar	Permitted in moderation. No more than 2 servings/d including nonfat sweets. A serving is equal to 1 tablespoon, or 12 g. Total of no more than 24 g/d.
Caffeine	All sources of caffeine are eliminated, including regular and decaffeinated coffees and teas, chocolate, cocoa, and regular or decaffeinated dark colas, *with the exception of green tea.* Caffeine's effect on the central nervous system interferes with the mind–body connection and therefore meditation and relaxation. *Why is green tea an exception?* Evidence from recent studies on tea shows that the health benefits of green tea outweigh the risks for most individuals. Green tea contains various powerful antioxidants called polyphenols, especially the flavonoids such as catechins, which may reduce the risk of many chronic diseases. *Individuals with arrhythmia and elevated stress levels should still avoid caffeinated beverages.* Green tea contains some caffeine but the content is lower than that found in coffee, black or oolong teas, and caffeinated cola soft drinks. It should be *limited to no more than 2 cups per day.* In addition, decaffeinated green tea can be consumed. Be sure to purchase green tea that has been decaffeinated with the "effervescence" method (uses water and carbon dioxide), which preserves most of the polyphenols present in regular green tea. Naturally caffeine-free herbal teas, grain-based coffees (i.e., Postum, Caffix, and Roma), carob powder, Sprite, 7-Up, or Ginger Ale are also good alternatives.
Sodium	Moderate salt use, unless medically indicated otherwise.
Alcohol	Allowed in small amounts but not encouraged. If consumed, enjoy 1 serving a day: 1.5 oz liquor, 4 oz wine, or 12 oz beer.
Soy	One serving per day of a "full-fat" soy food. A full-fat soy food is one that contains greater than 3 g of fat per serving, with none coming from added fats or oils.

(continued)

TABLE 4.11	Nutritional Guidelines of the Dean Ornish Diet (continued)
Supplements	A low-dose multivitamin and mineral supplement with B_{12} (without iron, if not of childbearing age), fish oil, and, possibly upon the advice of a physician, calcium supplements. Antioxidant vitamins and folic acid are optional and are based on health history and nutritional intake of these nutrients.

Used with permission from Preventive Medicine Research Institute, www.pmri.org, accessed December 20, 2008. Dean Ornish, MD.

Moderate cardiovascular endurance exercise, stress management and relaxation techniques, as well as support groups are also part of the program. The Lifestyle Heart Trial, using the Ornish program, was one of the first studies to demonstrate that lifestyle changes can stabilize or reverse atherosclerosis (47,50).

TABLE 4.12	Macronutrient Content of the Step 1 NCEP Diet Versus the Indo-Mediterranean Diet	
Nutrient	**AHA Step 1 Diet**	**Indo-Mediterranean Diet**
Total energy (kCal)	2,089	2,015
Carbohydrate (% kCal)	56.0	59.4
Complex (% kCal)	38.7	48.1
Total fiber (g/d)	25.9	48.1
Soluble fiber (g/d)	13.6	25.0
Protein (% kCal)	14.9	14.2
Fat (%kCal)	29.1	26.3
Saturated fat (% kCal)	12.1	8.2
PUFA (% kCal)	7.4	8.1
MUFA (% kCal)	9.6	10.0
n-3 fatty acids (% kCal)	0.78	1.79
Cholesterol (mg/d)	207.0	125.0
Salt (g/d)	9.5	8.4
Fruits, vegetables, nuts, and legumes (g/d)	231.0	573.0
Whole grains (g/d)	132.0	252.0
Oil (g/d)	15.2	31.0

NCEP, National Cholesterol Education Program; AHA, American Heart Association; PUFA, polyunsaturated fatty acid; MUFA, monounsaturated fatty acid.

The Indo-Mediterranean and Mediterranean Diets

Singh et al. (58) created a diet called the "Indo-Mediterranean Diet." The investigators randomized 1,000 participants with documented CAD or who were at high risk for CAD to either a step 1 diet (National Cholesterol Education Program) or the Indo-Mediterranean diet. The Indo-Mediterranean and step 1 dietary patterns are summarized in Table 4.12. Selected food content of the Indo-Mediterranean dietary pattern is provided later in this chapter. Figure 4.7 illustrates foods found in the Indo-Mediterranean diet.

Studies show that persons who eat a Mediterranean-type diet have lower rates of mortality from CVD, cancers, and all-causes (15,37,43,45,62,63). Several recent comparisons of the Mediterranean diet with the "Western" diet clearly demonstrate that it is effective for prevention of chronic disease (15,43,45,62). The American Association of Retired Persons Diet and Health study reported that older adults whose diet most closely matched a Mediterranean diet were 20% less likely to die of heart disease, cancer, or any cause over 5 years of follow-up (43). Trichopoulou et al. (62) recently demonstrated in an elderly population that substituting a high Mediterranean diet score was associated with increased survival across European populations. Heart attack survivors following a Mediterranean-type diet were significantly less likely to have a recurrent heart attack or stroke (15,63). In the Lyon Heart Trial, participants on the Mediterranean diet had a 71% lower risk of a recurrent heart attack compared with those on the AHA diet—step 1 diet (15). Finally, a recent study showed that the Mediterranean diet was more effective at reducing inflammation, blood glucose, and insulin resistance than either a low carbohydrate or step 1 AHA diet (57).

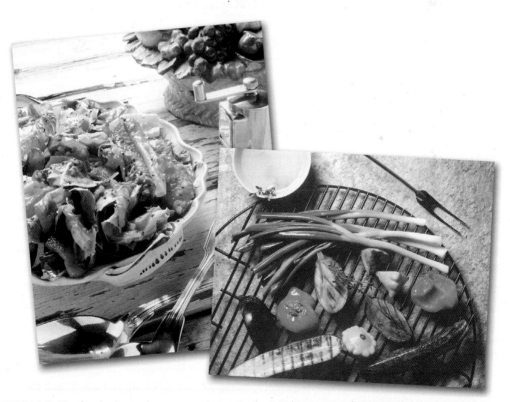

FIGURE 4.7 The foods shown here are common to the Mediterranean dietary pattern.

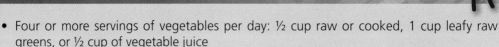

DID YOU KNOW?

Selected Food Content of the Indo-Mediterranean Dietary Pattern

- Four or more servings of vegetables per day: ½ cup raw or cooked, 1 cup leafy raw greens, or ½ cup of vegetable juice
- Four or more servings of fruit per day: ½ cup of fresh, frozen, or canned fruit; ¼ cup of dried fruit; one medium-sized fruit; or ½ cup of fruit juice
- Six or more servings of whole grains per day: 1 cup of dry breakfast cereal, ½ cup of cooked cereal, whole grain rice or pasta, or 1 slice of whole grain bread
- Two or more servings (4 oz/serving) of fish per week
- One serving of yogurt or cheese per day: 8 oz of yogurt or 2 oz of cheese
- One serving of beans or nuts per day: ½ cup cooked beans; 1.5 oz or a "handful" is a serving of nuts
- Limit alcohol to 1 drink for women and 2 for men; one drink is 5 oz of wine, 12 oz of beer, or 1.5 oz of liquor

FOOD PYRAMIDS

Food pyramids present a visual image of a healthy diet. Researchers from Tufts University Medical School created one of the first food pyramids for the U.S. Department of Agriculture (USDA). Several other food-guide pyramids have been created and proposed. We will discuss the USDA Dietary Guidelines and MyPyramid, as well as three other evidence-based pyramids in this section. Each is shown in the illustrations that accompany the discussion.

THE U.S. DEPARTMENT OF AGRICULTURE 2005 DIETARY GUIDELINES FOR AMERICANS

The 2005 USDA Dietary Guidelines for Americans provides science-based advice to promote health and to reduce the risk for chronic diseases through diet and physical activity (64). The intent of these guidelines is to summarize and synthesize available evidence regarding food components into recommendations for a pattern of eating that can be adopted by the public and result in improved health and a lower individual and population risk for preventable diseases. A basic premise of the USDA guidelines is that nutrient needs should be met primarily through consuming healthy nutritious foods and that fortified foods and dietary supplements may be useful sources of one or more nutrients that otherwise might be consumed in less than recommended amounts (64). The USDA guidelines address two healthy dietary patterns: (1) the USDA Food Guide (Fig. 4.8) and (2) the DASH diet (see the section on this diet). These guidelines are updated every 5 years and address recommendations for physical activity as well as diet across the lifespan. The next update is due to be published before the end of 2010. For more information visit the Web site (www.mypyramid.gov). The following box summarizes some of the key recommendations of the 2005 guidelines. Also reproduced in Figure 4.8 is the USDA pyramid referred to as "MyPyramid."

THE UNIVERSITY OF MICHIGAN HEALING FOODS PYRAMID

The Integrative Medicine Department at the University of Michigan developed the Healing Foods Pyramid (Fig. 4.9) (66). The primary purpose of this pyramid is to emphasize

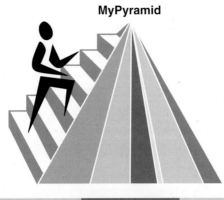

MyPyramid

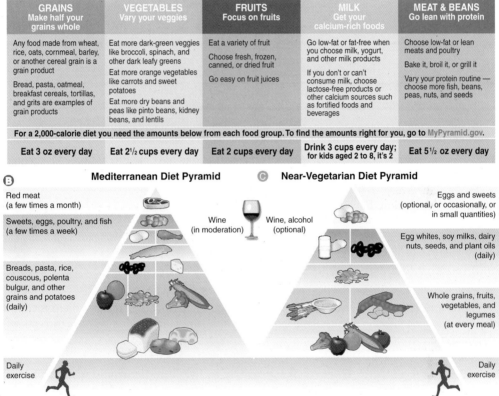

GRAINS Make half your grains whole	VEGETABLES Vary your veggies	FRUITS Focus on fruits	MILK Get your calcium-rich foods	MEAT & BEANS Go lean with protein
Any food made from wheat, rice, oats, cornmeal, barley, or another cereal grain is a grain product Bread, pasta, oatmeal, breakfast cereals, tortillas, and grits are examples of grain products	Eat more dark-green veggies like broccoli, spinach, and other dark leafy greens Eat more orange vegetables like carrots and sweet potatoes Eat more dry beans and peas like pinto beans, kidney beans, and lentils	Eat a variety of fruit Choose fresh, frozen, canned, or dried fruit Go easy on fruit juices	Go low-fat or fat-free when you choose milk, yogurt, and other milk products If you don't or can't consume milk, choose lactose-free products or other calcium sources such as fortified foods and beverages	Choose low-fat or lean meats and poultry Bake it, broil it, or grill it Vary your protein routine — choose more fish, beans, peas, nuts, and seeds
For a 2,000-calorie diet you need the amounts below from each food group. To find the amounts right for you, go to MyPyramid.gov.				
Eat 3 oz every day	Eat 2½ cups every day	Eat 2 cups every day	Drink 3 cups every day; for kids aged 2 to 8, it's 2	Eat 5½ oz every day

FIGURE 4.8 MyPyramid. From the USDA Center for Nutrition Policy and Promotion (available at: http://www.mypyramid.gov).

and advocate the use of functional foods for purposes of promoting healthy physiology. The box that follows Figure 4.9 illustrates the five key principles underlying the design of this pyramid.

The purpose and design of this pyramid is exceptional. The pyramid emphasizes

• the fundamental role of water in human health
• the rainbow of colors and essential nutrients found in fruits and vegetables
• whole grains that are excellent sources of healthful fiber and nutrients

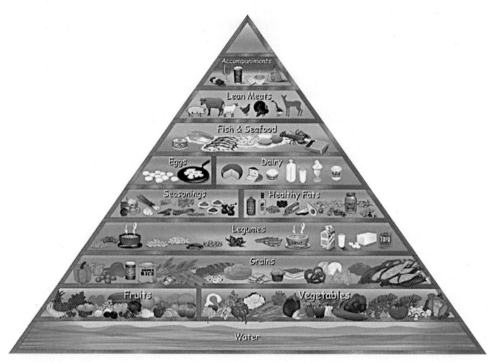

FIGURE 4.9 The Healing Foods Pyramid. Used with permission from the University of Michigan Integrative Medicine Institute.

DID YOU KNOW?

Summary of Key Recommendations of the 2005 USDA Dietary Guidelines

1. Consume various nutrient-dense foods and beverages within and among the basic food groups while limiting the intake of saturated and trans-fats, added sugars, cholesterol, salt, and alcohol
2. Adopt the My Pyramid (www.mypyramid.gov) or the DASH diet
3. To maintain a healthy body weight, balance calories from foods and beverages with calories expended
4. To prevent weight gain over time, make small decreases in food and beverage calories and increase physical activity
5. For a 2,000 calorie diet, consume 2 cups of fruit and 2.5 cups of vegetables per day from various sources
6. Consume 3 or more ounce equivalents of whole-grain products per day. In general, at least half of the grains should come from whole grains
7. Consume 3 cups of fat-free, low-fat milk, or equivalent milk products/day
8. Consume less than 10% of calories from saturated fat and less than 300 mg of cholesterol per day while keeping trans-fat consumption as close to zero as possible
9. Keep total fat intake to 20% to 35% of total calories per day
10. Choose fiber-rich fruits, vegetables, legumes, and whole grains
11. Consume less than 2,300 mg of sodium per day (1 tsp of salt)

DID YOU KNOW?
Basic Principles of the Healing Food Pyramid

- *Healing Foods*—only foods known to have healing benefits or essential nutrients are included
- *Plant-based choices*—the base of the pyramid and may be supplemented with small amounts of very lean animal foods
- *Variety and balance*—variety of colors, nutrients, portion size
- *Support healthful environment*—food choices reflect the health of ourselves and the earth
- *Mindful eating*—truly savor, enjoy, and focus on the variety of tastes and flavors in foods

- legumes that are excellent sources of protein, nutrients, and fiber
- healthy fats such as those found in olive and canola oil, fish, nuts, seeds, and soy
- egg whites that provide high-quality protein
- low-fat dairy that is rich in high-quality protein, calcium, and vitamin D
- lean meats, poultry, and fish as a complement to other foods
- fish and other seafood that is high in omega-3 fatty acids
- seasonings such as herbs, onions, garlic, pepper, others that add flavor
- dark, flavonol-rich chocolate that is high in cocoa (70% or more)
- moderation in alcohol and tea intake, both of which have health benefits

THE HEALTHY EATING PYRAMID

The Healthy Eating Pyramid was designed by Walter Willet, MD, and colleagues at the Harvard School of Public Health (www.healthyeatingpyramid). This pyramid emphasizes exercise and weight control at its base. Foods at the foundation of the pyramid are fruits, vegetables, whole grains, legumes, and healthy fats; they comprise the largest sections of the pyramid and, thus, are emphasized in a healthy lifestyle. Figure 4.10 and the box that follows provide more detail regarding this pyramid.

THE ORNISH PYRAMID

The Ornish pyramid presents the program's essential dietary and lifestyle recommendations. The foundation of this pyramid comes from whole, unrefined grains such as whole wheat and brown rice, fresh fruits and vegetables, and legumes (beans, peas, lentils), including soy. These foods provide a great variety of disease-fighting substances found only in plant-based foods (phytochemicals), which may help prevent chronic diseases such as heart disease and cancer (50). The bottom two layers of the pyramid, with the addition of 1 to 2 servings of egg whites and nonfat dairy products, characterize a stricter version of the diet, meant for people who have heart disease. The Ornish Pyramid can be viewed online at www.pmri.org or can be seen in Figure 4.11.

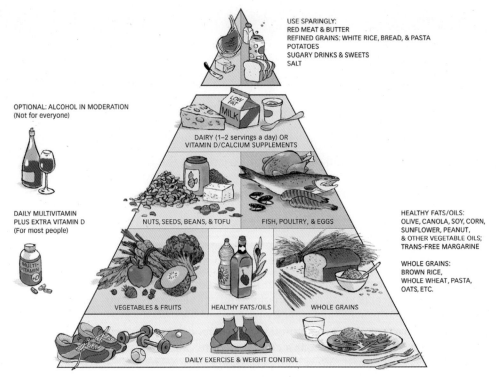

USE SPARINGLY:
RED MEAT & BUTTER
REFINED GRAINS: WHITE RICE, BREAD, & PASTA
POTATOES
SUGARY DRINKS & SWEETS
SALT

OPTIONAL: ALCOHOL IN MODERATION
(Not for everyone)

DAIRY (1–2 servings a day) OR
VITAMIN D/CALCIUM SUPPLEMENTS

DAILY MULTIVITAMIN
PLUS EXTRA VITAMIN D
(For most people)

NUTS, SEEDS, BEANS, & TOFU   FISH, POULTRY, & EGGS

HEALTHY FATS/OILS:
OLIVE, CANOLA, SOY, CORN,
SUNFLOWER, PEANUT,
& OTHER VEGETABLE OILS;
TRANS-FREE MARGARINE

WHOLE GRAINS:
BROWN RICE,
WHOLE WHEAT, PASTA,
OATS, ETC.

VEGETABLES & FRUITS   HEALTHY FATS/OILS   WHOLE GRAINS

DAILY EXERCISE & WEIGHT CONTROL

FIGURE 4.10 The Healthy Eating Pyramid. Used with permission from the Department of Nutrition, Harvard School of Public Health, Harvard University.

Healthy individuals, who want to prevent chronic disease and achieve or maintain a healthy weight, can utilize the top layers of the pyramid. These foods include the following:

- Higher-fat foods, such as nuts and avocados and plant oils low in saturated fat and high in omega-3 fatty acids (e.g., canola oil).
- Fish, which can also be enjoyed in small amounts, especially the varieties rich in omega-3 fatty acids, such as salmon, mackerel, and herring and trout.
- Nonfat dairy products and egg whites, which can be included to provide excellent-quality protein and important vitamins.
- Lean poultry, which can be added occasionally if a vegetarian diet is not acceptable, since the white meat of poultry provides very little additional fat or saturated fat.

Simple, refined carbohydrates such as sugars and white flour are strictly limited in this diet since they are not whole foods.

Red meat and trans fatty acids are excluded. Red meat is high in saturated fat and has been linked to an increased risk of heart disease and cancer. Trans fatty acids are even worse than saturated fat in increasing the risk for heart disease and are excluded.

The Ornish approach embraces a dietary pattern and overall lifestyle that offers a spectrum of choices. If food choices are viewed as part of a spectrum, then the Ornish plan offers a wide selection of foods. Relative to the degree that clients move in this direction, they will feel better, be more likely to lose weight, and more likely to optimize known markers of health.

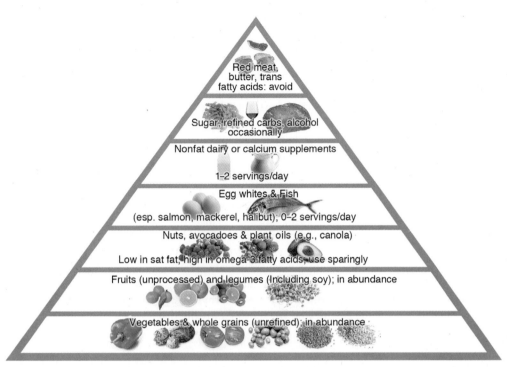

FIGURE 4.11 The Preventive Medicine Research Institute Food Guide Pyramid. Used with permission from the Preventive Medicine Research Institute (Available at: http://www.pmri.org; Dean Ornish, MD, President).

DID YOU KNOW?

Five Principles of the Healthy Eating Pyramid

1. **Start with exercise:** A healthy diet is built at the base of regular exercise, which keeps calories in balance and weight in check.
2. **Focus on food, not grams:** The Healthy Eating Pyramid doesn't worry about specific servings or grams of food, so neither should you. It's a simple, general guide to how you should eat, when you eat.
3. **Go with plants:** Eating a plant-based diet is healthiest. Choose plenty of vegetables, fruits, whole grains, and healthy fats, such as olive and canola oil.
4. **Cut way back on American staples:** Red meat, refined grains, potatoes, sugary drinks, and salty snacks are part of American culture, but they're also unhealthy. Go for a plant-based diet rich in nonstarchy vegetables, fruits, and whole grains. And if you eat meat, fish and poultry are the best choices.
5. **Take a multivitamin, and maybe have an alcoholic drink:** Taking a multivitamin can be a good nutrition insurance policy. Moderate drinking (no more than 1 for women and 1–2 for men per day) for many people can have real health benefits, but it's not for everyone. Those who don't drink shouldn't feel that they need to start.

Used with permission—Copyright © 2008 Harvard University. For more information about The Healthy Eating Pyramid, please see The Nutrition Source, Department of Nutrition, Harvard School of Public Health, http://www.thenutritionsource.org, and Eat, Drink, and Be Healthy, by Walter C. Willett, MD, and Patrick J. Skerrett (2005), New York: Free Press/Simon & Schuster Inc. (25).

THE BOTTOM LINE

These pyramids share many common characteristics. They emphasize increased consumption of plant-based foods, including fruits, vegetables, legumes, and other high-fiber complex carbohydrates. They recommend lower consumption of saturated and trans-fat by decreasing red meat, high-fat (whole milk) dairy products, and processed foods while increasing the intake of mono- and polyunsaturated fats from whole foods. Each dietary pattern described also recommends 2 to 3 servings of cold-water fish (salmon, mackerel, tuna, sardines, trout, other) per week.

Several alternative dietary patterns have been presented in this chapter that are supported by good nutritional, epidemiological, and clinical science. The pyramids are all based on science and unaffected by businesses and other organizations with a stake in the message. Both the Healing pyramid and the Ornish pyramid include many of the same aspects that the Healthy Eating pyramid does. The Healing pyramid emphasizes "functional foods" (similar to the PD), whereas Ornish and Pritikin programs emphasize a very low-fat, plant-based, high complex carbohydrate vegetarian diet. All these pyramids fit easily within the principles of a healthy dietary pattern. Implementing the principles of these pyramids as part of a comprehensive healthy lifestyle will conform to the essential principles of promoting health and preventing chronic diseases.

OMEGA-3 POLYUNSATURATED FATTY ACIDS

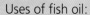

Consumption of omega-3 fatty acids is associated with numerous cardiovascular health benefits, including reduced triglycerides, atherosclerosis, ventricular arrhythmias, myocardial infarction, stroke, and sudden death (24,33,38). Lee et al. (38) and Harris et al. (37) summarized the cardioprotective effects of omega-3 fatty acids from fish sources and their recommendations are included in the following box.

Fish-oil supplements vary in the available amount of two primary omega-3 fats—eicosapentaenoic acid and docosahexaenoic acid. A dosage that includes approximately 600 mg of eicosapentaenoic acid and 400 mg of docosahexaenoic acid per day is recommended. This dosage can usually be obtained in 3 g of fish oil in capsule form. Strict

---

DID YOU KNOW?

Recommendations for Omega-3 Fatty Acids and Cardio Protection (24,45)

Uses of fish oil:

- Benefit is derived from either dietary fish sources or supplements
- 1 g/d for those with CVD and ½ g/d for those without CVD
- 3 to 4 g/d lowers triglycerides by 20% to 50%
- Two cold-water fish meals per week provide 400 to 500 mg of fish oils per day
- Salmon, blue-fin tuna, herring, mackerel, rainbow trout are good sources

Note: The FDA warning about the mercury content of fish is specific about which fish not to eat, including "king mackerel." When selecting fish, it is best to be aware of this warning, which can be found at http://www.cfsan.fda.gov/~dms/admehg3.html.

vegetarians may opt to take flaxseed oil capsules or preferably use ground flaxseed to obtain the benefits of the whole food. However, the omega-3 fatty acids in flaxseed are not as bioavailable as those in fish oil (24). *There is an additional precaution*: People who have recurrent angina, congestive heart failure, or evidence that the heart is not receiving enough blood flow during exercise *should consult their physician before taking fish oil*. Taking fish oil may *increase* the risk of sudden cardiac death for people with these conditions (8).

CONCLUSION: THE OPTIMAL CARDIOVASCULAR DISEASE PREVENTION DIET

Clearly, populations that live long lives and are free of premature CAD and other chronic disease consume diets that have the following common characteristics (6,21,46):

- high in complex carbohydrate and fiber and low in GI/GL.
- low-to-zero intake of carbohydrates with a high GI/GL.
- high in plant protein and in plant-based foods.
- low in saturated fat, trans-fat, and animal protein.

Table 4.13 summarizes the comparative effects of these diets on cardiovascular risk factors, and Table 4.14 provides recommendations for the optimal CVD prevention diet. Combined with regular physical activity, maintaining a normal body weight, not using tobacco products, and drinking moderate amounts of alcohol, 85% of atherosclerotic CVD can be prevented.

In summary, it is important to address the scope of practice as it relates to nutrition advice provided by exercise professionals. In general, the breadth and depth of training and education in nutrition is significantly less for most exercise professionals compared

TABLE 4.13 The Effect of These Diets on Cardiovascular Disease Risk Factors						
Diet	Total	LDL	HDL	Triglycerides	Blood Pressure	Blood Sugar
Typical Western	Inc	Inc	?/Inc	Inc	Inc	Inc
DASH	Dec	Dec	?/Dec	Dec/same	Dec	?/Dec
Omni Hi Pro	Dec	Dec	Dec	Dec	Dec	?/Dec
Omni Hi Unsat	Dec	Dec	Inc	Dec	Dec	Dec
Portfolio	Dec	Dec	Same	Dec	Dec	?
Pritikin*	Dec	Dec	Same	Dec	Dec	Dec
Ornish*	Dec	Dec	Dec	Dec	Dec	Dec
Indo-Mediterranean	Dec	Dec	Inc	Dec	Dec	Dec
New American Diet	Dec	Dec	Same	Dec	Dec	Dec

LDL, low-density lipoprotein; HDL, high-density lipoprotein; DASH, dietary approaches to stop hypertension; Dec, decrease; Inc, increase; ?, uncertain.
*Pritikin and Ornish Diets also emphasize exercise and weight loss.

TABLE 4.14   Optimal Cardiovascular Disease Prevention Plan*

Nutrient	Recommendation Per Day
Total fat (% kCal)	15%–30%
Saturated fat (% kCal)	<7%
Trans fat (% kCal)	<0.5%
MUFA/PUFA (% kCal)	10%–25%[1]
Dietary cholesterol (mg/d)	<100
Dietary fiber (g/d)	>35
Soluble fiber (g/d)	15–20
Sodium (mg/d)	<2,300[2]
Nuts and seeds	2 oz/d[3] 4–7 d/wk
Legumes	½–1 cup cooked 4–7 d/wk[4]
Omega-3 fish	6 oz[5] 2–3 d/wk
Berries	¼ C[6] 4–7 d/wk
Whole grains	4–5 servings/d[7]
Fruits/vegetables	6–9 servings/d[8]
Low-fat dairy or dairy substitute (e.g., soy)	2–3 servings/d[9]
Consider:	
Consider 25 g of soy protein—daily	
1.5–3.3 g of plant stanols/sterols—daily	

Adapted with permission from Roitman JL, LaFontaine TP. Efficacy of secondary prevention and risk factor reduction. In: *AACVPR Cardiac Rehabilitation Resource Manual*, by the American Association of Cardiovascular and Pulmonary Rehabilitation. Champaign, IL: Human Kinetics, 2006.

*Recommendations of the authors of this book:

1. Eicosapentaenoic, dehydropentanoic, and alpha linolenic acid emphasized.
2. DASH diet studies show persons with hypertension or prehypertension may benefit from 1,500 mg or less per day.
3. Almonds, walnuts, pecans, peanuts, flaxseed, cashews, macadamia, other.
4. Black, pinto, chickpeas, peas, anasazi, kidney, red, other: ½–1 cup cooked, ¼–½ cup dry.
5. Emphasize wild salmon, mackerel, sardines, tuna, trout: 4–6 oz, 2–3 days per week.
6. All berries are high in micronutrients, antioxidants, fiber: ¼ cup fresh.
7. Oats, wheat, barley, bulgur, couscous, quinoa, millet, rye, other (avoid processed grains): 1 slice bread, ½ cup cooked cereal, ½ cup dry cereal, ½ cup whole grain salad.
8. Medium-size fruit, ½ cup fresh fruit, ½ cup canned fruit in own juice, ¼ cup dried fruit, ½ cup fruit juice, 1 cup raw vegetable salad, ½ cup steamed vegetables, ½ cup vegetable juice.
9. 1% or less fat dairy or dairy products, 1 cup liquid, 1 cup yogurt, 1 oz cheese, ½ cup cottage cheese.

with a registered and/or licensed dietician. For example, there are only a few distinct American College of Sports Medicine knowledges and skills relating to nutrition and weight management for the American College of Sports Medicine Certified Health Fitness Specialist certification compared with 101 nutrition-related competencies for the Committee on Accreditation for Dietetics Education (which establishes curriculum for dieticians) (56). Essentially it is within the scope of an exercise professional; however, an exercise professional can explain only the basic principles of nutrition and weight management, as he or she generally does not possess the knowledge and abilities to assess a client's dietary status and outline a specific plan to improve nutrition-related biomarkers such as blood lipids or glucose. The reader is advised to review the article in the reference list by Sass et al. for more information regarding the scope of nutritional advice that an exercise professional can and should be capable of providing clients (56).

DIGGING DEEPER

During the past 10 years it has become increasingly clear that the dietary pattern necessary to prevent heart disease is very similar to that required to prevent other chronic disease. Recently, AHA and the American Diabetes Association produced a joint statement calling for a collaborative effort to prevent CVD and diabetes mellitus, particularly type 2 diabetes (18). These diseases are known to be associated with similar risk factors such as physical inactivity, obesity, dyslipidemia, and hypertension.

Recently, the AICR and WCRF published a joint report titled "Food, Nutrition, Physical Activity, and the Prevention of Cancer: A Global Perspective" (73). This report is one of the most extensive and well-documented reports ever published on prevention of disease (cancer) with nutrition and physical activity. Because of the dramatic advancements in the science of lifestyle factors and cancer, this document, first published in 1997, was revised and updated in 2007. An authoritative team of experts reviewed an extensive amount of relevant research using meticulous and well-defined guidelines in order to produce a comprehensive set of recommendations on food, nutrition, physical activity, and the prevention of cancer.

The process of developing this report took 5 years and culminated in progressive and detailed recommendations for the prevention of cancers. In reviewing the key recommendations, it is apparent that there is much overlap between the effects of nutrition and physical activity in the prevention of the chronic diseases that we have discussed and also in their role in the prevention of cancer.

This report is too lengthy (more than 400 pages and more than 1,500 references) to summarize in its entirety here. We can, however, extract some of the pertinent research to highlight three important issues related to nutritional status and cancer prevention. The role of overweight and obesity; red and processed meats, fruits, and vegetables; and dietary pattern will be discussed in this section.

The authors and the writing team of this report define the weight of the evidence relative to its importance in prevention. The terms *convincing* and *probable* are used relative to the evidence in this document. Both terms are based on strong research findings, and in the case of *convincing*, the authors state that the evidence suggests that these findings are not likely to be reversed by subsequent studies. In this document, *probable* means that the evidence "justifies goals and recommendations designed to reduce the incidence of cancer," another category based on strong evidence for the effect.

(continued)

Body Composition

The connection (causal?) between body composition and cancer, specifically, overweight and obesity, as well as waist circumference is well established. The authors of the document state it best by saying, "Anything that modifies the risk of weight gain, overweight, and obesity also modifies the risk of those cancers whose risk is increased by weight gain." Thus, the implication is that there are many nutritional relationships, such as the energy density of foods, as well as factors such as physical inactivity, that increase the risk of various cancers.

The association between those risks and the cancers is shown in Table 4.15. Interestingly, the writing group for this comprehensive document uses the word "cause" in relation to these behaviors and the cancers for which they increase risk. Thus, the relationship between being overweight, obese, and waist circumference (or waist–hip ratio) is established as "causative" for some cancers.

Meat and Processed Meat

A second area of interest, because of the link to the chronic diseases that have been discussed in this book, is dietary meat. The report states that there is *convincing* evidence for the association of red- and processed-meat intake and colorectal cancer. This evidence comes from both cohort and case–control studies. A dose–response effect has been demonstrated. In addition, though processed meat has not been specifically defined, in this report it means meats that have been preserved by "smoking, curing or salting, or by the addition of preservatives." This definition generally (though not always) includes ham, bacon, pastrami/salami, sausage, hot dogs, and other meats to which nitrates or nitrites are added as preservatives.

Fruits and Vegetables

The preventive benefits of fruits and vegetables are addressed and extensively documented. Interestingly the writing team found no *convincing* evidence for the relationship between the consumption of fruits and vegetables and cancer. They did, however, describe a *probable*, causal relationship between these factors. Thus, the relationship between consumption of fruits and vegetables and many types of cancer is strong enough to warrant the recommendations for increasing fruit and vegetable consumption for preventing cancer.

They do report that it is *probable* that the consumption of "nonstarchy" vegetables may protect against various cancers, including "mouth, larynx, pharynx, esophagus, and stomach." In addition, fruits may be protective against lung cancer.

Several other sections under the fruit and vegetable category provide interesting and intriguing information. For example, preparation of vegetables (i.e., cooking) is a subject of a brief discussion. Many forms of cooking reduce the nutrient content of vegetables, and raw consumption is a trend in some dietary patterns. However, cooking vegetables with both carotene (e.g., carrots and other yellow and orange vegetables) and lycopene (tomatoes) makes the nutrients in those vegetables biologically more available during digestion and thus increases their potential disease-preventing effects. Garlic has many known and touted health benefits. Peeling and crushing garlic releases an enzyme called *allinase* that may have some health benefits. Heating garlic reduces this enzyme and, therefore, its beneficial properties. However, if the peeled and crushed garlic is left to sit for about 15 minutes, those agents are not inactivated by cooking. Thus, preparation of food (specifically fruits and vegetables) may affect the potential benefits of the food.

Dietary Pattern

Finally, they address the relationship between dietary pattern and cancer. The report divides dietary pattern into three classifications as follows: "Traditional and Industrial," "Cultural," and "Other." We have discussed dietary patterns extensively in this chapter and those discussed here would fall into the "Traditional and Industrial" category according to this report. They discuss each of these separately in their summary for this section of the report.

The report concludes this section with a statement that it is not possible to make a "firm judgment" on any relationship between dietary pattern and risk of cancer. The Mediterranean pattern was related to some reduced risk of colorectal cancer in women, but not men. Several large cohorts with the Western dietary pattern, including the Health Professionals' Follow-up study and the Nurses Health Study, demonstrated no associations between Western dietary pattern and breast, prostate, or pancreatic cancer.

However, the research they report on "dietary pattern" is specifically exactly that. That is, they report many studies that used "dietary pattern" and not specific nutrients to test the effect of that specific pattern on the incidence and risk of cancer. These recommendations are summarized in the following box. It is notable that all of these are related to dietary pattern and, in fact, can be used to establish a "pattern" that is associated with reduced risk of cancer.

The AICR and WCRF expert panel also recognized that these recommendations would likely help in the prevention of other chronic diseases. The authors of this text believe that this document provides the most comprehensive and optimal set of recommendations for the prevention of not only cancers but also CVD, dyslipidemia, hypertension, and type 2 diabetes mellitus.

TABLE 4.15	**Body Fatness and the Risk of Cancer***			
	Decreases Risk		**Increases Risk**	
	Exposure	**Cancer Site**	**Exposure**	**Cancer Site**
Convincing			Body fatness	Esophagus[†] Pancreas Colorectum
				Breast (postmenopause)
				Endometrium Kidney
			Abdominal fatness	Colorectum
			Red meat[‡]	Colorectum
			Processed meat[§]	Colorectum

(continued)

TABLE 4.15	Body Fatness and the Risk of Cancer* (continued)			
	Body Fatness	Breast (Premenopause)	Body Fatness	Gallbladder
Probable			Abdominal fatness	Pancreas
				Breast (postmenopause)
				Endometrium
			Adult weight gain	Breast (postmenopause)
	Nonstarchy vegetables[ll]		Mouth, pharynx, larynx, esophagus, stomach	
	Allium vegetables[ll]		Stomach	
	Garlic[ll]		Colorectum	
	Fruits[ll]		Mouth, pharynx, larynx, esophagus, lung, stomach	
	Foods containing folate[¶]		Pancreas	
	Foods containing carotenoids[¶]		Mouth, pharynx, larynx, lung	
	Foods containing beta-carotene[¶]		Esophagus	
	Foods containing Lycopene[¶,Π]		Prostate	
	Foods containing vitamin C[¶,**]		Esophagus	
	Foods containing selenium[¶]		Prostate	

Adapted with permission from the Second Report of the World Cancer Research Fund (www.wcrf.org) and the American Institute for Cancer Research (www.aicr.org). "Food Nutrition, Physical Activity, and the Prevention of Cancer: A Global Perspective."

*In the judgment of the Panel, the factors listed below modify the risk of cancer. Judgments are graded according to the strength of the evidence.

[†]For esophageal adenocarcinomas only.

[‡]The term "red meat" refers to beef, pork, lamb, and goat from domesticated animals.

[§]The term "processed meat" refers to meats preserved by smoking, curing, or salting, or addition of chemical preservatives.

[ll]Judgments on vegetables and fruits do not include those preserved by salting and/or pickling.

[¶]Includes both foods naturally containing the constituent and foods that have the constituent added (see chapter 3.5.3).

[Π]Mostly contained in tomatoes and tomato products. Also fruits such as grapefruit, watermelon, guava, and apricot.

[**]Also found in some roots and tubers—notably potatoes. See chapter 4.1.

DID YOU KNOW?

Dietary recommendations of the Second Report of the AICR/WCRF

1. Body fatness: achieve a body weight between 21 and 23 BMI and avoid weight gain and increases in waist circumference throughout adulthood.
2. Limit consumption of energy-dense foods and avoid sugary drinks and consume fast foods sparingly and preferably not at all.
3. Eat mostly foods of plant origin, limit refined starchy processed foods, and consume unprocessed whole grains and/or legumes with every meal and at least five servings of nonstarchy vegetables and fruits every day.
4. Limit intake of red meat, no more than 18 oz per week, and avoid processed meats entirely.
5. Limit alcoholic drinks to no >1 per day for most women and no >2 per day for most men.
6. Limit consumption of salt, particularly processed foods with added salt to ensure an intake of no >2,400 mg of sodium per day.
7. Dietary supplements are not recommended for cancer prevention. Aim to meet nutritional needs through diet alone.

Significant RESEARCH

The two readings selected for these recommendations are reviews of nutrition as it relates to prevention of chronic disease. The first, by Dr. James O'Keefe and his colleagues, is an article by a physician who both practices (Preventive Cardiology) and does research. Dr. O'Keefe is a highly respected practitioner (45). The second article by Drs. Roberts and Barnard addresses exercise and diet and their effects on chronic disease (54). This is a more challenging article about this subject, but is comprehensive enough that it is also highly recommended.

Diet and Postprandial Lipemia

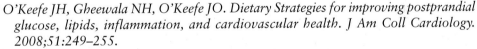

O'Keefe JH, Gheewala NH, O'Keefe JO. *Dietary Strategies for improving postprandial glucose, lipids, inflammation, and cardiovascular health. J Am Coll Cardiology. 2008;51:249–255.*

Dr. O'Keefe and his colleagues have written an excellent summary/review article about the effects of specific nutrients and enhancing dietary pattern on preventing chronic disease. Despite the daunting title, this article really discusses the relationship of specific nutrients and macronutrients with the aim of enhancing cardiovascular health. This comprehensive article reviews the use of nutrition and dietary pattern approaches to decreasing the postprandial and inflammatory effects associated with hyperglycemia and hyperlipemia (as they relate to diet). O'Keefe provides brief, but clear explanations of specific dietary strategies and nutrients that they relate to hyperglycemia, hyperlipemia, and inflammation. He then makes an extremely interesting and provocative statement, which we fully agree with and have rarely seen made by physicians: "however, resorting to drug therapy for an epidemic caused by a maladaptive diet is less rational than simply realigning our eating habits with our physiological needs."

(continued)

The article discusses a number of different dietary approaches to modifying the pathology referred to earlier. The authors present information regarding a wide spectrum of foods and dietary approaches to improving metabolic health, including discussion of the role of nuts, olive and fish oil, type of carbohydrate, caloric restriction, exercise, and the Mediterranean diet pattern. All of this is in the context of research literature and the efficacy of these approaches. It is a well-written, interesting article that the readers of this text are encouraged to review and absorb.

Prevention of Chronic Disease with Exercise and Diet

Roberts CK, Barnard RJ. Effects of exercise and diet on chronic disease. J Appl Physiol. 2005;98:3–30.

Drs. Roberts and Barnard have written a comprehensive and extensively documented review article about exercise, diet, and prevention of chronic disease. It is a detailed review of literature that is relatively intense and challenging to read, but the effort is worthwhile. The article is based largely on research conducted at the Pritikin Longevity Center (51). It is somewhat technical, though not overly so. It is full of detailed and well-documented scientific information. We do not make this point to warn off readers, but offer it as a caution about how to read the article. The interested reader is best served to filter the information that is beyond their need (and, perhaps understanding) and to read for the wider purpose, which is to glean information that is practical, useful, and understandable.

The authors cover aggressive and comprehensive dietary changes and exercise on the most common chronic diseases, including CAD, hypertension, diabetes, and cancer. Each chronic disease is discussed with respect to the research conclusions about the influence and efficacy of diet and exercise for modifying and, in some cases, reversing the disease process. Although much of the research on the Pritikin diet was single group and nonrandomized, Roberts and Barnard make an excellent case for optimal implementation of these two health behaviors for preventing chronic disease.

REFERENCES

1. Akesson A, Weismayer C, PK Newby, et al. Combined effect of low-risk dietary and lifestyle behaviors in primary prevention of myocardial infarction in women. Arch Intern Med. 2007;167:2122–2127.

2. Anand SS, Islam S, Rosengren A, et al. Risk factors for myocardial infarction in women and men: Insights from the INTERHEART Study. Eur Heart J. 2008;29:932–940.

3. Appel LJ, Brands MW, Daniels SR. Dietary approaches to prevent and treat hypertension: a scientific statement from the American Heart Association. Hypertension. 2006;47:296–308.

4. Appel LJ, Sacks FM, Carey VJ, et al. Effects of protein, monounsaturated fat, and carbohydrate intake on blood pressure and serum lipids: results of the OmniHeart randomized trial. JAMA. 2005;294:2455–2464.

5. Bassuk SS, Manson JE. Lifestyle and risk of cardiovascular disease and Type 2 diabetes in women: a review of epidemiologic findings. Am J Lifestyle Med. 2008;2:191–213.

6. Blue Zone Website [Internet]. Available at: http://www.bluezones.com. Accessed February 15, 2010.

7. Brennan SA, Cantwell MM, Cardwell CR, et al. Dietary patterns and breast cancer risk: a systematic review and meta-analysis. Am J Clin Nutr. 2010;doi:10-3945/ajcn.2009.28796.

8. Burr ML, Ashfield-Watt PAL, Dunstan FDJ, et al. Lack of benefit of dietary advice to men with angina: results of a controlled trial. Eur J Clin Nutr. 2003;57:193–200.

9. Carlson JJ, Monti V. The role of inclusive dietary patterns for achieving secondary prevention cardiovascular nutrition guidelines and optimal cardiovascular health. J Cardiopulm Rehabil. 2003;23:322–333.

10. Castelli W, Garrison RJ, Wilson PW, et al. Incidence of coronary heart disease and lipoprotein cholesterol levels. JAMA. 1986;256:2835–2838.

11. Chiuve SE, Rexrode KM, Spiegelman D, et al. Primary prevention of stroke by healthy lifestyle. Circulation. 2008;118:947–954.

12. Connor SL, Connor WE. The New American Diet. Fireside, New York, NY, 1991.

13. Connor SL, Gustafson JR, Artaud-Wild SM, et al. The cholesterol/saturated-fat index: an indication of the hypercholesterolemic and atherogenic potential of food. Lancet. 1986;319:1229–1232.

14. Dawber TR, Kannel WB, Revotskie N, et al. Some factors associated with the development of coronary heart disease; six years' follow-up experience in the Framingham Study. Am J Public Health. 1959;49:1349–1356.

15. de Longeril M, Salen P, Martin JL, et al. Mediterranean diet, traditional risk factors, and the rate of cardiovascular complications after myocardial infarction: final report of the Lyon Diet Heart Study. Circulation. 1999;99:779–785.

16. de Souza RJ, Swain JF, Appel LJ, et al. Alternatives for macronutrient intake and chronic disease: a comparison of the OmniHeart diets with popular diets and with dietary recommendations. Am J Clin Nutr. 2008;88:1–11.

17. Eckel RH, Kahn R, Robertson RM, et al. Preventing cardiovascular disease and diabetes: a call to action from the American Diabetes Association and the American Heart Association. Circulation. 2006;113:2943–2946.

18. Ehrman JK, ed. ACSM's Resource Manual for Guidelines for Exercise Testing and Prescription. 6th Ed. Baltimore, MD: LWW, 2010.

19. Ford ES, Li C, Zhao G, et al. Trends in the prevalence of low risk factor burden for cardiovascular disease among United States adults. Circulation. 2009;120:1181–1183.

20. Framingham Heart Study Web Site. Available at: www.nhlbi.nih.gov/about/framingham/. Accessed December 30, 2008.

21. Fraser GE. Vegetarian diets: what do we know of their effects on common chronic diseases? Am J Clin Nutr. 2009;89(Suppl):1S–6S.

22. Fung TT, Willett WC, Stampfer MJ, et al. Dietary patterns and risk of coronary heart disease in women. Arch Intern Med. 2001;161:1857–1862.

23. Gastrich MD, Lasser NL, Wren M, et al. Dietary complex carbohydrates and low glycemic index/load decrease levels of specific metabolic syndrome/cardiovascular disease risk factors. Top Clin Nutr. 2008;23:76–96.

24. Harvard School of Public Health Web Site. Available at: http://www.hsph.harvard.edu/nutrition-source/what-should-you-eat/pyramid/. Accessed March 6, 2009.

25. Heidemann C, Schulze MB, Franco OH, et al. Dietary patterns and risk of mortality from cardiovascular disease, cancer, and all causes in a prospective cohort of women. Circulation. 2008; 118:230–237.

26. Howard BV, Van Horn L, Hsia J, et al. Low-fat dietary pattern and risk of cardiovascular disease: the Women's Health Initiative Randomized Controlled Dietary Modification Trial. JAMA. 2006;295:655–666.

27. Hu FB. Dietary pattern analysis: a new direction in nutritional epidemiology. Curr Opin Lipidology. 2002;13(1):3–9.

28. Hu FB, Rimm EB, Stampfer MJ, et al. Prospective study of major dietary patterns and risk of coronary heart disease in men. Am J Clin Nutr. 2000;72:912–921.

29. International Food Information Council Website. Available at: http://www.foodinsight.org/. Accessed February 5, 2009.

30. Iqbal R, Anand S, Ounpuu S, et al. Dietary patterns and risk of acute myocardial infarction in 52 countries: results of the INTERHEART study. Circulation. 2008;118:1929–1937.

31. Jenkins DJA, Josse AR, Wong JMW, et al. The portfolio diet for cardiovascular risk reduction. Curr Atheroscler Rep. 2007;9:501–507.

32. Kandasamy N, Joseph F, Goenka N. The role of omega-3 fatty acids in cardiovascular disease, hypertension, and diabetes mellitus. Br J Diabetes Vasc Dis. 2008;8:121–128.

33. Keys A. Coronary heart disease in seven countries. 1970. Nutrition. 1997;13:250–252.

34. Khaw KT, Wareham N, Bingham S, et al. Combined impact of health behaviours and mortality in men and women: the EPIC Norfolk prospective population study. PLoS Med. 2008:5:e12–e18.

35. King DE, Mainous AG, Geesey ME. Turning back the clock: adopting a healthy lifestyle in middle age. Am J Med. 2007;120:598–603.

36. Knoops KT, de Groot LC, Kromhout D, et al. Mediterranean diet, lifestyle factors, and 10-yr mortality in elderly European men and women. JAMA. 2004;292:1433–1439.

37. Kris-Etherton PM, Harris W, Appel LJ. Fish consumption, fish oil, omega-3 fatty acids, and cardiovascular disease. Circulation. 2002;106:2747–2757.

38. Lee JH, O'Keefe JH, Lavie CJ, et al. Omega-3 fatty acids for cardioprotection. Mayo Clin Proc. 2008;83:324–332.

39. Lichtenstein AH, Appel LJ, Brands M, et al. American Heart Association Diet and Lifestyle Recommendations Revisions 2006. Circulation. 2006;114:82–96.

40. Lopez-Garcia E, Schulze MB, Fung TT, et al. Major dietary patterns are related to plasma concentrations of markers of inflammation and endothelial dysfunction. Am J Clin Nutr. 2004;80:1029–1035.

41. Maruthur NM, Wang NY, Appel LJ. Lifestyle interventions reduce coronary heart disease risk. Circulation. 2009;119:2026–2031.

42. Miller ER, Erlinger TP, Appel LJ. The effects of macronutrients on blood pressure and lipids: an overview of the DASH and OmniHeart Trials. Curr Atheroscler Rep. 2006;8:460–465.

43. Mitrou PN, Kipnis V, Thiebaut ACM, et al. Mediterranean dietary pattern and prediction of all cause mortality in a US population. Arch Intern Med. 2007;167:2461–2468.

44. Nettleton JA, Steffen LM, Mayer-Davis E, et al. Dietary patterns are associated with biochemical

markers of inflammation and endothelial activation in the Multi-Ethnic Study of Atherosclerosis (MESA). Am J Clin Nutr. 2006;83:1369–1379.

45. O'Keefe JH, Gheewala NH, O'Keefe JO. Dietary Strategies for improving post-prandial glucose, lipids, inflammation, and cardiovascular health. J Am Coll Cardiol. 2008;51:249–255.

46. Okinawa Project Website [Internet]. Available at: http://www.okicent.org/index.html. Accessed April 21, 2010.

47. Ornish D, Scherwitz LW, Billings JW, et al. Intensive lifestyle changes for reversal of coronary heart disease. JAMA. 1998;280:2001–2007.

48. Panagiotakos DB, Kokkinos P, Manios Y, et al. Physical activity and markers of inflammation and thrombosis related to coronary heart disease. Atherosclerosis. 2004;176(2):303–310.

49. Pollan M. In Defense of Food. The Penguin Press, USA: 2007. ISBN-13: 9781594201455.

50. Preventive Medicine Research Institute Web Site Available at: www.pmri.org. Accessed December 20, 2008.

51. Pritikin Longevity Center + Spa Website. [Internet]. Available at: www.pritikin.com. Accessed March 15, 2010.

52. Reedy J, Mitrou PN, Krebs-Smith SM, et al. Index-based dietary patterns and risk of colorectal cancer. Am J Epidemiol. 2008;168:38–48.

53. Reeves MJ, Rafferty AP. Healthy lifestyle characteristics among adults in the United States 2000. Arch Intern Med. 2005;165:854–857.

54. Roberts CK, Barnard RJ. Effects of exercise and diet on chronic disease. J Appl Physiol. 2005; 98:3–30.

55. Sacks FM, Svetkey LP, Vollmer WM, et al. Effects on blood pressure of reduced sodium and the Dietary Approaches to Stop Hypertension (DASH). diet. N Engl J Med. 2001;344:3–10.

56. Sass C, Eickhoff-Shemek JM, Manore MM, et al. Crossing the line: understanding the scope of practice between registered dietitians and health/fitness professionals. Health Fit J. 2007;11:12–19.

57. Shai I, Schwarzfuchs D, Henkin Y, et al. Weight loss with a low carbohydrate, Mediterranean, or low fat diet. NEJM. 2008;359:229–241.

58. Singh RB, Dubnov G, Niaz MA. Effect of an Indo-Mediterranean diet on progression of coronary artery disease in high-risk patients: a randomized single-blind trial. Lancet. 2002;360: 1455–1461.

59. Stamler J, Neaton JD. The Multiple Risk Factor Intervention Trial (MRFIT). Importance then and now. JAMA. 2008;300:1343–1345.

60. Stamler J, Wentworth D, Neaton JD. Is the relationship between serum cholesterol and risk of premature death from coronary heart disease continuous and graded: findings in 356,222 primary screenees in the Multiple Risk Factor Intervention Trial (MRFIT). JAMA. 1986;2823–1828.

61. Swain JE, McCarron PB, Hamilton EF, et al. Characteristics of the diet patterns tested in the optimal macronutrient intake trial to prevent heart disease (OmniHeart): options for a heart healthy diet. J Am Diet Assoc. 2008;108:257–265.

62. Trichopoulou A, Orfanos P, de-Bueno NT, et al. Modified Mediterranean diet and survival: epic-elderly prospective cohort study. B M J. 2005;330:991–998.

63. Tuttle KR, Shuler LA, Packard DP, et al. Comparison of low-fat versus Mediterranean-style dietary intervention after first myocardial infarction (from the Heart Institute of Spokane Diet Intervention and Evaluation Trial). Am J Cardiol. 2008;101: 1523–1530.

64. United States Department of Agriculture. Dietary Guidelines for Americans. 2005. Available at: http://www.cnpp.usda.gov/DGAs2005Guidelines.htm. Accessed June 2010.

65. United States Department of Agriculture Web site [Internet]. Washington, DC. Available at: http://fnic.nal.usda.gov/nal_display/index.php?info_center=4&tax_level=3&tax_subject=358&topic_id=1610&level3_id=5947&level4_id=0&level5_id=0&placement_default=0. Accessed April 20, 2010.

66. University of Michigan Integrative Medicine Web Site. Available at: http://www.med.umich.edu/umim/clinical/pyramid/index.htm or http://www.med.umich.edu/umim/. Accessed December 16, 2008.

67. van Dam RM. New approaches to the study of dietary patterns. Br J Nutr. 2005;93:573–574.

68. van Dam RM, Li T, Spiegelman D, et al. Combined impact of lifestyle factors on mortality: prospective cohort study in the US women. B M J. 2008;337:1440–1447.

69. van Dam RM, Rimm EB, Willett WC, et al. Dietary patterns and risk for Type 2 diabetes mellitus in U.S. men. Ann Intern Med. 2002;136:201–209.

70. van Dam RM, Willett WC. Unmet potential for cardiovascular disease prevention in the United States. Circulation. 2009;120:1171–1173.

71. Villegas R, Salim A, Flynn A, et al. Prudent diet and risk of insulin resistance. Nutr Metab Cardiovasc Dis. 2004;14:334–343.

72. Willett W. Nuritional Epidemiology. 2nd Ed. New York, NY: Oxford University Press, 1998.

73. World Cancer Research Fund and the American Institute for Cancer Research. Food Nutrition, Physical Activity, and the Prevention of Cancer: a Global Perspective. Washington DC, AICR, 2007. Available at: www.dietandcancerreport.org/.

74. Yusuf S, Hawken S, Qunpuu S, et al. Effect of potentially modifiable risk factors associated with myocardial infarction in 52 countries (The INTERHEART Study and Control Study). Lancet. 2004;364:937–952.

CHAPTER 5

Atherosclerosis and Other Occlusive Vascular Diseases

ABBREVIATIONS

ACS	Acute coronary syndrome	IL-6	Interleukin 6
ACSM	American College of Sports Medicine	LTPA	Leisure time physical activity
		PA	Physical activity
AHA	American Heart Association	PAD	Peripheral artery disease
CAD	Coronary artery disease	PF	Physical fitness
CRF	Cardiorespiratory fitness	PGC	Perixosome-proliferatory-activated receptor-γ-coactivator
CRP	C-reactive protein		
CVD	Cardiovascular disease	TNF-α	Tumor necrosis factor α
EPCs	Endothelial progenitor cells	VO$_2$max	Maximum oxygen consumption

Chapter 2 discusses some chronic vascular diseases and though this discussion may be repetitive, it is primarily focused on atherosclerosis or coronary artery disease (CAD), which is the major form of cardiovascular disease (CVD). We will touch briefly on other related occlusive vascular diseases. Generally speaking, these are chronic diseases that are pathophysiologically identical. However, there are differences with respect to the anatomic site, signs, symptoms, and limitations, and they may be associated with different functional and activity restrictions.

CAD causes heart attacks, whereas peripheral artery disease (PAD) causes intermittent claudication (see box titled "Intermittent Claudication" on the next page) and other circulatory problems such as carotid artery disease and stroke. CAD is specific to coronary arteries. As such, it is the causative factor in most cases of heart attacks (myocardial infarction) and ultimately most cases of congestive heart failure. It is not directly implicated in some cardiovascular diseases such as valvular disease and structural heart disease and in many cardiac dysrhythmias (see Fig. 5.1).

EPIDEMIOLOGY OF CVD

The American Heart Association (AHA) estimates that more than 80 million adults have some form of CVD (1). Recent reports from the Centers for Disease Control and Prevention indicate that death rates from CVD have decreased by more than 25% since 1999. See Table 5.1 for the prevalence rates of various types of CVD (23). It is projected that these rates will be down almost 35%. The decrease in death rate is lower for women and for African Americans, a disparity that is, perhaps, partially explained by differences in

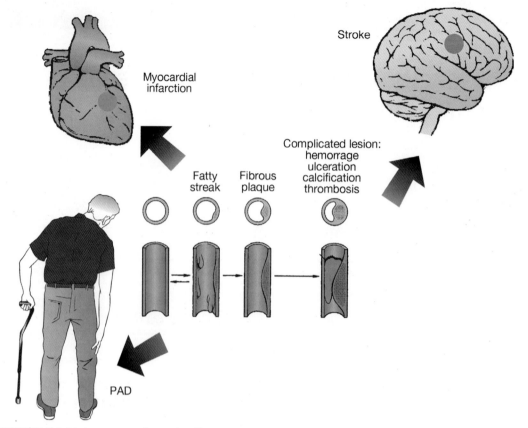

FIGURE 5.1 Various types of vascular disease. PAD, peripheral artery disease.

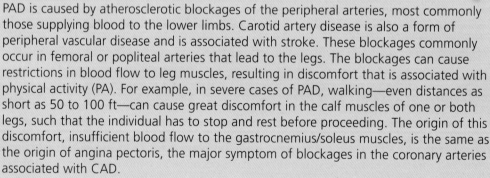

DID YOU KNOW?

Intermittent Claudication

PAD is caused by atherosclerotic blockages of the peripheral arteries, most commonly those supplying blood to the lower limbs. Carotid artery disease is also a form of peripheral vascular disease and is associated with stroke. These blockages commonly occur in femoral or popliteal arteries that lead to the legs. The blockages can cause restrictions in blood flow to leg muscles, resulting in discomfort that is associated with physical activity (PA). For example, in severe cases of PAD, walking—even distances as short as 50 to 100 ft—can cause great discomfort in the calf muscles of one or both legs, such that the individual has to stop and rest before proceeding. The origin of this discomfort, insufficient blood flow to the gastrocnemius/soleus muscles, is the same as the origin of angina pectoris, the major symptom of blockages in the coronary arteries associated with CAD.

This condition (actually a symptom) is called *intermittent claudication*. The term "intermittent" is added because the claudication is not a constant discomfort, like arthritic pain may be, but rather occurs only intermittently, usually during walking.

TABLE 5.1	Prevalence of Various Types of CVD in the United States (23)	
Type of CVD	**Prevalence in Population**	**Important Comments**
High blood pressure (Htn)	Htn: 74.5 million Pre-Htn: 65 million	Defined as follows: • SBP >140 mm Hg or DBP >90 mm Hg • Taking anti-Htn medication • Told by physician
CAD	17,600,000	Clinically diagnosed
Heart attack	8,500,000	1.25 million new and recurrent cases of myocardial infarction each year; almost 50% will die
Angina pectoris (symptomatic CAD)	10,200,000	
Heart failure (CHF)	5,800,000	More than 280,000 with CHF as the cause of death or as an underlying cause of death; CHF is much more prevalent in African Americans than in Caucasian Americans
Stroke	6,400,000	About 795,000 new and recurrent cases of stroke per year; one every 40 seconds
Congenital heart defects	650,000–1,300,000	Usually found and corrected in childhood

CVD, cardiovascular disease; Htn, hypertension; SBP, systolic blood pressure; DBP, diastolic blood pressure; CAD, coronary artery disease; CHF, coronary heart failure.

access to acute cardiac care as well as "usual" health care. Differences in risk factors and susceptibility among these populations may also be responsible (23).

Nearly 2,400 Americans die each day from CVD, and 151,000 individuals younger than 65 die annually from CVD—the equivalent of more than 400 per day. More than 33% of the deaths occur at ages younger than 77.5, the average life expectancy (23). Twenty percent of the deaths in 2005 were from CAD, and in 2010, it is estimated that more than 785,000 people will have first heart attacks and another 470,000 will have a recurrent event (23). The indirect and direct cost of CVD in the United States in 2008 was estimated to be $503 billion. See Figure 5.2 for an illustration of the extent of the problem of CVD in the United States.

PATHOPHYSIOLOGY OF ATHEROSCLEROSIS

Blockages (called plaque) in coronary arteries define CAD, which is the primary cause of heart attack (acute myocardial infarction) and acute coronary syndrome (ACS). This type of vascular disease is also primarily responsible for strokes (cerebrovascular accidents),

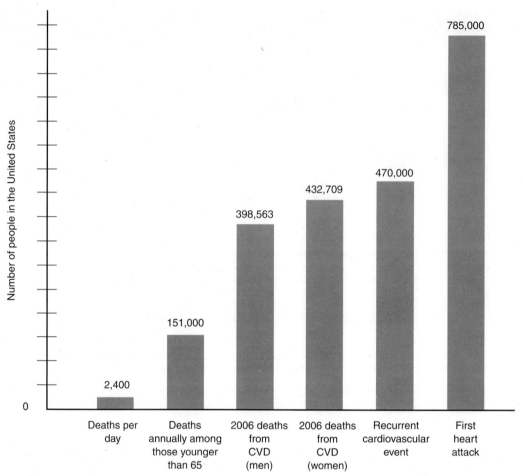

FIGURE 5.2 Cardiovascular disease is the #1 killer of Americans. CVD, cardiovascular disease.

transient ischemic attacks, and intermittent claudication (see box titled "Intermittent Claudication" earlier).

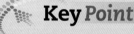

Key Point

Atherosclerosis is in the category of "occlusive vascular disease" and usually refers to blockages within the arteries of the heart. Occlusive vascular disease can occur in almost any artery in the body and often affects the legs (peripheral vascular disease), brain (strokes), kidneys, and other organ systems (see Fig. 5.1).

CAD is a distinct and separate category of CVD. It is an accumulation of various cellular materials including cholesterol, fat, monocytes, fibrous material, smooth muscle, and so forth. This "plaque" collects under the inner lining of the artery (called the endothelium). The atherosclerotic disease process that forms plaque is progressive, meaning that it continues over time (see Fig. 5.3). The plaque may ultimately result in a partial (50%–75% or less in many cases) or sometimes complete (95%–100%) obstruction of the lumen (opening) of the artery. In addition, inflammation and vascular dysfunction are key abnormalities that constitute part of the pathophysiology of CAD and other occlusive vascular diseases (21,22). (For a more complete and

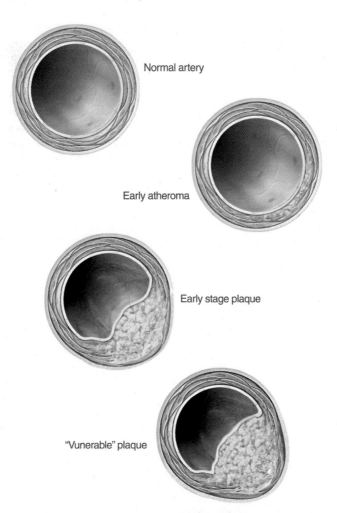

Normal artery

Early atheroma

Early stage plaque

"Vunerable" plaque

FIGURE 5.3 Atherosclerosis involves development and progression of plaque on a continuous basis. Some are small enough that they do not cause either signs (abnormal exercise test results or electrocardiographic changes) or symptoms (angina or other discomfort related to the blockage) and may not restrict blood flow.

detailed description of this disease process, please see Chapter 2, Pathophysiology of Chronic Vascular Disease.)

THE FORMATION OF ATHEROSCLEROTIC PLAQUE

Plaque, as stated earlier, forms within the intima under the endothelium, the inside cellular layer of the artery. The plaque usually begins in childhood as a *fatty streak* (see Figs. 5.3 and 5.4). This fatty streak may be caused by some initial injury to the intima that leads to inflammation or dysfunction of the endothelium. It is uncertain whether the initial injury causes the inflammation and/or dysfunction or whether the inflammation causes the initial injury, with subsequent vascular dysfunction. At the present time, it appears that some initial inflammatory mechanism causes vascular dysfunction and other pathophysiological changes, which allows plaque to develop (2,21).

Atherosclerotic Vascular Disease: Atherosclerosis is defined by the formation of "plaque" under the lining of the vessel, called the endothelium. Blockages in the artery may limit blood flow to distal tissue.

PAD: Blockages may occur in the arteries that supply tissues outside the central organs and brain with oxygen and nutrients. Examples are femoral and popliteal arteries of the leg that supply blood to the leg muscles, as well as the renal arteries that supply blood to the kidneys. PAD is most common in legs and causes "claudication"—discomfort or pain in the muscles with limited blood flow.

CAD: The disease is defined by blockages (plaque) in the walls of arteries that supply oxygen and nutrients to heart muscle (myocardium).

Cerebrovascular Disease: Atherosclerotic disease of the arteries in the head or neck that supply oxygen and nutrients directly to the brain. Most commonly associated with stroke or transient ischemic attack.

> ## Key Point
>
> The initial injury to an artery that ultimately results in the development and progression of atherosclerosis may be related to direct or indirect exposure to environmental influences such as high-fat dietary pattern, tobacco smoke, and sedentary lifestyle at very early ages.

Lifestyle (environmental) factors such as first- or second-hand cigarette smoke, high levels of low-density lipoprotein ("bad cholesterol"), and a high level of saturated and/or trans fat in the diet may cause or be associated with the initial inflammation. Many of the known risk factors for heart disease cause inflammation and endothelial dysfunction (see Figs. 5.5 and 5.6). A positive family history (parents, grandparents, or siblings) predisposes individuals to endothelial dysfunction and, thus, to the formation of fatty streaks (38). However, it has also been shown that a low-risk lifestyle for CAD can significantly decrease the risk associated with a family history of CAD (2).

PLAQUE PROGRESSION

Fatty streaks develop over time to become collections of various types of cells that, if they progress, may eventually narrow and obstruct the artery and restrict blood flow. As plaques progress and grow, they become complex collections of phagocytic cells (containing fat droplets), low-density lipoproteins, smooth muscle cells, white blood cells, scar tissue, calcium, and other substances. Plaques may progress to significant blockages that cause symptoms in months to years (21).

Initially plaque pushes the walls of the artery outward. Therefore, early plaque formation may not restrict blood flow at all and may not be visible with coronary catheterization, even though significant plaque (total plaque burden) is present (see Fig. 5.3). Eventually, as the plaque grows it may partially block the opening of the artery (the lumen) and begin to restrict blood flow. Plaque that has progressed over time eventually

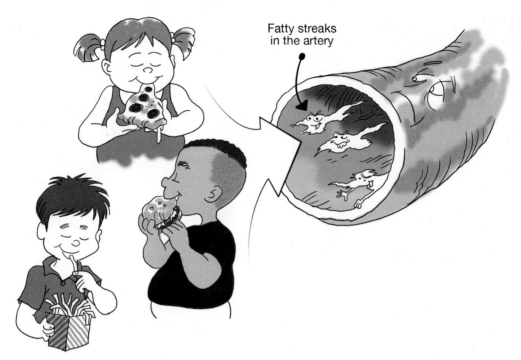

FIGURE 5.4 Exposure to risk factors (health behaviors) at young ages promotes the development and growth of atherosclerotic plaque. The initial stage of plaque development is the fatty streak stage illustrated above.

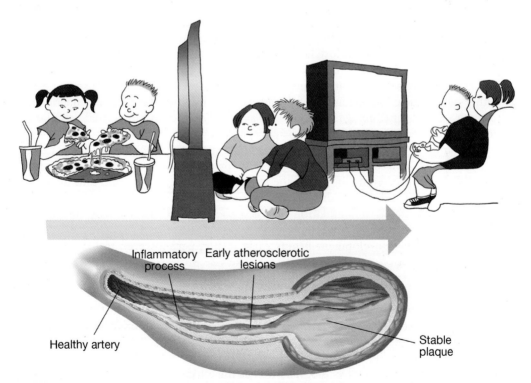

FIGURE 5.5 The progression of atherosclerosis is partially dependent on the lifestyle behaviors that are associated with the risk factors for heart disease.

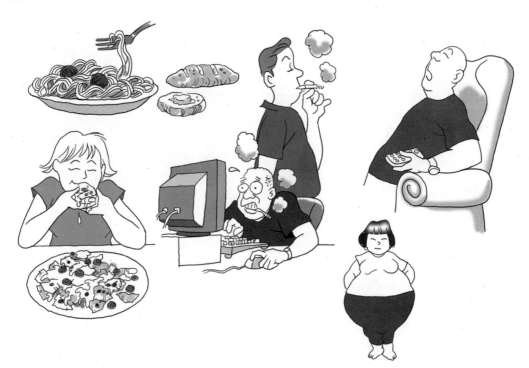

FIGURE 5.6 Lifestyle and risk factors directly influence the development and progression of atherosclerosis.

forms a fibrous cap covering the material inside. This cap, at later stages, may be protective from plaque rupture, the primary event in a heart attack. Newer plaques, however, with a developing, but thin, fibrous cap are more prone to rupture. Almost 75% of cases of plaque rupture (and therefore heart attacks or "acute coronary syndromes") occur in plaques that obstruct the artery less than 50% (see Fig. 5.3) (21,22).

Plaque progression is enhanced, interestingly, by the presence of plaque itself. Substances within the plaque cause the lining of the artery (the endothelium) to be dysfunctional and unstable. A well-functioning endothelium is extremely important to normal vascular function (see Chapter 2). In dysfunctional arteries, inflammatory substances, present during the initiation of plaque growth, enhance and promote further plaque growth. Thus, the problems that cause atherosclerosis to develop also promote the disease process and further contribute to its worsening. If we add the influence of the high trans and saturated fat and other *atherogenic* (substances that cause atherosclerosis) foods, as well as a sedentary lifestyle and the systemic inflammation that is associated with overweight and obesity, it becomes clear that lifestyle is the major culprit in CAD (see Fig. 5.7).

Because plaque development begins early in life, perhaps even in infancy, primary prevention in youth is extremely important. Exercise professionals must be aware of the risk and be familiar with the preventive measures that address not only CAD but all vascular diseases. The role of diet and exercise is especially important in youth, because these are the formative years for health behaviors, as well as the early days of the disease process. Instilling positive health behaviors, that is, "the optimal preventive lifestyle," becomes of paramount importance beginning early in life (see Fig. 5.8).

For more detailed information on the pathophysiology of CAD, please see Chapter 2. Knowing about the pathophysiology, as well as the effects of exercise on that pathophysiology (see Chapter 3), will enable exercise professionals to better address these conditions when working with clients who are affected by CAD and other CVDs. It will also allow

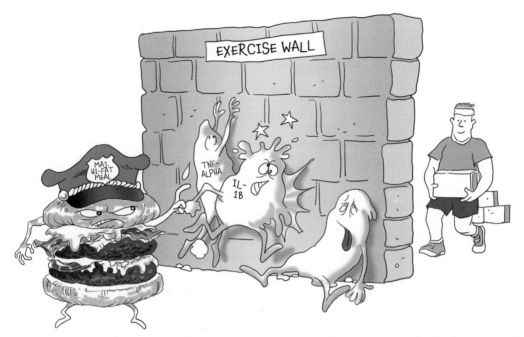

FIGURE 5.7 Positive lifestyle behaviors are anti-inflammatory and help to prevent the development and growth of atherosclerotic plaque.

exercise professionals to understand and translate the beneficial (scientific) effects of exercise to clients.

As we stated in Chapter 1 (Epidemiology and Risk Factors), many of the risk factors for atherosclerosis are modifiable. Table 5.2 summarizes the risk factors for CAD and the optimal levels recommended for preventing this disease.

EXERCISE AND HEART DISEASE

Exercise and physical activity (PA) affect many, if not most, of the pathophysiological conditions that underlie CAD. Chapter 3 addresses the pathophysiology and the effects of exercise in detail, so we will only briefly summarize them here.

EXERCISE AND INFLAMMATION

Inflammation is a primary component of the pathophysiology that causes formation of atherosclerotic plaque in CAD (12). A low-grade systemic inflammation can be demonstrated by the presence of chemical "markers" such as C-reactive protein (CRP) in the blood. In addition to being markers of inflammation, many of these substances are pro-inflammatory (promote inflammation). Anti-inflammatory substances (physiologically and biochemically) are produced by many cells, and exercise facilitates the production and effectiveness of these substances (36). CRP decreases with exercise training regardless of weight loss or other changes in risk factors associated with elevated CRP (such as diabetes and obesity) (9,34,36).

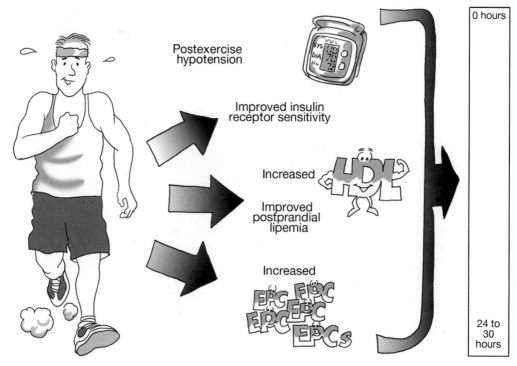

FIGURE 5.8 There are many subacute and chronic benefits to regular exercise that promote prevention of atherosclerosis and other chronic disease. EPCs, endothelial progenitor cells; HDL, high-density lipoprotein.

However, either high-intensity or long-duration exercise (or a combination of both) causes acute increases in inflammatory markers, such as CRP. These changes are *transient* or temporary and are unlikely to have any long-term effects that promote chronic disease processes (36). Appropriate prescription of intensity and duration of exercise can avoid harmful, though temporary, inflammatory effects, as can increased fitness level (6,9,36). We urge caution in prescribing intense exercise in individuals with CAD or other chronic diseases that are associated with this systemic inflammation. Note also that the beneficial, anti-inflammatory effects of exercise occur subsequent to each exercise session and are relatively temporary; thus they are "subacute" (see Chapter 3) (9,36).

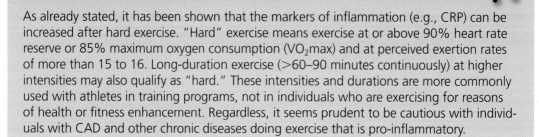

DID YOU KNOW?
Hard Exercise and Inflammation

As already stated, it has been shown that the markers of inflammation (e.g., CRP) can be increased after hard exercise. "Hard" exercise means exercise at or above 90% heart rate reserve or 85% maximum oxygen consumption (VO_2max) and at perceived exertion rates of more than 15 to 16. Long-duration exercise (>60–90 minutes continuously) at higher intensities may also qualify as "hard." These intensities and durations are more commonly used with athletes in training programs, not in individuals who are exercising for reasons of health or fitness enhancement. Regardless, it seems prudent to be cautious with individuals with CAD and other chronic diseases doing exercise that is pro-inflammatory.

TABLE 5.2	Summary of Specific Optimal Risk Factor Recommendations for Prevention of CAD
Risk Factor	**Recommendation**
Smoking	Complete cessation of all tobacco use and exposure
Obesity	• Isocaloric diet if BMI is <25.0 • Hypocaloric diet if BMI is >25.0 or waist circumference is >40 inches for men and >35 inches for women
Exercise and physical activity	• Weekly caloric expenditure of ≥2,000 kcal in exercise and high levels of physical activity • 2 d/wk high-intensity exercise (>75% HRR or VO$_2$R) • Resistance training 2–3 d/wk
Hypertension	• BP <120/80 mm Hg • Sodium intake <1,600 mg/d
Lipids	• All lipids at ATP III goals
Diet	• Fat = 15%–25% of total calories • Sat fat <5% • MUFA = 5%–12% • PUFA = 5%–10% (omega-3 fatty acids) • Cholesterol <150 mg/d • Fiber intake = >30 g/d • Include functional foods, e.g., stanols and increased soluble fiber • Omega-3 intake = 1 g/d (EPA, DHA) in addition to 1 g/d of ALA
Stress	• Acquire and practice some kind of stress management skill 5–7 d/wk • Therapy and counseling as indicated and required • Remain socially connected, avoid isolation • Control anger, hostility
Emerging risk factors	• Assess hsCRP, Lp(a), and Hcy in premature CAD, or in high-risk individuals with >2 RFs • Recommend daily multiple vitamin tablet; consider vitamin D supplementation

Adapted with permission from Roitman JL, LaFontaine TP. Efficacy of secondary prevention and risk factor reduction. In: *AACVPR Cardiac Rehabilitation Resource Manual*, by the American Association of Cardiovascular and Pulmonary Rehabilitation. Champaign, IL: Human Kinetics, 2006.

BMI, body mass index; HRR, heart rate reserve; VO$_2$R, oxygen uptake reserve; ATP, adenosine triphosphate; EPA, eicosapentaenoic acid; DHA, docosahexaenoic acid; ALA alpha-linoleic acid; hsCRP, high-sensitivity c-reactive protein; Lp(a), lipoprotein a; Hcy, homocysteine; CAD, coronary artery disease; RF, risk factor.

EXERCISE AND ENDOTHELIAL PROGENITOR CELLS

EPCs have been discussed previously in both Chapters 2 and 3, but the topic is reviewed briefly here. EPCs are actually "stem cells" that are produced in the bone marrow, and they promote the growth and repair of the endothelium when it is not functioning properly or when it is damaged (40).

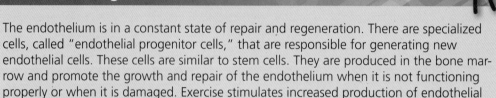

DID YOU KNOW?
Endothelial Progenitor Cells

The endothelium is in a constant state of repair and regeneration. There are specialized cells, called "endothelial progenitor cells," that are responsible for generating new endothelial cells. These cells are similar to stem cells. They are produced in the bone marrow and promote the growth and repair of the endothelium when it is not functioning properly or when it is damaged. Exercise stimulates increased production of endothelial progenitor cells (EPCs).

Exercise promotes the production and release of EPCs. These cells are active in repairing the endothelium when it becomes dysfunctional under the influence of inflammatory conditions or in the presence of traditional risk factors such as smoking, high dietary fat intake, and hypertension. The endothelium is continually trying to "repair" itself, or to improve its functional status. EPCs are critical to the repair process. In addition to promoting endothelial repair, exercise helps to "stabilize" the endothelium by enhancing the nitric oxide system. The nitric oxide system is another critical component of normal endothelial function (17,44).

A final important fact is that the stimulation of EPCs, as well as the improvement in endothelial function, is a subacute effect of exercise. It occurs subsequent to individual bouts of exercise and though it may also improve chronically, each single exercise bout improves endothelial function and stimulates the production of EPCs (17,18,39,44). The importance of this is that daily exercise and PA are crucial to obtaining many of the beneficial effects of an active lifestyle and a regular exercise program. Optimally, exercise and PA, including leisure time physical activity (LTPA), should be performed every day for the best health and quality-of-life outcomes, as well as for optimal prevention of chronic disease.

DID YOU KNOW?
Nitric Oxide: The "Ultimate" Vasodilator

We discussed nitric oxide in Chapter 2. It is a substance that is released from the intima of arteries, which causes arterial dilation. This is especially important to normal vascular function, since arteries need to expand when increased blood supply is required, for example, for increased activity, or even digestion of food. If an artery is not functioning properly because of inflammation, nitric oxide will not be released normally and the vessel does not expand appropriately in response to increased metabolic demands. In fact, it has been demonstrated that dysfunctional arteries (especially coronary arteries) may constrict rather than expand when conditions require more blood flow.

EXERCISE AND HEART DISEASE

A lengthy, detailed discussion of the effects of exercise on the pathophysiology and the risk factors for heart disease can be found in Chapter 3. It is clear that exercise has positive effects on nearly all of the modifiable risk factors. These benefits come from both chronic (long-term) and subacute effects of exercise.

In this section, the discussion is focused on exercise, PA, and their effects on the risk for heart disease—more specifically, how exercise can affect both primary and secondary prevention of atherosclerosis and the optimal exercise program for preventing new and recurrent atherosclerosis-related events. Preventing disease or risk factors in people who do not yet have a clinical diagnosis (or signs and symptoms) is called *primary prevention*. Preventing recurrent events and/or death in people who already have the disease is called *secondary prevention*.

There are several ways to approach this issue. We will first discuss physical inactivity and PA (also see "Digging Deeper" discussion in Chapter 3). Then we will focus on physical fitness (PF) and increases in fitness.

INACTIVITY AND ACTIVITY

Dr. Jeremy Morris and Dr. Ralph Paffenbarger were two of the pioneer researchers in the field of epidemiology of exercise. Initially, they investigated occupational activity and its relationship with chronic disease and mortality. Morris (26) studied busmen in London, England. Ticket takers (conductors) were very active walking up and down the aisles and stairs of the double-decker buses all day, whereas drivers were more sedentary, since they spent most of their day sitting. Paffenbarger studied longshoremen who worked in several job classes ranging from sedentary to very active (31). Both researchers found that those in the most active jobs had the lowest death rates from heart and other vascular disease. In fact, Paffenbarger also reported that those who changed from more active to less active jobs as they were "promoted" increased their risk of death from CAD (31).

Later, Dr. Henry Taylor (41) studied railroad men and demonstrated a "dose–response" effect between active and sedentary jobs and mortality. A "dose–response" effect means that as the amount of exercise increased (frequency, duration, and intensity combined), the protective effect of exercise increased. Compared with the least active group, the most active group had the lowest death rate (2.0 times lower), while the moderately active group had a death rate that was 1.5 times lower. The most sedentary group had a death rate more than 100% higher than that of the least active group (41). Later, Paffenbarger also studied a large group of college alumni and demonstrated a similar dose–response effect (31,33).

So far, the information that we have discussed shows that more active people are less likely to die of heart attack or other CVDs. In addition, we know that if we compare levels of activity, increasing volume of PA leads to increased protection from CAD (31,32). Thus, it is clear that increased PA is inversely associated with CAD and death from heart attack. It is also clear that decreasing one's level of job-related or leisure time activity is associated with increased death from heart disease and stroke. Similarly, this has been shown to be true with exercise and other types of chronic disease (4,13).

Dr. Steven Blair and his colleagues using data from the Aerobics Center Longitudinal Study have contributed another important piece of information to the question of PA, cardiorespiratory fitness (CRF), and the risk of heart disease. Up to this point, we have not discussed research showing that increasing the fitness level decreases the chances of death from CAD. Chapter 3 contains a detailed discussion of CRF, PA, and mortality. The previous discussion involved occupational PA or LTPA and their association with CAD. Blair and his colleagues showed that men who improve measured fitness level (metabolic equivalents on a standard treadmill test) decrease their risk of death from CAD by almost 50% (3,4). In fact, one of Blair's most interesting findings is that men who raised their fitness level by a small amount (moving from the lowest to the next lowest level of fitness reduced risk by 44%) received the greatest proportional benefit (4,24).

Women were underrepresented in earlier studies, but they have been included in more recent research. Their results are similar to men. Increased levels of PA, as well as increased levels of CRF, decrease the chances of having CAD as well as dying from the disease (19,20,24). There is another interesting piece of information that fits into this puzzle. Men who have a high maximum oxygen consumption but who are not physically active do not obtain the equivalent "protective" effect. When CRF and PA are combined the protective effect becomes more prominent with increased CRF and PA (14).

Recently, a group of researchers published a meta-analysis (see box titled "Meta-Analyses" below) with more than 880,000 people on PA and the risk of death from heart disease, as well as from all causes. This study confirmed that "activity" (unfortunately, they did not distinguish between CRF and PA) was associated with a 33% and a 35% reduction in death from all causes and heart disease, respectively (28). Consistent with other research, they also concluded that studies that *measured* the CRF level demonstrated that this variable is an even more powerful predictor in studies in which it was measured than in those studies that did not measure it (3,27). This result has been confirmed by other researchers and by statements from national organizations, such as the American College of Sports Medicine (ACSM) and AHA (13).

Finally, many of these studies statistically adjust for the other risk factors such as smoking, cholesterol, and blood pressure. Although this statistical adjustment results in a slight decrease in the *protective power* of PA and CRF, it does not affect the overall relationship. Thus we can conclude that PA and CRF are directly associated with protection from CAD (13,28). See Chapter 3 for a complete discussion of PA versus PF and protection from CAD.

Another study assessed various risk factors for CAD and their association with the amount of weekly exercise (expressed as caloric expenditure) in women (25). The study authors

DID YOU KNOW?
Meta-Analyses

A meta-analysis is a specific type of research that combines several studies in order to increase the statistical power of the analysis. Meta-analyses have become increasingly common in epidemiological research so that more and more subjects can be included in the data on particular topics, such as PF, PA, and heart disease. There is even one prestigious journal that solicits and publishes these meta-analyses for many topics in science and medicine. *The Cochrane Reviews* can be found at www.cochrane.org/reviews/.

It is necessary to use some caution when reading and using these types of study to interpret relationships such as exercise and chronic disease. One major problem is that the authors of a meta-analysis can choose to include (or remove) any study or group of studies based on research criteria that they select. The best of this type of research is strict with the criteria used to either include or eliminate particular studies. Once strict inclusion criteria have been selected, the results can be very powerful and may also be biased by those criteria.

combined risk factors and exercise (using statistical analysis) in an attempt to determine the mechanism through which exercise lowers the risk for heart attack. They concluded that the most powerful effects were on the risk factors associated with inflammation and clotting of blood. The next most powerful effects were on blood pressure. Thus, this study confirms the effects of PA on mortality and attempts to clarify the source of these effects (25).

As we have previously stated, it is known that exercise is protective for those who already have atherosclerosis. Several studies and meta-analyses investigating participation in Cardiac Rehabilitation have been performed. These studies indicate that patients who undergo Cardiac Rehabilitation reduce their death rates from heart attack and all-cause death by 31% and 27%, respectively (15,30). We should add that these reductions in death rates seem to be partially related to the exercise that is central to these programs but that changes in risk factors (e.g., lipids, blood pressure, and even pharmaceutical preventive measures—aspirin, statins) could also have a significant impact on this reduction (29,42).

How Much Exercise Is Optimal?

There is some relative agreement about how much exercise is required to obtain this protective effect. Generally, it is agreed that 2,000 kcal/week or more in excess energy expenditure (above daily resting) is required for the protective effect (10,20,32). However, there is some disagreement about whether PA or CRF is the most important factor. (See Chapter 3 for a more detailed discussion of PA versus PF and protection from heart and other chronic disease.)

This does not really tell us much about how much exercise is optimal, other than the total amount of calories that we need to burn every week. Exercise must be prescribed in terms of frequency (sessions per week), intensity, time (duration per session), and type so that people can easily understand exactly what they need to do. Once again, the research allows us be somewhat more precise about the amount of exercise that is required for a protective effect in individuals with atherosclerosis, although there is not total agreement among experts.

It must be specified that both CRF and PA are important to optimal prevention of atherosclerosis. Although it is possible, for example, to obtain the entire 2,000 kcal that seem to be required through exercise alone, we believe that the optimal program to maintain the benefits that are accrued from exercise must also include high amounts of PA (LTPA) every day (13). In this case, PA above a "sedentary" level (sitting or lying, for example) may prolong the beneficial, subacute changes that accrue from each exercise session. LTPA may also contribute to metabolic effects (enhanced glucose and fat metabolism), and it certainly expends more calories than remaining sedentary. The logical conclusion, as stated above, is that high amounts of PA combined with regular cardiorespiratory endurance exercise is optimal.

> **Key Point**
>
> A weekly caloric expenditure in PA and exercise exceeding 2,000 kcal is generally accepted as the level required for prevention of heart (and other chronic) disease.

Frequency

This may be the easiest of the four factors to prescribe. The ACSM statement (as well as most others) specifies that 30 minutes of exercise should be done *every day or almost every day*. Although this is not sufficiently precise for our purposes, it does serve as a good guide. Daily exercise and activity is optimal for a number of reasons.

Perhaps the most important reason is that many of the most important and preventive benefits of exercise accrue from each exercise session (subacute benefits). Such subacute benefits of exercise as positive changes in inflammation, lipids and postprandial lipemia, insulin sensitivity, and blood pressure are just a few of them. (See Chapter 3 for a more detailed discussion of these changes.) Because many of these benefits last less than 12 to 24 hours, daily exercise and activity are important to maintaining them.

DURATION

The total volume of exercise required (weekly caloric expenditure) is approximately 2,000 kcal/week. The duration of exercise required to expend 2,000 kcal is approximately 4 to 6 hours per week for most individuals, depending on the intensity of the exercise and the weight of the individual. Therefore, the 30 minutes of "almost daily" exercise and activity that is recommended in the ACSM/AHA guidelines would be insufficient for most people to expend the required 2,000 calories (43). Rather, it would require a range of 35 to 55 minutes on most days of the week for most persons to reach the 2,000 kcal per week goal. Thus, our recommendation is 45 to 60 minutes of exercise per day along with high daily levels of LTPA, for example, 8,000–12,000 steps per day, not including structured exercise.

INTENSITY

The appropriate intensity of exercise depends on the purpose or intended outcome. In Table 5.3 (and in Chapter 3), we categorize exercise into CRF exercise and light-to-moderate exercise. The intensity of each of these types of exercise differs. CRF exercise is performed between 60% and 85% oxygen uptake reserve, by definition and standard guidelines (43). This is the type of exercise that is most effective to raise the CRF level. Light-to-moderate exercise, by definition, is lighter, less intense exercise (40%–60% VO_2R or heart rate reserve). While these may be effective in increasing the fitness level and producing health benefits, a daily dose of CRF exercise is likely to be associated with more frequent exercise-related overuse injuries. Most individuals prefer and respond better to a mix of higher (no more than every other day) and more moderate-intensity exercise.

TYPE

The type of exercise for CRF exercise is described as large muscle group, repetitive exercise that can be performed for periods of time ranging from 10 to 60 minutes continuously or more. The purpose of using this type of exercise for CRF is to increase physiological demands on the cardiovascular and musculoskeletal systems sufficiently to raise the heart rate, blood pressure, blood flow, and associated energy metabolism so that a relative "overload" on the system produces adaptation. The sum of this adaptation is increased CRF.

Table 5.3 describes the optimal exercise prescription for primary and secondary prevention of atherosclerosis. Prescribing exercise (for anyone) requires some flexibility in addressing these factors. Changing one (e.g., duration) may require adjustment in another. For example, increasing duration past 60 minutes for, say, a long bike ride usually necessitates

TABLE 5.3	Optimal Exercise Prescription for Disease Prevention
Frequency	
CRF exercise	3–4 d/wk
Resistance exercise	2–3 d/wk
LMEx/	3–4 d/wk (opposite cardiorespiratory endurance exercise)
LTPA	many times during every day
Duration	
CRF exercise	minimum of 30 minutes of continuous exercise
LMEx/LTPA	minimum of 30 minutes
Intensity	
CRF exercise	60%–85% VO_2R (HRR)
LMEx/LTPA	40%–70% VO_2R (HRR)
Mode	
CRF exercise	Repetitive, large muscle group exercise, e.g., walking, jogging, and swimming
LMEx/LTPA	Any other activity including team sports, recreational activities, job-related or household activities are in this category

LMEx, Light-to-moderate exercise; LTPA, leisure time physical activity; CRF, cardiorespiratory fitness; VO_2R, oxygen uptake reserve; HRR, heart rate reserve.

decreasing intensity so that the entire 60 minutes can be completed. This is generally true for the variables in an exercise prescription and adjustments across several may be necessary to accommodate individual differences.

DIGGING DEEPER

Exercise and Inflammation

The inflammatory process involves production of many substances produced in most cells of the body. These substances are regulatory, some are proinflammatory or anti-inflammatory, and some are both (5,9,34,35). The balance of inflammation is maintained very closely in a highly complex system. The genomic expression of substances that maintain and support that balance makes a complete understanding even more daunting. Entire books are dedicated to this topic and we cannot do justice to it in this brief summary. Rather, this is an attempt to explain some of the research demonstrating the inflammatory and the anti-inflammatory effects of exercise as they relate to the protective effect of PF and PA.

The connection between low-level systemic inflammation and pathophysiology of chronic disease is well established (5). We have discussed it in detail in Chapter 2 and earlier in the explanation of the development and progression of atherosclerosis. The connection

(continued)

between the lifestyle (risk factors) and the pathophysiology of the atherosclerotic process is also well documented and has been previously discussed. Finally, we have also briefly discussed the protective, as well as the mediating, effects of exercise and PA on chronic disease in Chapter 3. All of these connecting lines are well established.

In an attempt to enhance understanding of this topic, this discussion will focus on three important substances and the mechanisms involved in inflammation. These substances are interleukin (IL) 6, perixosome-proliferatory-activated receptor-γ-coactivator (PGC) 1α, and tumor necrosis factor (TNF) α. These substances have common characteristics and functions that will allow simplification of this discussion, but because of the extreme complexity of this topic, it is neither close to being fully understood nor sorted out by researchers. The box titled "Inflammatory Substances and Their Function" on this page defines each of these components. Later, we will also be required to introduce other substances that are critical components of the discussion of exercise as an anti-inflammatory behavior.

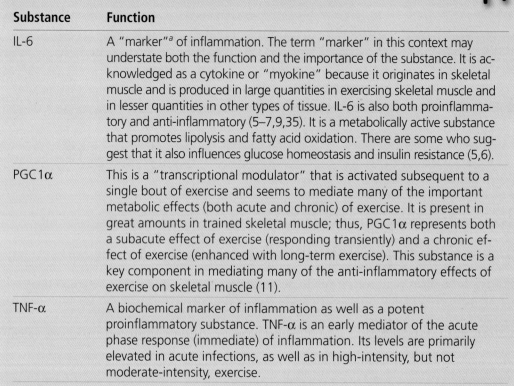

DID YOU KNOW?

Inflammatory Substances and Their Function

Substance	Function
IL-6	A "marker"[a] of inflammation. The term "marker" in this context may understate both the function and the importance of the substance. It is acknowledged as a cytokine or "myokine" because it originates in skeletal muscle and is produced in large quantities in exercising skeletal muscle and in lesser quantities in other types of tissue. IL-6 is also both proinflammatory and anti-inflammatory (5–7,9,35). It is a metabolically active substance that promotes lipolysis and fatty acid oxidation. There are some who suggest that it also influences glucose homeostasis and insulin resistance (5,6).
PGC1α	This is a "transcriptional modulator" that is activated subsequent to a single bout of exercise and seems to mediate many of the important metabolic effects (both acute and chronic) of exercise. It is present in great amounts in trained skeletal muscle; thus, PGC1α represents both a subacute effect of exercise (responding transiently) and a chronic effect of exercise (enhanced with long-term exercise). This substance is a key component in mediating many of the anti-inflammatory effects of exercise on skeletal muscle (11).
TNF-α	A biochemical marker of inflammation as well as a potent proinflammatory substance. TNF-α is an early mediator of the acute phase response (immediate) of inflammation. Its levels are primarily elevated in acute infections, as well as in high-intensity, but not moderate-intensity, exercise.

IL-6, interleukin 6; PGC1α, perixosome-proliferatory-activated receptor-α-coactivator; TNF-α, tumor necrosis factor α.

[a]A "marker" for inflammation is a substance in the blood (or other tissue) that can be measured and is associated with an inflammatory response.

IL-6 is produced in large amounts during and subsequent to single bouts of both moderate and vigorous exercise (7,45). Chronically increased levels of IL-6 have been shown to be related to some cancers and are predictive of obesity and type 2 diabetes (7,11). Coupled with increased c-reactive protein (CRP—another "marker" of inflammation) it has been shown to be predictive of morbidity (5,8). Thus, it may be proinflammatory.

However, IL-6 also has significant and important anti-inflammatory effects (5). It inhibits the production of TNF-α, stimulates the adreno–pituitary axis (the home of the immune response in the central nervous system and endocrine systems), and stimulates production of several other anti-inflammatory cytokines (e.g., IL-10 and IL-1Ra). It appears that, in this context, IL-6 may well be one of the primary *anti-inflammatory* substances that are connected with the protective effect of moderate exercise (5,9,11,35). In moderate exercise, IL-6 is produced in large amounts in skeletal muscle (it is a "myokine") and is circulated in the blood. The amount of IL-6 produced is proportionate to the intensity, duration, and frequency of the exercise and is not limited (as was previously thought) to eccentric contractions (7). Rather, it is produced with concentric contractions of moderate force prevalent in cardiovascular endurance exercise (5).

TNF-α is a cytokine that mediates the immune response by initiating the acute inflammatory phase (21). Its levels are elevated in chronic infections such as those caused by Chlamydia, upper respiratory tract infection, and dental infection. Increased circulating levels of TNF-α are associated with obesity (weight loss reverses the elevation) and insulin resistance. It is also associated with dysfunction of the renin–angiotensin system in hypertension and thus is implicated in the inflammation that accompanies that chronic disease (5,6). Finally, it is associated with the stimulation and production of vascular adhesion molecules that are prominent in promoting the atherosclerotic process (12,21). TNF-α levels are elevated after high-intensity exercise, but not after moderate- or low-intensity exercise (9,16,45). Thus, elevation in levels of TNF-α demonstrates an inflammatory response to exercise.

Finally, PGC1α is one of the most important substances relative to the anti-inflammatory effects of exercise. PGC1α is a "transcriptional" activator that drives the production of substances in skeletal muscle related to energy metabolism, specifically aerobic metabolism in the case of this substance. It is generated by a single bout of exercise (cardiovascular endurance) and seems to regulate metabolic activity in skeletal muscle during exercise and chronically increases the metabolic capabilities of regularly exercised skeletal muscle. PGC1α is, therefore, also increased in chronically exercised skeletal muscle and is present in increased quantities in muscle tissue of trained individuals. It is associated with and has been demonstrated to mediate many of the enhanced metabolic capacities of endurance-trained skeletal muscle.

Muscle cells produce inflammatory myokines that are actively suppressed by increased quantities of PGC1α (11). Thus, an intensified inflammatory response may be moderated by the PGC1α associated with endurance exercise. Conversely, a sedentary lifestyle decreases the amount of PGC1α in skeletal muscle, further promoting the low-level systemic inflammation. One final note is that PGC1α appears to be protective against muscle atrophy (wasting) that is found in various chronic diseases, as well as the frailty associated with inactivity and aging (11).

In summary, high-intensity exercise associated with inflammation is associated with increased levels of TNF-α. IL-6 is produced in large amounts in moderate exercise and inhibits TNF-α as well as engages the adreno–pituitary axis, thus moderating inflammation. The mediator of the process may well be PGC1α, which activates the transcription of genes that are anti-inflammatory and protective of muscle mass. Therefore, regular, daily exercise can protect from inflammation and decrease levels of inflammatory substances.

Significant RESEARCH

Two important articles fit this category for the topic of atherosclerosis. Both are by the same author, Dr. Peter Libby who is an excellent scientific writer (as well as researcher). The first is a very important review/topical article from *Scientific American* that may have been the first to outline the mechanisms of inflammation as a primary and, perhaps, causative factor in atherosclerosis. Dr. Peter Libby wrote this article in 2002 based on more than 15 years of research leading to the conclusion that a low-level systemic inflammatory process is formative and primary in the atherosclerotic process.

The Physiology of Atherosclerosis

Libby P. Atherosclerosis: the new view. Sci Am. 2002;286:47–53.

Libby's article traces the history of the atherosclerotic process from the mistaken belief that fat builds up directly on the walls of coronary arteries ultimately leading to a heart attack, to the accepted and much more physiologically accurate construct about the development of atherosclerosis. He describes the endothelium as a living and functioning layer of cells (an "organ"), rather than the inert lining of a tube; the presence of cytokines and other substances that drive the formation of plaque from inside and outside the intima; and the inflammatory process as a driving factor in the whole atherogenic process. Finally, he describes the importance of inflammation on plaque stability, the precipitating factor in almost all heart attacks. This is an article that explains the process of atherogenesis in an understandable and clear way.

The Physiology and Biochemistry of Inflammation

Libby P, Ridker P, Hansson GK. Inflammation in atherosclerosis: from pathophysiology to practice. J Am Coll Cardiol. 2009;54(23):2129–2138.

The first of these two articles is really a seminal article in the literature. Dr. Libby summarizes literature that had been reported for a number of years into a readable and understandable explanation of the physiology and anatomy of the development (atherogenesis) and progression of atherosclerotic plaque. The material can be challenging at times, but articles in *Scientific American* are aimed at informed readers of science, not necessarily experts in a given field. This article puts into perspective what was known about this topic in the early part of the 2000s. It is an excellent summary that guides the reader through the process with some depth, but with enough simplicity and clarity to make it suitable for most who will expend some effort to understand.

The second and more recent article provides an update to the process of inflammation and atherosclerosis. Dr. Libby outlines the native and adaptive inflammatory processes, their role in atherogenesis, and the complexity of the role of inflammation markers. This is, as mentioned above, a transformative article for understanding the process of inflammation, atherosclerosis, and the protective role of exercise and PA.

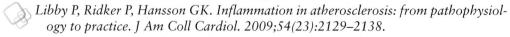

SUMMARY

Atherosclerosis is an occlusive vascular disease that can affect most arteries. It is related to inflammation, and, in fact, it may be initiated by the inflammatory response to environmental factors (often called "risk factors") such as dietary, saturated, and/or trans fat or exposure to tobacco smoke. These factors may cause the genetic expression of the pathophysiology that causes the initiation of arterial plaque. It is clear that the disease process may be interrupted and reversed with optimal lifestyle behaviors including healthy diet and daily PA and exercise.

REFERENCES

1. American Heart Association Web Site [Internet]. Dallas, TX: American Heart Association. Available at: http://www.americanheart.org/presenter.jhtml?identifier=1200026. Accessed July 15, 2008.
2. Berenson GS, Wattigney WA, Tracy RE, et al. Atherosclerosis of the aorta and coronary arteries and cardiovascular risk factors in persons aged 6 to 30 years and studied at necropsy (The Bogalusa Heart Study). Am J Cardiol. 1992;70: 851–858.
3. Blair SN, Cheng Y, Holder JS. Is physical activity or physical fitness more important in defining health benefits? Med Sci Sports Exerc. 2001;33(6, Suppl):s379–s399.
4. Blair SN, Kohl HW, Barlow RS, et al. Changes in physical fitness and all-cause mortality: a prospective study of healthy and unhealthy men. JAMA. 1995;273:1093–1098.
5. Bruunsgaard H. Physical activity and modulation of systemic low-level inflammation. J Leukoc Biol. 2005;78:819–835.
6. Edwards KM, Ziegler MG, Mills PJ. The potential anti-inflammatory benefits of improving physical fitness in hypertension. J Hypertens. 2007;25 (8):1533–1542.
7. Febbraio MA, Pedersen BK. Muscle-derived interleukin-6: mechanisms for activation and possible biological roles. FASEB J. 2002;16:1335–1347.
8. Ford ES. Does exercise reduce inflammation? Physical activity and C-reactive protein among U.S. adults. Minerva Endocrinol. 2002;27(3): 209–214.
9. Gleeson M. Immune function in sport and exercise. J Appl Physiol. 2007;103(2):693–699.
10. Hambrecht R, Niebauer J, Marburger C, et al. Various intensities of leisure time physical activity in patients with coronary artery disease: effects on cardiorespiratory fitness and progression of coronary atherosclerotic lesions. J Am Coll Cardiol. 1993;22:468–477.
11. Handschin C, Spiefelman BM. The role of exercise and PGC1a in inflammation and chronic disease. Nature. 2008;454(24):463–469.
12. Hansson GK. Inflammation, atherosclerosis and coronary artery disease. N Engl J Med. 2005;352: 1685–1695.
13. Haskell WL, Lee IM, Pate RR, et al. Physical activity and public health: updated recommendation for adults from the American College of Sports Medicine and the American Heart Association. Med Sci Sports Exerc. 2007;39(8):1423–1434.

14. Hein HO, Suadicani P, Gyntelberg F. Physical fitness or physical activity as a predictor of ischaemic heart disease? A 17-year follow-up in the Copenhagen Male Study. J Int Med. 1992;232(6): 471–479.
15. Jolliffe J, Rees K, Taylor RRS, et al. Exercise-based rehabilitation for coronary heart disease. Cochrane Database Syst Rev. 2001;(1):CD001800. DOI: 10.1002/14651858.CD001800.
16. Kasapis C, Thompson PD. The effects of physical activity on serum C-reactive protein and inflammatory markers. J Am Coll Cardiol. 2005;45(10): 1563–1569.
17. Laufs U, Werner N, Link A, et al. Physical training increases endothelial progenitor cells, inhibits neointima formation, and enhances angiogenesis. Circulation. 2004;109:220–226.
18. Laughlin HM. Physical activity in prevention and treatment of coronary disease: the battle line is in exercise vascular cell biology. Med Sci Sports Exerc. 2004;36(3):352–362.
19. Lee IM, Rexrode KM, Cook NR, et al. Physical activity and coronary heart disease in women: is "no pain, no gain" passe? JAMA. 2001;285(11): 1447–1454.
20. Lee IM, Skerrett PJ. Physical activity and all-cause mortality: what is the dose-response relation? Med Sci Sports Exerc. 2001;33:S459–S471.
21. Libby P. Atherosclerosis: the new view. Sci Am. 2002;286:47–53.
22. Libby P, Ridker P, Hansson GK. Inflammation in atherosclerosis: from pathophysiology to practice. J Am Coll Cardiol. 2009;54(23):2129–2138.
23. Lloyd-Jones D, Adams RJ, Brown TM, et al. Heart disease and stroke statistics—2010 update: a report from the American Heart Association. AHA Statistical Update. Circulation. 2010;121(7):e46–e215.
24. Manson JE, Greenland P, LaCroix AZ, et al. Walking compared with vigorous exercise for the prevention of cardiovascular events in women. N Engl J Med. 2002;347:716–725.
25. Mora S, Cook N, Buring JE, et al. Physical activity and reduced risk of cardiovascular events: potential mediating mechanisms. Circulation. 2007;116(19): 2110–2118.
26. Morris JN, Kagan A, Pattison DC, et al. Incidence and prediction of ischaemic heart disease in London busmen. Lancet. 1966;2:553–559.
27. Myers J, Kaykha A, George S, et al. Fitness versus physical activity patterns in predicting mortality in men. Am J Med. 2004;117:912–918.

28. Nocon M, Hiemann T, Muller-Riemenschneider F, et al. Association of physical activity with all-cause and cardiovascular mortality: a systematic review and meta-analysis. Eur J Cardiovasc Prev Rehabil. 2008;15(3):239–246.

29. O'Connor GT, Buring JE, Usuf S, et al. An overview of randomized trials of rehabilitation with exercise after myocardial infarction. Circulation. 1989;80:234–244.

30. Oldridge NB, Guyatt GH, Fisher ME, et al. Cardiac rehabilitation after myocardial infarction: combined experience of randomized clinical trials. JAMA. 1988;260:945–950.

31. Paffenbarger RSJ, Laughlin ME, Gima AS, et al. Work activity of longshoremen as related to death from coronary heart disease and stroke. N Engl J Med. 1970;282:1109–1114.

32. Paffenbarger RSJ, Lee IM. A natural history of athleticism, health and longevity. J Sports Sci. 1998;16(Suppl):S32–S45.

33. Paffenbarger RSJ, Wing AL, Hyde. Physical activity as an index of heart attack risk in college alumni. Am J Epidemiol. 1978;252:161–175.

34. Panagiotakos DB, Kokkinos P, Manios Y, et al. Physical activity and markers of inflammation and thrombosis related to coronary heart disease. Prev Cardiol. 2004;7(4):190–194.

35. Pedersen BK. Il-6 signalling in exercise and disease. Biochem Soc Trans. 2007;35(5):1295–1297.

36. Plaisance EP, Grandjean PMW. Physical activity and high-sensitivity C-reactive protein. Sports Med. 2006;36(5):443–458.

37. Roitman JL, TP LaFontaine. Secondary prevention of coronary artery disease. In: AACVPR Cardiac Rehabilitation Resource Manual. Champaign, IL: Human Kinetics, 2005, pp. 27–42.

38. Schachinger F, Britten MB, Elsner M, et al. A positive family history of premature coronary artery disease is associated with impaired endothelium-dependent coronary blood flow regulation. Circulation. 1999;100:1502–1508.

39. Steiner S, Niessner A, Ziegler S, et al. Endurance training increases the number of endothelial progenitor cells in patients with cardiovascular risk and coronary artery disease. Atherosclerosis. 2005;181:305–310.

40. Szmitko PE, Fedak PWM, Weisel RD, et al. Endothelial progenitor cells: new hope for a broken heart. Circulation. 2000;107:3093–3100.

41. Taylor HL, Klepetar E, Keys A, et al. Death rates among physically active and sedentary employees of the railroad industry. Am J Public Health. 1962;52:1697–1707.

42. Taylor RS, Brown A, Ebrahim S, et al. Exercise-based rehabilitation for patients with coronary heart disease: systematic review and meta-analysis of randomized controlled trials. Am J Med. 2004;116(10):682–692.

43. Thompson W, ed. ACSM's Guidelines for Exercise Testing and Prescription. 8th Ed. Baltimore, MD: Lippincott Williams & Wilkins, 2009.

44. Wahl P, Bloch W, Schmidt A. Exercise has a positive effect on endothelial progenitor cells, which could be necessary for vascular adaptation processes. Int J Sports Med. 2007;28(5):374–380.

45. Woods JA, Vieira VJ, Keylock KT. Exercise, inflammation and immunity. Immunol Allergy Clin North Am. 2009;29:381–393.

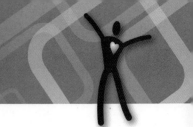

CHAPTER 6

Overweight and Obesity

ABBREVIATIONS

ACSM	American College of Sports Medicine	GPS	Global positioning system
BMI	Body mass index	LTPA	Leisure time physical activity
EE	Energy expenditure	MetS	Metabolic syndrome
EI	Energy intake	PA	Physical activity
GI	Glycemic index	WHR	Waist-to-hip ratio

O besity develops slowly over a relatively long period of time and persists. Given the notable lack of long-term success in weight loss programs, obesity almost always persists for long periods of time and often recurs throughout life. Approximately 20% of people who attempt weight loss in any given year are able to lose and maintain a 10% loss of body weight for a year (58). Obesity has an inherent pathophysiology that is similar to the other chronic diseases discussed in this book. The disease process may resolve and go away with appropriate and sustained lifestyle treatment. Lifestyle, drugs, and surgical treatment modalities are complementary in more severe cases (body mass index [BMI] >35.0), but optimal lifestyle management is the most effective treatment (58).

DID YOU KNOW?
Overweight Versus Obesity (38)

When using the terms "overweight" and "obesity" in this chapter, we will use the following conventions:

1. **Overweight:** This will refer to those who have a BMI between 25.0 and 29.9. The research information about the risk of being overweight is much less definitive than being, by definition, obese.
2. **Obesity:** This will refer specifically to individuals with a BMI of ≥30.0 who are, by standard definition (of the Centers for Disease Control and Prevention), obese. More specifically, the following definitions are generally accepted:
   • Stage 1 obesity: 30.0–34.9
   • Stage 2 obesity: 35.0–39.9
   • Stage 3 obesity: >40.0

Obesity is an epidemic in the United States and worldwide. Figure 6.1 shows the increased incidence of obesity in the United States over the past 10 years (17). The *Journal of the American Medical Association* recently reported that the incidence of obesity was approximately 36% in women and 34% in men, while the incidence of overweight and obesity was 64% in women and 72% in men (17). Several important facts are apparent from the figure. In 1985, the highest rate of obesity among states that reported data was 10% to 14% of the population, but not all states were reporting data. In 1995, when every state reported data, 10% to 14% of the population was overweight or obese in every state. Fully 50% of states had obesity rates at 15% to 19% of the population. It is important to note that the chart (and these data) is self-report data, which are generally known to be underestimates of actual numbers of overweight and obese people.

In 1999, more than 64% of the U.S. population was overweight or obese; by 2004, the overweight or obese population was more than 66% of the total population (see Fig. 6.1). That amounts to almost 150 million people! The numbers for children are lower, but still discouraging since the rate of increase parallels that of adults. The population of obese and overweight children of all ages has increased steadily since 1999 (see Table 6.1).

The data for ethnic groups are even more discouraging. By 2004, over 75% of African American women were overweight or obese (17,18). Almost 75% of Hispanic men and women older than 20 years are overweight or obese. More than 65% of white men and almost 80% of African American women are overweight or obese (BMI >25.0) (7,8,17).

Finally, the increasing prevalence of overweight and obese individuals is not confined to the United States, though U.S. adults and particularly youth have shown the greatest increase during the past 20 years. Almost 1 billion people in the world are overweight; one-third of them (300 million people) are considered obese by World Health Organization standards (see Fig. 6.2). The rates range from less than 5% of the population of China and most of Asia to more than 75% of those in urban Samoa.

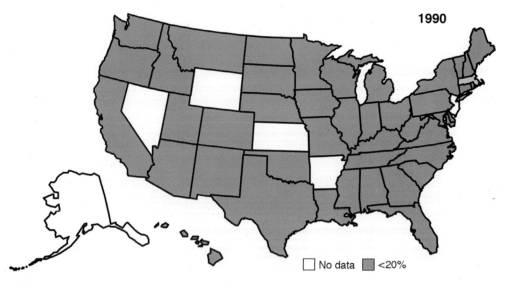

FIGURE 6.1 The incidence and prevalence of obesity in the United States (and the world) has grown exponentially since the mid-1980s. The map here shows obesity trends among U.S. adults from 1990, 1999, and 2008, from the centers for Disease Control and Prevention's Behavioral Risk Factor Surveillance system. (*Fig. 6.1 continued on page 135.*)

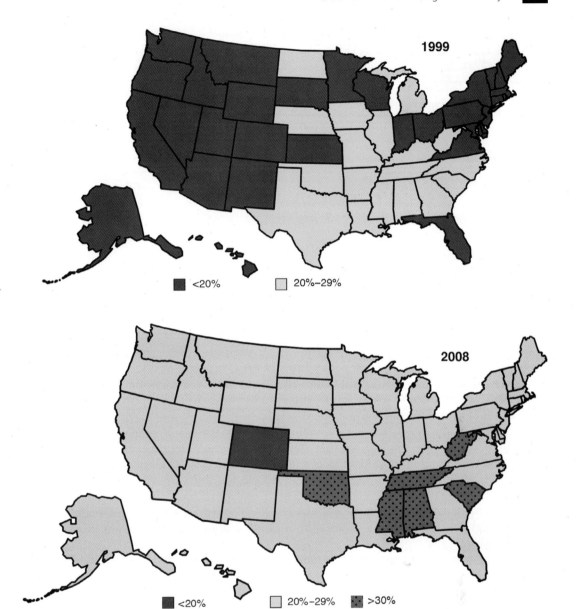

FIGURE 6.1 (*continued*)

TABLE 6.1	Incidence of Obesity in the United States (17,18)			
	1999	1999	2008	2008
Age	Men	Women	Men	Women
20–39	23.7	28.4	27.5	34
40–59	28.8	37.8	34.3	38.2
>60	31.8	35	37.1	33.6

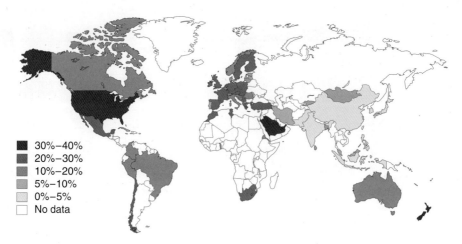

FIGURE 6.2 Although the United States has the most serious and widespread problem with obesity, the international problem is also serious and of epidemic proportions.
Source: World Health Organization. Global strategy on diet, physical activity, and health. Overweight and obesity. Available at: http://www.who.int/dietphysicalactivity/publications/facts/obesity/en/. Accessed June 27, 2008.

Interestingly, though the rate is very low in China, the rates of obesity increase to more than 20% in many of the large cities of China. Finally, though the United States has only 2% of the world's population, it has 15% of the overweight and obese adults, an astounding and concerning statistic (51,59).

The reasons for increasing international obesity levels are complex. In fact, obesity often exists among populations that are *undernourished*. The reason most often given is excess consumption of foods high in calories, saturated fats, and refined carbohydrates, especially simple sugars, the so-called high-calorie, low nutrient-density foods. This means they have high caloric content coupled with little nutritional value and generally large amounts of fat and/or sugars and processed carbohydrates. Combined with a lack of physical activity (PA), the result is high rates of obese and overweight people in the population (59).

The contribution of obesity to the epidemic numbers of persons with hypertension, type 2 diabetes, and the metabolic syndrome is astounding. In fact, the Centers for Disease Control and Prevention recently estimated that in the United States, there are currently 24 million people with diabetes and another 57 million people with "prediabetes." Almost 25% of the adult population has or is at risk for having type 2 diabetes (8–10).

Exercise professionals must be knowledgeable about obesity, type 2 diabetes, and MetS. In addition, exercise professionals must be prepared to effectively coach these individuals toward enhanced health and fitness, thereby assisting them to prevent, improve, and/or resolve the pathophysiology of these diseases. Successful implementation of programs addressing these conditions may, in fact, be the customer base of the fitness and wellness industry for the next 25 years.

Key Point

Overweight and obesity are at epidemic proportions in the United States. The connection between adipose tissue and the pathophysiology of chronic disease is well established and the epidemic is likely to lead to continued increases in rates of type 2 diabetes and other chronic diseases in the coming decades.

PATHOPHYSIOLOGY OF OBESITY

The same low-level systemic inflammatory syndrome that has been previously discussed is inherent to the development and presence of excess adipose tissue (overweight and obesity) (21,32). In fact, some attribute the initial inflammatory insult to adipokines produced in adipose tissue. Thus, logically, adipose tissue produces adipokines, which further promote the pathophysiology of obesity. Additional adipose tissue produces even more adipokines. The vicious cycle of adipose tissue, adipokines, and altered metabolic states is set in motion.

Adipokines are produced and secreted by adipose tissue (adipocytes) and they may well be the underlying cause of the systemic, low-level inflammation, though this remains speculative (see Fig. 6.3) (21,32,53). Table 6.2 introduces some of the *adipokines* and their function. Ten to 15 years ago, adipocytes were thought to function as simple storage depots for fat. Adipokines are known to be proinflammatory and negatively affect fat and glucose metabolism, immune function, vascular function, insulin secretion, and many other physiological functions (4,20,21,32).

Many adipokines directly affect inflammation, metabolism, and insulin secretion and sensitivity (see Table 6.2). In fact, they may cause the underlying inflammatory condition associated with obesity and particularly abdominal obesity. In other cases, adipokines are used to "detect" inflammation (inflammatory markers; see Chapter 2). Several of these adipokines, such as interleukin-6 and tumor necrosis factor-α are "proinflammatory"; that is, they actually promote inflammation. In addition, many adipokines cause various negative and positive influences on insulin secretion, sensitivity and insulin resistance, hunger, appetite, and energy

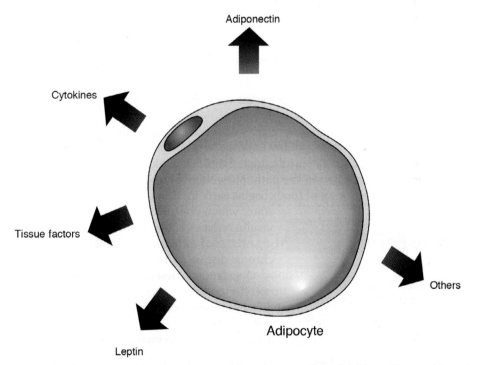

FIGURE 6.3 Adipokines are produced and secreted by adipocytes (fat cells). They affect a wide variety of cellular and physiological processes including hunger, glucose, and fat metabolism and many are proinflammatory.

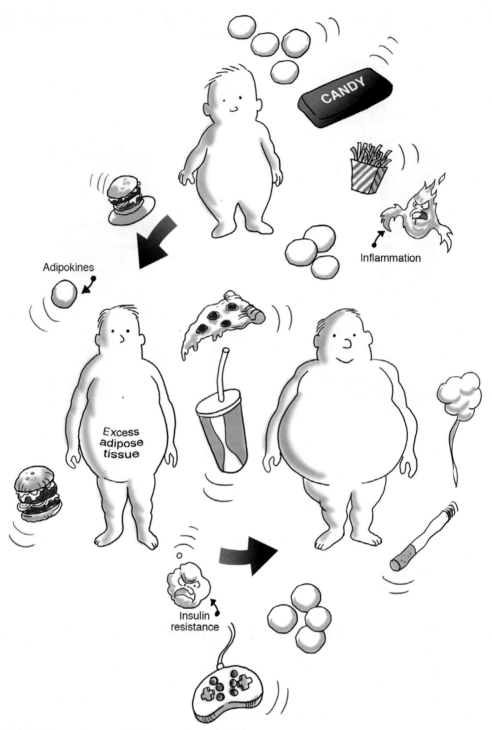

FIGURE 6.5 Exposure to multiple, negative environmental variables associated with overweight and obesity that promote inflammation, insulin resistance, and the other pathophysiology of chronic disease begins early in life.

TABLE 6.3	Assessing Obesity (37–40,52)	
Measure	**Method**	**Standards**
Percentage of body fat	Measure specific sites for skinfold thickness to estimate subcutaneous and total body fat, as well as lean tissue. The most accurate estimates come from formulas that are specific to age and sex.	Recommendations (by age): *Men:* 18–34 years: 8%–22% >35 years: 10%–25% Obese >25% *Women:* 18–34 years: 20%–35% 35–55 years: 23%–38% 55 years: 25%–38% Obese >38%
Body mass index (BMI)	Combines height and weight. BMI is the body weight (kg) divided by the square of the height (m). $BMI = weight\ (kg)/height^2\ (m)$ Or $BMI = (weight\ (lb) \times 703)/height^2\ (inch)$	Underweight <18.5 Normal weight = 18.5–24.9 Overweight = 25.0–29.9 Obesity = >30.0
Waist circumference	The circumference of the waist at the level of the iliac crest.	*Men:* 40 inches *Women:* <35 inches
Waist-to-hip ratio (WHR)	Waist circumference divided by hip circumference. Measure waist as above. Measure hips at the widest point (including buttocks in the measurement).	*Men:* Low risk <0.95 Moderate risk = 0.96–1.0 High risk >1.0 *Women:* Low risk <0.80 Moderate risk = 0.81–0.85 High risk >0.85

to the pathophysiology of several chronic diseases (12–15). Table 6.3 outlines several accepted methods for measuring and defining overweight and obesity.

WEIGHT LOSS AND MAINTENANCE

Weight loss and weight maintenance have become obsessions that consume large amounts of time and money; some estimates put this at almost $100 billion (10). The number of overweight and obese Americans are staggering. One other particularly interesting number is that approximately one-third of Americans are on a weight loss diet of some kind at any given time (48). Finally, somewhere between 5% and 20% of everyone on a weight loss program are able to sustain the weight loss for more than 12 months or to maintain significant weight loss over periods of longer than 1 year (1,47,58).

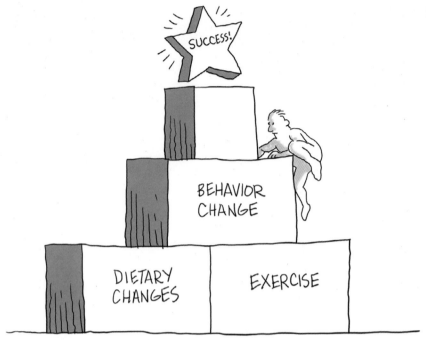

FIGURE 6.6 Successful weight loss programs combine dietary pattern changes (including caloric restriction), exercise and physical activity, and behavioral change.

In the following section, we will discuss weight loss programs and the research concerning exercise and daily PA, diet, and behavior change. Most effective weight loss and maintenance programs combine all three of these strategies and when used separately, none is as effective as any combination of the three methods (see Fig. 6.6). It is also particularly pertinent to emphasize that individual preference and situation is extremely important in guiding successful weight loss and maintenance. Exercise professionals must be aware of the individual needs, preferences, and goals of clients in coaching them toward successful weight control programs.

DIET AND WEIGHT LOSS

There are countless weight loss diets, programs, and fad diets available for anyone who wants to lose weight. Consumers (or clients) may be unaware of the drawbacks or disadvantages of many of these programs. Many are based on false scientific premises that were developed solely to sell products. Others were developed on the basis of valid scientific information that is inappropriately interpreted and/or utilized. Some are entirely valid scientifically and behaviorally but are virtually impossible to maintain and adhere to over long periods of time; therefore, they are not practical for most people.

Diets aimed at weight loss require common characteristics to be effective. Those characteristics include adequate caloric intake to sustain daily activities and exercise, various foods that satisfy individual preferences (rather than elimination of whole food groups or significantly increased consumption of specific food groups at the expense of others), and, finally, a dietary pattern that can be maintained for life. Unfortunately, most popular fad diets do not conform to these basic principles and they are very difficult to adhere to over the long term; thus, they are not practical or viable alternatives.

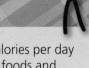

DID YOU KNOW?
Categories of Weight Loss Diets (1)

Low-calorie diets: Characterized by caloric restriction of 800 to 1,200 calories per day for women and 1,200 to 1,400 calories per day for men. The quality of foods and the number of calories consumed is extremely important. In general, these diets are composed of low caloric density foods such as fruits and vegetables.

Low-fat (high-carbohydrate) diets: Characterized by restriction of daily calories from fat. Often <15% to 20% and sometimes as low as <10% of calories from fat. Attention must be given to the type of fat consumed; that is, monounsaturated, polyunsaturated should be predominant in these diets.

Low-carbohydrate (high-fat) diets: Restriction of carbohydrates to <60 g/day or <10% of total calories. Strict limitations on refined carbohydrates (processed grain used in pasta, white bread, and sugar) along with high protein and, sometimes, high fat are common characteristics of these diets.

Weight loss programs must be based on individual preferences, individual metabolism and physiology, and sound behavioral change principles and practices. Without a combination of all three, the likelihood of long-term maintenance of weight loss (prevention of weight regain) is significantly diminished. Knowledge of individual food preferences and eating patterns are of vital importance in helping clients to choose an effective weight loss plan.

Diets for weight loss can be categorized into three broad groups (see Chapter 4 for a more detailed discussion of "healthy" diets). These groups are as follows:

1. low-calorie balanced diets;
2. low-fat diets; and
3. low-carbohydrate diets.

Although there are variations of these, this is a convenient way to look at the effectiveness of a particular dietary pattern for weight loss. We will not review very low-calorie diets (defined as a caloric intake of <800 calories per day) because of the need for ongoing medical assessment to safely and effectively comply with these diets. They are more aligned with the "medical" model; therefore, these are outside the realm of this book.

Low-Calorie Diets

All diets that address weight loss and/or weight maintenance must effectively restrict calories to establish a negative caloric balance. This category is added because there are, in fact, low-calorie, balanced nutrient diets that have been demonstrated to be successful with weight loss and maintenance. These diets have also been called "hypoenergetic, balanced diets" because they attempt to remain balanced between carbohydrates, protein, and fat (1).

These diets restrict calories to 800 to 1,200 calories per day (for women) or 1,200 to 1,400 calories per day (for men) and generally do not limit or emphasize any particular food group. This category includes diets such as the American Heart Association Step 1 diet and some weight watcher's plans. The consensus is that the foods in these diets should be high fiber and low glycemic index (GI) for increased effectiveness and health benefits. Low-calorie diets have been found to be effective in short-term and long-term weight loss for a significant portion of those who can maintain them (37).

Low-Carbohydrate Diets

Although these diets are often cited as the most effective type of diet for rapid weight loss, they are generally not recommended and we certainly do not recommend them as a "healthy dietary pattern." For most consumers, this simply means "low carbs" (no bread, white rice, potatoes, and other high-GI carbohydrates) and high protein (increased meat, cheese, and other high-fat dairy). These low-carbohydrate diets have been shown to be effective for weight loss but are not recommended by the American Dietetic Association or other major professional organizations (20,43,46,49).

In some people, this type of diet may be effective for short-term weight loss, as well as for modifying diet-related risk factors including lipids, insulin sensitivity and resistance, and glucose and fat metabolism (20,43,46,49). However, many of the foods included in these diets are proinflammatory, they are processed and refined, and they are in direct contradiction to the healthy dietary patterns described in Chapter 4 on nutrition. In the long term, they simply cannot be sustained and are not optimal for preventing chronic disease.

Many of the low-carbohydrate diets are high protein and may also be high in saturated and trans fats (e.g., Atkins). Consequently, these diets are not recommended for anyone with chronic disease or even risk factors for chronic disease. That fact argues for limited use of these diets in any weight loss program. The goal of any weight loss program should be to guide clients toward healthy, sustained lifestyle change. These diets promote the pathophysiology of chronic disease processes. Changing them to low-GI diets can help to make them healthier. Choosing carbohydrates that are higher in fiber and lower in refined sugars is an excellent way to make them healthier.

Low-Fat Diets

Low-fat diets (and very low-fat diets) that restrict fat calories to 10% to 25% or less of total calories or less can also be effective for weight loss. (See Chapter 4 for definitions of low-fat vs. high-fat diets.) Diets such as Ornish or Pritikin are examples of these. Their effects on weight loss are significant and they have also been shown to significantly lower total cholesterol and low-density lipoprotein, improve insulin sensitivity, and reduce inflammation (49). These diets have also been demonstrated to increase triglyceride and decrease high-density lipoprotein levels. These effects are not positive for pathophysiology of chronic disease. The optimal program for weight loss and weight loss maintenance also involves daily exercise. Exercise has been shown to prevent this rise in triglycerides and also to increase high-density lipoprotein levels (28,30). In addition, many consider these diets to be so restrictive in fat calories that adherence and compliance become problems for many individuals who follow them.

Caloric Balance

A common strategy for weight loss and weight maintenance uses caloric balance as the principle factor in prescribing a combination of exercise and calorie restriction. For example, combining 250 calories per day in exercise-related energy expenditure (EE) with 250 calories per day in calorie restriction produces a total energy deficit of 500 calories per day. Theoretically, this is equivalent to a weight loss of 1 lb per week. Although it seems logical on the surface, physiological and biochemical issues have an impact on the real-life application of this principle; thus, it does not necessarily happen "as calculated." However, the principle of using this kind of negative energy balance clearly works and is necessary for an effective weight loss or weight control program.

DID YOU KNOW?
Principles of Energy Balance (24)

- Some people may be genetically prone to obesity; thus, there are difficulties using traditional methods of producing a negative energy balance for intake and expenditure with food and exercise.
- The total change in energy balance, called *"energy flux,"* may be important to the effectiveness of changing energy balance. A greater energy flux may ensure more success than a smaller energy flux. Those individuals with the greatest energy flux (combination of intake and expenditure) may be able to lose more weight. Higher levels of activity may allow people to regulate energy intake (EI) more effectively. On the other hand, individuals with a low energy flux (small changes in energy balance) may not be able to restrict calories enough to successfully lose or maintain weight loss.
- Dietary pattern may variably affect weight loss depending on whether a person is in negative, positive, or equivalent energy balance. Eating a high-fat diet when energy balance is positive (intake > expenditure) can cause greater amounts of weight gain than eating a high-carbohydrate diet.
- When a negative energy balance is present, there is little difference in weight loss associated with high-protein, low-fat, or low-carbohydrate diets.
- It seems possible that small increases in PA can prevent weight gain, but that relatively large increases in PA are necessary to *prevent weight gain after weight loss*.
- The challenge of maintaining a weight loss is more difficult because losing weight causes decreased energy requirements both at rest and during exercise. Therefore, after a weight loss, maintaining that loss may require increased EE.
- Systematic changes in the environment—both the "food" environment and the exercise/activity environment that support sustaining PA—are critical to changing weight.

An effective weight loss program requires a negative caloric balance. In other words, caloric expenditure must exceed calorie intake to lose weight and must equal calorie intake to maintain weight. **There must be a negative energy balance for weight loss to occur and there must be an equivalent energy balance to maintain weight.** Unfortunately, this is not always as simple as it seems. One of the premier researchers in weight loss has recently written about this and his findings and recommendations are summarized in the box above (24).

Thus, diet composition and caloric balance are related to weight loss and weight gain. Restricting calorie intake during periods of attempted weight loss is critical to establishing the negative energy balance. In addition, when intake and expenditure are equal, the macronutrient composition of the calories consumed is important to the effectiveness of the weight loss maintenance. The exercise professional must be attentive to both factors if successful weight loss and weight maintenance are to be part of the repertoire.

EXERCISE AND WEIGHT LOSS

There is little question that increased PA is necessary to establish the negative energy balance required to achieve successful weight loss. No other method of increasing calorie expenditure is as powerful or as effective. Research demonstrates that weight loss programs

Critical Nutritional Principles of Weight Loss Programs

1. Caloric restriction should be moderate (250–500 per day) and should aim at reducing saturated fat and refined carbohydrates. In general, greater restriction in carbohydrates leads to greater weight loss early in a program but not necessarily in the long term (20,25).
2. Fat restriction should center on foods containing saturated and trans fat. A nutritional plan should include foods containing monounsaturated and polyunsaturated fat for their health benefits. Using the types of fat produces positive changes in nutritionally related risk factors including blood lipids, glucose and fat metabolism, and inflammatory state.
3. Carbohydrate restriction should center on simple sugars and refined and processed carbohydrates. Restricting these requires, by default, consuming mostly complex and high-fiber carbohydrates. This is the healthier dietary pattern and one that helps with hunger and satiety.
4. Very low-calorie diets (<800 calories per day) should not be used without the ongoing supervision of a physician. Extreme calorie restriction can blunt the results of weight loss programs for all but the most obese (37).
5. Any diet should limit the consumption of high caloric density foods because they are often high in fat or simple carbohydrates and also because high caloric density foods are almost always low-volume foods. Hunger may be a constant problem in these diets.

using activity alone are not as effective as weight loss programs using diet alone. However, in both of these types of programs, the total amount of weight loss is only on the order of a few pounds over the long term (12 months) (57). It has also been shown that prescribing and maintaining higher activity levels after weight loss is helpful in maintenance of weight loss (50). Basic logic tells us that both calorie restriction and increased exercise and LTPA are the most effective combination.

One important point to consider is that even though it is possible to lose a modest amount of weight using PA alone, it is sometimes difficult for overweight people (especially extremely obese people) to perform sufficient amounts of PA to lose weight, if it is the lone change in lifestyle (i.e., without caloric restriction). Thus, one approach early in weight loss programs for extremely obese clients is the use of medically controlled, very low-calorie diets used in combination with low-intensity, low-impact activities (13). We will not discuss these diets in this book, but rather discuss principles for overweight and obese individuals who do not fall in the "superobese" category (BMI ≥40.0).

The real question for the exercise professional is *How much and what kind of exercise is most effective?* Answers to that question, though not simple, can be reduced to a single crucial matter—increased calorie expenditure through PA (to help create a negative energy balance) contributes to weight loss and particularly to the maintenance of weight loss—it may be most important that *some type* of PA is included, rather than *what type* it is. Several sources indicate that 2,000 calories in energy expenditure per week by exercise is necessary for losing weight (15,25,26). It may take greater calorie expenditure, perhaps 2,500 to 3,500 PA-related calories per week, to maintain that weight loss (23). This may be partially explained by the loss of lean mass (muscle) during a weight loss program that interestingly may be somewhat limited by adding resistance

DID YOU KNOW?
Very Low-Calorie Diets (55)

Very low-calorie diets restrict calories to less than 800 per day and are usually (and should be) medically supervised. These diets include some kind of daily source of nutrients that is usually a drink (a "shake") that includes a daily dose of vitamins and minerals and some fiber. They are restricted from other food intake for a specified period of time (up to 6–8 weeks) and then slowly put back on "real food" after this early intense period of low-calorie "fasting." These diets are uncommon and are not recommended without supervision, and the track record for long-term weight loss is not very good.

training to the PA associated with such programs. Losing lean mass decreases basal metabolic rate; thus, the overall loss of muscle mass combined with lower total body weight decreases resting metabolism and the energy cost of activities when compared with the overweight or obese condition. Simply put, both resting and exercise/activity EE are lower after successful weight loss.

The question of how much exercise and activity is necessary to promote and sustain weight loss is important. The consensus is that the 2,000-calorie figure stated above, now expressed in terms of minutes (300 per week), is the threshold (15). One large database of individuals who have lost significant amounts of weight and maintained that weight loss for more than 5 years cites high levels of PA as one of the

> ## Key Point
> Combining exercise and diet in a weight loss program is the most effective method for losing weight for most people.

common characteristics of this group. However, there is a significant range of PA level in these individuals. Most (75%) have been able to maintain high PA levels that initially helped them succeed in their weight loss programs (5,57). These "high" PA levels (some individuals report >400 kcal/day) illustrate the importance of increased PA in the long-term maintenance of weight loss.

Another recent epidemiological study of more than 35,000 women found that only normal weight women in the most active group (>21.5 MET hours per week of activity) were able to avoid weight gain during the 13 years of follow-up (32). This level of exercise is nearly 60 minutes per day. Thus, weight gain is difficult without high levels of PA (32,50,57,58). [*Note*: a "MET-hour" is a unit that quantifies both intensity (MET) and duration (hours) into a single number that is often used to compare various levels of exercise. For example, three MET-hours are equivalent to performing an exercise of three METs for 60 minutes].

Recently, there has been much discussion of the relative benefits of LTPA versus "exercise" in weight loss and maintenance program. Clearly, we know that most people do not exercise by American College of Sports Medicine (ACSM) guidelines for frequency, duration, and intensity. That is, most individuals do not participate in a regular form of activity designed to increase physical fitness (one definition of "exercise"). The inclusion of LTPA into the caloric balance equation adds an additional variable to increase energy flux.

There are many ways to assess LTPA. Some are described in the box on the next page. One of the simplest ways is to count steps; in fact, campaigns promoting "10,000 steps per day" are widespread. It appears that the 10,000 steps per day recommendation is consistent

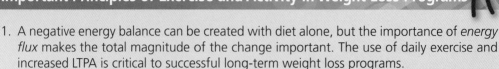

DID YOU KNOW?

Important Principles of Exercise and Activity in Weight Loss Programs

1. A negative energy balance can be created with diet alone, but the importance of *energy flux* makes the total magnitude of the change important. The use of daily exercise and increased LTPA is critical to successful long-term weight loss programs.
2. Public health recommendations for exercise are equivalent to about 200 to 250 calories per day in EE. These are guidelines for promoting health but are not necessarily adequate or effective for weight loss programs. A more appropriate and effective amount may be 300 to 400 calories per day or more in exercise and PA.
3. Routine and consistency are important to success. Developing habits requires repetition of the desired behavior for many months before it is actually a habit. Encourage and support daily exercise and PA.
4. Measuring the activity is good feedback and can be valuable for assessing progress. Encourage the purchase of an accurate step counter (pedometer) for ongoing assessment of exercise and activity behavior. Visual records and feedback may be an additional motivator for some.

with the public health recommendations for exercise (54). In addition, for weight loss and prevention of weight regain, most recommend this in addition to 30 minutes or more of daily exercise (23,24). Step counting is an excellent way to assess exercise and activity habits of individuals as well as a way to help individuals increase activity levels. Determining a baseline and then helping people increase daily steps in small increments can be a successful method for increasing activity in weight control programs (23).

The Initial Exercise Prescription for Weight Loss

There is one additional important factor that must be considered when using exercise and PA in weight loss programs. It has been demonstrated in many different settings that overweight and obese people are less tolerant of weight-bearing exercise and sustain exercise-related injuries more often than individuals at their healthy weight. It is also clear that higher intensity, duration, and frequency of exercise also causes more injury than less frequent, shorter-duration, and lower-intensity exercise, especially when initiating exercise programs in deconditioned individuals (15). Thus, exercise prescription for unfit or low fit individuals who are significantly overweight becomes a balancing act between offering an effective dose of

DID YOU KNOW?

Energy Flux (24)

The term *energy flux* is discussed in the box above. It is defined as the total daily caloric deficit from the combined decrease in caloric intake (dietary calories) and increased PA (daily exercise plus PA). According to James Hill, the greater the energy flux, the more effective the weight control program.

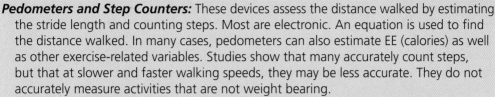

DID YOU KNOW?
Methods for Assessing Leisure Time Physical Activity

Pedometers and Step Counters: These devices assess the distance walked by estimating the stride length and counting steps. Most are electronic. An equation is used to find the distance walked. In many cases, pedometers can also estimate EE (calories) as well as other exercise-related variables. Studies show that many accurately count steps, but that at slower and faster walking speeds, they may be less accurate. They do not accurately measure activities that are not weight bearing.

Accelerometers: These are small devices similar to step counters that are designed to measure acceleration. They accumulate "acceleration units" that are converted into EE in various categories of intensity by mathematic algorithms. Accelerometers have been shown to be reasonably accurate in estimating activity levels and EE of a wide range of activities. Like pedometers, they are less accurate at the extremes of activity.

Global Positioning System (GPS) Devices: A more recent addition to the marketplace is a device that works by using GPS. These are accurate as long as they are able to maintain contact with a satellite. They can estimate calorie expenditure accurately because they actually measure the distance and speed traveled using GPS technology. These devices allow storage of information for record keeping. Expense is the primary obstacle, but as prices decrease, they will become more prevalent.

exercise and preventing exercise-related injuries along with cultivating the compliance that will ensure success.

The exercise professional must use initial caution when prescribing exercise programs in overweight and obese individuals. Intensity and duration of exercise should be progressed gradually. The individual's need to see progress toward the weight loss goals may complicate the situation. In most cases, lower-intensity exercise must be used because of deconditioning. Often the use of short-duration (10–15 minutes), intermittent exercise, or short-duration exercise more than two or more times per day is a solution to this problem. The importance of ensuring success in the early part of an exercise program for overweight/obese, deconditioned individuals cannot be understated.

THE OPTIMAL LIFESTYLE PROGRAM FOR OVERWEIGHT AND OBESITY

The pathophysiology of obesity is amenable to change with exercise and nutritional intervention (24). The systemic low-level inflammation, the negative influence of adipokines, and the metabolic abnormalities associated with increased adipose tissue are moderated by weight loss (41,60). In fact, achieving the optimal body weight, BMI or WHR, may completely normalize the metabolic abnormalities associated with obesity. The optimal program requires changes in dietary pattern and adherence to a regular, structured exercise program as well as increased LTPA.

Increased monounsaturated and polyunsaturated fat, fiber, and complex carbohydrates are at the core of this dietary pattern (refer back to Fig. 4.7). Decreased saturated and trans fat, simple sugars, and other refined carbohydrates as well as decreased calorie intake are

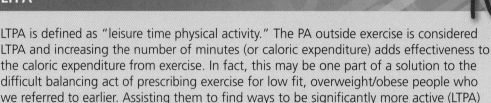

LTPA is defined as "leisure time physical activity." The PA outside exercise is considered LTPA and increasing the number of minutes (or caloric expenditure) adds effectiveness to the caloric expenditure from exercise. In fact, this may be one part of a solution to the difficult balancing act of prescribing exercise for low fit, overweight/obese people who we referred to earlier. Assisting them to find ways to be significantly more active (LTPA) can increase the daily energy flux without adding the stress of increased frequency, duration, or intensity that is related to noncompliance and injury.

additional recommended changes. See Chapter 4 for a detailed discussion and description of the optimal nutritional pattern.

The optimal exercise pattern is summarized in the box below. Simply put, regular daily exercise that expends >300 to 400 calories per day, along with additional LTPA (e.g., steps, walking stairs, chores, recreational activities) is optimal for achieving and maintaining ideal weight and body composition. Be aware that the amount of exercise and activity necessary to *achieve weight loss* may differ from that necessary to *maintain weight loss* (24).

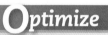

Exercise Prescription

The table below highlights the optimal exercise for weight loss and/or prevention of weight regain.

Frequency	7 d/wk
Intensity	Light to moderate—heart rate in the range of 40%–60% maximum heart rate reserve; rating of perceived exertion in the 11–13 range (on a 6–20 scale).
Duration	60–90 min/d; may be divided into multiple shorter sessions but not less than 15 minutes and to at least one session longer than 30 minutes after satisfactory progress.
Type	Walking, running, biking, swimming,* or aerobics classes are all acceptable examples of modalities. Resistance training should be used as an adjunct but in addition to the cardiorespiratory endurance exercise or as part of a circuit resistance training program.
Calorie expenditure	Calorie expenditure should equal >2,000 kcal/wk outside normal daily activities. LTPA should be added to the exercise program in amounts equaling the calorie expenditure during exercise. We also recommend a step counter to quantify daily activity with a goal of >10,000 steps/day outside exercise. Total steps including exercise and activity should be 11,000–14,000.

*Initially weight-bearing activities may be difficult, may cause injury, and may not be ideal for obese and very obese participants or clients.

LTPA, leisure time physical activity.

DIGGING DEEPER

Exercise and Appetite

The notion that using exercise may be ineffective for weight loss because it increases appetite is not new (9,34). The question of appetite, EI, EE, and energy balance is complicated and difficult. There are various pertinent questions, but the answers to most remain unresolved. In this "Digging Deeper" section, we will consider two major subdivisions of the topic: (a) the coupling of EI and EE and (b) the influence of exercise on appetite-related hormones. The consensus is that exercise alone is unlikely to stimulate increased appetite during a weight loss program that involves both diet and exercise. Although this is controversial, it is not an appropriate reason to remove exercise from the energy balance equation in weight loss programs. It is also important to understand that the eating- and activity-related environments and individual physiology contribute to eating behavior. Therefore, exercise is not and should not be the sole factor used to produce a negative energy balance.

A recent study by King et al. (27) shows that two processes may drive appetite regulation in response to exercise. King supervised 12 weeks of exercise in obese men and women. Satiety (satisfaction from a meal) and subjective hunger were measured using accepted scales, and food intake was directly measured at four intervals during the 12-week period. King and colleagues (27) analyzed individuals who had expected and less-than-expected weight loss according to the calculated EE from the exercise program ("nonresponders" and "responders"). Satiety was assessed after a "fixed breakfast" was fed to the subjects four times during the 12-week period (27).

Both groups lost significant amounts of weight. Satiety was increased after the training program; thus, exercisers felt progressively more satisfied after the meal as their exercise program progressed through the 12-week period. Fasting and total daily hunger increased in the nonresponders. Thus, a two-part mechanism was hypothesized. Nonresponders lost less weight than did responders, perhaps because their hunger level and, therefore, their EI after exercise increased in response to the exercise. Both groups lost significant amounts of weight, and both groups demonstrated increased satiety throughout the course of the study in response to the exercise program (27).

The majority of this type of research shows that exercise does not increase appetite or EI. In fact, high-intensity exercise has been shown to produce a temporary decrease in appetite, but that effect is unlikely to result in significant long-term effects on EI (35). It may be that the "coupling" between EI and EE is a more important factor in the efficacy of weight loss programs using exercise than isolated changes in appetite. King et al.'s study (27) above partially confirms this notion, by demonstrating a two-stage mechanism— hunger and satiety have an impact on EI.

Dr. Jean Mayer (35), a world-renowned nutritional researcher, was among the first to demonstrate this uncoupling of EI and EE in a classic epidemiological study. His study examined EI and EE in a population of workers in India who had been previously classified with respect to job class and EE. Workers in the most sedentary job classes were the heaviest and had the highest EIs compared with workers throughout a range of occupations from "light" to "very heavy" EE. Mayer et al. (35) concluded that EI "increases with activity only within a certain zone" that he called "normal activity." The most sedentary workers (below the normal zone) had the highest EI and the lowest EE, thus were heaviest. In 1956, Mayer hypothesized the inappropriate coupling of EI and EE in people with low PA.

(continued)

The effect of exercise on appetite-related hormones is also only partially answered, but there is pertinent information. Several substances including ghrelin and leptin are important. They belong to two classes of compounds that "signal" the brain about nutritional status. The first, ghrelin, serves as an acute signal coming from the gut and provides information about nutritional intake as food in consumed. The second, leptin, provides a chronic signal from adipose tissue about the ongoing status of these energy stores (34). The hormonal regulation, then, is built on immediate feedback from the gut during eating and chronic feedback from adipose tissue regarding long-term stores of energy.

Initial studies about exercise and this system yield little in the way of conclusive evidence. Leptin and ghrelin may increase, decrease, or not change in response to exercise. Indeed, one conclusion is that neither leptin nor ghrelin changes in response to exercise without accompanying weight loss (34). However, there are different biochemical forms of ghrelin, and early research did not separate these substances. Recently, it has been demonstrated that two forms of ghrelin (acylated and deacylated ghrelin) respond to exercise in a positive way with respect to exercise and weight loss (3). These results confirm the work of King et al. (27) that we discussed on the previous page.

To add confusion and complexity to this picture (if that is possible), it appears that men and women respond to exercise differently with respect to hunger and these hormones (22). Men seem to adjust EI and EE concurrently. That is, the exercise response in men shows that they do not exhibit an increased hunger response if the EI is balancd by EE. Women demonstrate the opposite effect—hunger is stimulated after exercise and EI is increased (22). In addition, there are differences with respect to whether energy balance is reestablished after exercise or not, making the picture even more complex. Church et al. (9) confirmed this in an earlier study with women exercising at different EEs when he found that women exercising at the highest intensity (12 kcal/kg/minute) had less-than-expected weight loss.

The current status of this research (hormonal responses and exercise) leaves a gaping hole in what is known about exercise, appetite, and weight loss that has yet to be resolved. It is safe to say that regular exercise and PA should play a significant role in a weight loss program, as should caloric restriction through diet (15).

Significant RESEARCH

Two articles have been selected for this section. The first article by Lee explains the connection between adipose tissue and inflammation in a very clear and relatively simple way. The second is a "Position Stand" (an "official statement" from ACSM). The team of authors who wrote this statement is composed of experts on weight control and exercise. It is comprehensive, extremely well documented, and extensive in its discussion of weight loss and weight maintenance.

The Pathophysiology of Obesity

Lee Y-H, Pratley RE. Abdominal obesity and cardiovascular disease risk: the emerging role of the adipocyte. J Cardiopulm Rehab Prev. 2007;27(1):2–10.

Dr. Lee lays out the connection between the low-level systemic inflammation that is present in obese individuals in a very clear and concise way. He defines obesity and then connects it as a risk factor in several chronic diseases including hypertension, type 2 diabetes, and MetS, among others. The ensuing discussion of the physiology and pathophysiology of adipose tissue lays out the connections between the secretion and action of the adipokines and the inflammation and other pathophysiology (e.g., insulin resistance) that is inherent in obesity secondary to the excess adipose tissue. Logically, the next step is to explain the adipokines themselves and how they drive these pathophysiological processes linked to the chronic disease.

Lee does all of these in a very orderly, clear, and relatively simple fashion. Although the article is somewhat dated due to the volume of research that this topic has generated in the following time period, it certainly introduces this fundamental issue and basis for this topic. This is an excellent article that provides a clear introduction to this difficult topic.

The Role of PA in Weight Loss and Maintenance

Donnelly JE, Blair SN, Jakicic JM, et al. ACSM's position stand on appropriate physical activity intervention strategies for weight loss and prevention of weight regain for adults. Med Sci Sports Exerc. 2009;41(2):459–471.

This paper is a comprehensive review of exercise and PA and their role in weight loss and prevention of weight regain. Donnelly and his coauthors, each an expert in the subject, use an evidence-based approach to examining this topic. Each statement is simple (PA will prevent weight gain), then the evidence is "graded" (A, B, etc.) for strength. The statement above, for example, is "evidence category A," meaning the strength of that evidence denotes the highest level of confidence in the quality of the research. Thus, each statement is accompanied by this level of evidence statement that allows the reader to judge the strength of the research upon which the statement is based.

The major statements include the following topics:

- PA to prevent weight gain
- PA for weight loss
- PA for weight maintenance after weight loss
- Lifestyle PA to counter energy imbalance present in most obese adults
- PA and diet restriction
- PA will increase weight loss
- Resistance training for weight loss

A formal position statement is made for each of these topics and graded for evidence to support the statement (all statements are positive with respect to the outcome; e.g., "lifestyle PA is useful for weight management. Evidence category B.") What follows is a comprehensive discussion that summarizes the significant literature for each statement. Several paragraphs follow each of these statements. Individual studies are usually not explained; rather the research is categorized for design, subject population, or other common characteristics relative to the statement and the outcomes reported. A summary paragraph concludes each section that restates the conclusion and gives a brief synopsis of the material.

A brief, but comprehensive, discussion of PA and risk factors for chronic disease concludes the article. The authors agree in general with the ACSM recommendation of "150 minutes/week of moderate-intensity PA to prevent significant weight gain," but appropriately caution that this amount of exercise is likely to result in only "modest" weight loss and that the dose–response effect (and the literature) shows that >2,000 kcal/week, the equivalent of 250 to 300 minute/week, is likely to be more effective. We highly recommend reading and using the information in this well-written and documented ACSM position stand.

REFERENCES

1. Aggoun Y. Obesity, metabolic syndrome, and cardiovascular disease. Ped Res. 2007;61(6): 653–659.
2. Anderson JW, Konz EC, Frederich RC, et al. Long-term weight-loss maintenance: a meta-analysis of US studies. Am J Clin Nutr. 2001;74:579–584.
3. Bahia L, Aguiar LG, Villela N, et al. Relationship between adipokines, inflammation, and vascular reactivity in lean controls and obese subjects with metabolic syndrome. Clinics. 2006; 61(5):433–440.
4. Broom DR, Stensel DJ, Bishop NC, et al. Exercise-induced suppression of acylated ghrelin in humans. J Appl Physiol. 2007;102:2165–2171.
5. Calabro P, Limongelli G, Pacileo G, et al. The role of adiposity as a determinant of an inflammatory milieu. J Cardiovasc Med. 2008;9(5):450–460.
6. Catenacci VA, Ogden LG, Stuht J, et al. Physical activity patterns in the National Weight Control Registry. Obesity. 2008;16(1):153–161.
7. Centers for Disease Control and Prevention Web Site [Internet]. Atlanta, GA: Centers for Disease Control and Prevention. Available at: http://www.cdc.gov/nccdphp/dnpa/obesity/. Accessed June 27, 2008.
8. Centers for Disease Control and Prevention Web Site [Internet]. Atlanta, GA: Centers for Disease Control and Prevention. Available at: http://www.cdc.gov/nccdphp/dnpa/obesity/trend/maps/index.htm. Accessed June 27, 2008.
9. Centers for Disease Control and Prevention Web Site [Internet]. Atlanta, GA: Centers for Disease Control and Prevention. Available at: http://www.cdc.gov/media/pressrel/2008/r080624.htm. Accessed June 27, 2008.
10. Centers for Disease Control and Prevention Web Site [Internet]. Atlanta, GA: Centers for Disease Control and Prevention. Available at: http://www.cdc.gov/nchs/pressroom/07newsreleases/obesity.htm. Accessed June 27, 2008.
11. Church TS, Martin CK, Thompson AM, et al. Changes in weight, waist circumference and compensatory responses with different doses of exercise among sedentary, overweight postmenopausal women [published online ahead of print February 18, 2009]. PLoS One. 2009;4(2): e4515. doi: 10.1371/journal.pone. 0004515.
12. de Koning L, Merchant AT, Pogue J, et al. Waist circumference and waist-to-hip ratio as predictors of cardiovascular events: meta-regressional analysis of prospective studies. Eur Heart J. 2007; 28:850–856.
13. Delbridge E, Proietto J. State of the science: VLED (Very Low Energy Diet) for obesity. Asia Pac J Clin Nutr. 2006;15(Suppl):49–54.
14. Despres JP, Lemieux I, Bergeron J et al. Abdominal obesity and the metabolic syndrome: contribution to global cardiometabolic risk. Arterioscler Thromb Vasc Biol. 2008;28(6):1039–1049.
15. Dobbelsteyn CJ, Joffres MR, MacLean DR. A comparative evaluation of waist circumference, waist-to-hip ratio and body mass index as indicators of cardiovascular risk factors. The Canadian heart health surveys. Int J Obes Relat Metab Disord. 2001;25(5):652–661.
16. Donnelly J, Blair SN, Jakicic JM, et al. ACSM's Position Stand on appropriate physical activity intervention strategies for weight loss and prevention of weight regain for adults. Med Sci Sports Exerc. 2009;41(2):459–471.
17. Festa A, D'Agostino R, Williams K, et al. The relation of body fat mass and distribution to markers of chronic inflammation. Int J Obes Relat Metab Disord. 2001;25:1407–1415.
18. Flegal KM, Carroll MD, Ogden CL, et al. Prevalence and trends in obesity among US adults, 1999–2008. JAMA. 2010;303(3):235–241. doi: 10.1001/jama.2009.2014.
19. Flegal KM, Graubard BI, Williamson DF, et al. Cause-specific excess deaths associated with underweight, overweight, and obesity. JAMA. 2007;298(17):2028–2037.
20. Frühbeck G. The adipose tissue as a source of vasoactive factors. Curr Med Chem. 2004;2(3): 197–208.
21. Gardner CD, Kiazand A, Alhassan S, et al. Comparison of the Atkins, Zone, Ornish, and LEARN diets for change in weight and related risk factors among overweight premenopausal women: the A TO Z Weight Loss Study: a randomized trial. JAMA. 2007;297:969–977.
22. Gustafson B, Hammarstedt A, Andersson CX, et al. Inflamed adipose tissue: a culprit underlying the metabolic syndrome and atherosclerosis. Arterioscler Throm Vasc Biol. 2007;27(11): 2276–2283.
23. Hagobian TA, Sharoff CG, Stephens BR, et al. Effects of exercise on energy-regulating hormones and appetite in men and women. Am J Physiol Regul Integr Comp Physiol. 2009;296:R233–R242.
24. Hill JO. Understanding and addressing the epidemic of obesity: an energy balance perspective. Endocr Rev. 2006;27:750–761.
25. Hill JO, Wyatt HR. Role of physical activity in preventing and treating obesity. J Appl Physiol. 2005;99(2):765–770.
26. Institute of Medicine, Dietary Reference Intakes for Energy, Carbohydrate, Fiber, Fat, Fatty Acids, Cholesterol, Protein, and Amino Acids (Macronutrients). Washington, DC: National Academies Press, 2002.
27. Jakicic JM, Clark K, Coleman E, et al. American College of Sports Medicine Position Stand: appropriate intervention strategies for weight loss and prevention of weight regain for adults. Med Sci Sports Exerc. 2001;33:2145–2156.
28. King NA, Caudwell PP, Hopkins M, et al. Dual-process action of exercise on appetite control:

increase in orexigenic drive but improvement in meal-induced satiety. Am J Clin Nutr. 2009;90(4): 921–927.

29. Koutsari C, Hardman AE. Exercise prevents the augmentation of postprandial lipaemia attributable to a low-fat high-carbohydrate diet. Br J Nutr. 2001;86(2):197–205.

30. Koutsari C, Karpe F, Humphreys SM, et al. Exercise prevents the accumulation of triglyceride-rich lipoproteins and their remnants seen when changing to a high-carbohydrate diet. Arterioscler Thromb Vasc Biol. 2001;21(9):1520–1525.

31. Lee IM, Djoussé L, Sesso HD, et al. Physical activity and weight gain prevention. J Am Med Assoc. 2010;303(12):1173–1179.

32. Lee Y-H, Pratley RE. Abdominal obesity and cardiovascular disease risk: the emerging role of the adipocyte. J Cardiopulm Rehabil Prev. 2007;27(1):2–10.

33. Lenz A, Diamond FB. Obesity: the hormonal milieu. Curr Opin Endocrinol Diabetes Obes. 2008;15(1):9–20.

34. Liese AD, Schulz M, Moore CG, et al. Dietary patterns, insulin sensitivity and adiposity in the multi-ethnic Insulin Resistance Atherosclerosis Study population. Br J Nutr. 2004;92(6):973–984.

35. Martins C, Morgan L, Truby H. A review of the effects of exercise on appetite regulation: an obesity perspective. Int J Obes. 2008;32: 1337–1347.

36. Mayer J, Purnima R, Mitra KP. Relation between caloric intake, body weight, and physical work: studies in an industrial male population in West Bengal. Am J Clin Nutr. 1956;4:169–175.

37. National Health and Nutrition Examination Survey Web Site. Available at: http://www.cdc.gov/nchs/nhanes.htm. Accessed June 27, 2008.

38. National Heart, Lung and Blood Institute. Clinical Guidelines on the identification, evaluation and treatment of overweight and obesity in adults. The evidence report. NIH Publication No. 9804083; September 1998.

39. National Heart, Lung and Blood Institute Web Site. Available at: http://www.nhlbi.nih.gov/health/dci/Diseases/obe/obe_diagnosis.html. Accessed June 27, 2008.

40. National Heart, Lung and Blood Institute Web Site. Available at: http://www.nhlbisupport.com/bmi/. Accessed June 27, 2008.

41. Navab M, Gharavi N, Watson AD. Inflammation and metabolic disorders. Curr Opin Clin Nutr Metab Care. 2008;11(4):459–464.

42. Nicklas BJ, Ambrosius W, Messier SP, et al. Diet-induced weight loss, exercise, and chronic inflammation in older, obese adults: a randomized controlled clinical trial. Am J Clin Nutr. 2004; 79(4):544–551.

43. Nordmann AJ, Nordmann A, Briel M, et al. Effects of low-carbohydrate vs low-fat diets on weight loss and cardiovascular risk factors: a meta-analysis of randomized controlled trials. Arch Intern Med. 2006;166(3):285–293.

44. Nutrition recommendations and interventions for diabetes: a position statement of the American Diabetes Association. Diabetes Care. 2008; 31:S61–S78.

45. Rabe K, Lehrke M, Parhofer KG, et al. Adipokines and insulin resistance. Mol Med. 2008; 14(11–12):741–751.

46. Rucker D, Raj P, Li SK, et al. Long term pharmacotherapy for obesity and overweight: updated meta-analysis. BMJ. 2007;335:1194–1203.

47. Sacks FM, Bray GA, Carey VJ, et al. Comparison of weight-loss diets with different compositions of fat, protein, and carbohydrates. N Engl J Med. 2009;360(9):852–873.

48. Sarlio-Lähteenkorva S, Rissanen A, Kaprio A. A descriptive study of weight loss maintenance: 6 and 15 year follow-up of initially overweight adults. Int J Obes Relat Metab Disord. 2000; 24(1):116–125.

49. Serdula MK, Mokdad AH, Williamson DF, et al. Prevalence of attempting weight loss and strategies for controlling weight. JAMA. 1999;282(14): 1353–1358.

50. Strychar I. Diet in the management of weight loss. CMAJ. 2006;174(1):56–63.

51. Tate DF, Jeffery RW, Sherwood NE, et al. Long-term weight losses associated with prescription of higher physical activity goals. Are higher levels of physical activity protective against weight regain? Am J Clin Nutr. 2007;85(4):954–959.

52. Telford RD. Low physical activity and obesity: causes of chronic disease or simply predictors? Med Sci Sports Exerc. 2007;39(8):1233–1240.

53. Thompson WA, Ed. ACSM's Guidelines for Exercise Testing and Prescription. 8th Ed. Baltimore, MD: Lippincott Williams & Wilkins, 2010.

54. Tudor-Locke C, Hatano Y, Pangrazi R, et al. Revisiting "How many steps are enough?" Med Sci Sports Exerc. 2008;40(7S):S537–S543.

55. Turk MW, Yang K, Hravnak M, et al. Randomized clinical trials of weight loss maintenance: a review. J Cardiovasc Nurs. 2009;24(1):58–80.

56. Willett WC, Sacks F, Trichopoulou F, et al. Mediterranean diet pyramid: a cultural model for healthy eating. Am J Clin Nutr. 1995;61:1402S–1406S.

57. Wing RR. Physical activity in the treatment of the adulthood overweight and obesity: current evidence and research issues. Med Sci Sports Exerc. 1999;31(Suppl 11):s547–s552.

58. Wing RR, Phelan S. Long-term weight loss maintenance. Am J Clin Nutr. 2005;82(1):222S–225S.

59. World Health Organization Web Site [Internet]. Geneva, Switzerland: World Health Organization. Available at: http://www.who.int/dietphysicalactivity/publications/facts/obesity/en/. Accessed June 27, 2008.

60. You T, Nicklas BJ. Chronic inflammation: role of adipose tissue and modulation by weight loss. Curr Diabetes Rev. 2006;2(1):29–37.

Type 2 Diabetes Mellitus and Metabolic Syndrome

ABBREVIATIONS

BMI	Body mass index	MUFA	Monounsaturated
CAD	Coronary artery disease		fatty acid
CRF	Cardiorespiratory fitness	PA	Physical activity
CVD	Cardiovascular disease	PUFA	Polyunsaturated fatty acid
GI	Glycemic index	RM	Repetition maximum
GL	Glycemic load	RT	Resistance training
HDL	High-density lipoprotein	WHR	Waist-to-hip ratio
MetS	Metabolic syndrome		

Type 2 diabetes mellitus is a disease of insulin resistance, whereas metabolic syndrome (MetS) is a cluster of pathophysiological conditions related to insulin resistance. Insulin resistance, MetS, and type 2 diabetes are associated with physical inactivity, overweight and obesity, or the excess accumulation of body fat (adipose tissue). Excess fat located in the upper body—waist and trunk—is strongly associated with type 2 diabetes (18). As discussed throughout this book, the increasing prevalence of obesity in the United States has lead to increased incidence of MetS and type 2 diabetes, as well as of other types of chronic diseases (5,24,33). The pathophysiology of type 2 diabetes must be discussed in the context of its relationship to physical inactivity, overweight and obesity, and MetS; thus, we will discuss all three in this chapter, with a more detailed discussion of overweight and obesity in Chapter 6.

Nearly 24 million people in the United States have diabetes and 90% of these cases are of type 2 diabetes. The incidence of type 1 diabetes is low—less than 1% of the population. There are more than 6 million undiagnosed cases of type 2 diabetes. The incidence of type 2 diabetes is higher in men than in women, and among ethnic groups is highest among non-Hispanic African Americans (approximately 12%). Type 2 diabetes doubles in incidence between ages 20 (approximately 10%) and 60 (>20%) (51).

Almost 26% of Americans older than 20 years have impaired fasting glucose and 25% have MetS. These numbers suggest that more than 57 million people have prediabetes, a number that may be in excess of 100 million people within 20 years. Hispanic Americans have the highest rate of MetS among ethnic groups at 32%. The prevalence of type 2 diabetes in Pima Indians of the southwest United States is a startling 50%, and 95% of those with type 2 diabetes are obese (50–52).

A brief note about type 1 diabetes seems appropriate here. Type 1 diabetes has previously been called "juvenile" or "insulin-dependent diabetes." Type 1 diabetes is actually a disease unlike type 2 diabetes in etiology. Type 1 diabetes occurs when the insulin-producing beta cells of the pancreas are destroyed by an autoimmune process (59). As the destruction of these cells progresses, the ability of the pancreas to produce and secrete insulin becomes progressively diminished until exogenous insulin is required. Type 1 diabetes is usually diagnosed in adolescent years, but diagnosis is not uncommon in adulthood. Type 1 diabetes has many of the same complications and pathology in the end organ systems as type 2 diabetes.

PATHOPHYSIOLOGY AND RISK FACTO
FOR METABOLIC SYNDROME

MetS is defined by the characteristics shown in the box be   he National Cholesterol
Education Program specifies that if a person has three of the ti e risk factors, he or she has
MetS (see Fig. 7.1) (23). Those with MetS have a two- to threefold increased risk of having
type 2 diabetes and cardiovascular disease (CVD) as well as mortality from CVD (15,39).
The classification of these risk factors into MetS is not universally accepted; nonetheless,
MetS is related to obesity and type 2 diabetes and people with MetS are at an increased
risk for mortality and morbidity from coronary artery disease (CAD). One study
shows that 75% of men and women with MetS have four of these five risk factors for
CAD (71).

PATHOPHYSIOLOGY OF TYPE 2 DIABETES

Type 2 diabetes is characterized by nearly the same underlying pathophysiology as obesity,
prediabetes, and MetS. Systemic low-level inflammation and endothelial dysfunction—
along with insulin resistance (refer to Chapter 2 for discussions of common pathophysiology), hyperglycemia, abnormal blood lipids, abnormal insulin production and secretion,
central body fat, overweight, and obesity—are hallmarks of this disease (1,24,33). Elevated
triglyceride levels cause inflammation, resulting in both insulin resistance and endothelial
dysfunction (14,21). Thus, the pathophysiology for hyperglycemia, hyperinsulinemia, insulin resistance, MetS, prediabetes, and type 2 diabetes are set in motion (see Fig. 7.6). A
sedentary lifestyle further aggravates these conditions (13,20).

People with type 2 diabetes can have either hypoinsulinemia (producing and/or secreting
too little insulin) or hyperinsulinemia (producing and/or secreting too much insulin). Hyperinsulinemia is usually prevalent early in the course of the disease when increased blood
glucose levels coupled with some level of insulin resistance drive up insulin production and
secretion. As the insulin resistance increases (especially in skeletal muscle), resulting in even

---

DID YOU KNOW?
Metabolic Syndrome* Risk Factors (1,4)

Abdominal obesity (waist circumference)	Men >40 inches Women >35 inches
Hypertriglyceridemia	>150 mg% (or taking medication)
Low high-density lipoprotein cholesterol	Men <40 Women <50 (or on medication)
Elevated blood pressure	>130/>85 mm Hg (or taking medication)
Hyperglycemia	Fasting blood glucose >100
	Glycated hemoglobin >6.5 (or taking medication)

*Metabolic syndrome is defined as having three of the five risk factors described in the table above.

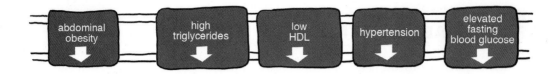

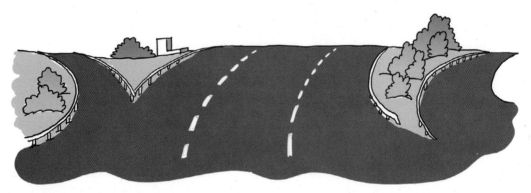

FIGURE 7.1 Metabolic syndrome is defined by the presence of three out of five "risk factors" as depicted above. HDL, high-density lipoprotein.

higher blood glucose levels, the cells in the pancreas that produce insulin can "fatigue" and begin to produce less insulin. Thus, hyperinsulinemia is an early sign of type 2 diabetes; hypoinsulinemia (lack of sufficient insulin) is a later sign (see the box below).

The insulin resistance is thought to be caused by the inflammatory processes (stimulated by proinflammatory adipokines) that cause the insulin receptors to become less sensitive (see above) (34,45). Inflammation and endothelial dysfunction (see Chapters 2 and 5), along with the metabolic abnormalities associated with insulin resistance, significantly impair lipid metabolism; thus, many people with type 2 diabetes also have abnormal blood lipid levels. High levels of triglycerides and low levels of high-density lipoproteins (HDLs) are especially prevalent among those with type 2 diabetes. The pathophysiology of type 2 diabetes is complex and, perhaps, still not sufficiently understood to allow a clear explanation (56).

DID YOU KNOW?

Hypoinsulinemia or Hyperinsulinemia?

How can both be signs of type 2 diabetes? Although this is not always the case, one may lead to the other. Simply stated, over time, the presence of too much insulin in the blood (overproduction by the beta cells of the pancreas), which is a result of insulin resistance, causes the pancreatic beta cells to become unable to produce sufficient insulin. In effect, they become "fatigued." This long-term hyperinsulinemia eventually leads to decreased ability of beta cells to produce insulin; thus, hypoinsulinemia is one outcome. The ability of the beta cells becomes compromised, and the lack of ability to produce insulin is the end result.

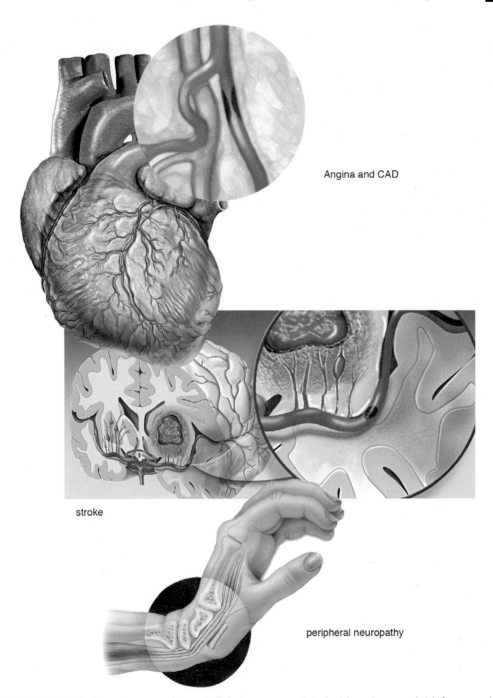

Angina and CAD

stroke

peripheral neuropathy

FIGURE 7.2 Metabolic syndrome and type 2 diabetes are associated with an increased risk for a number of accompanying comorbidities. CAD, coronary artery disease.

It is sufficient to say that insulin resistance is present in type 2 diabetes. Insulin resistance and type 2 diabetes develop slowly; progression of the initial, "nonclinical" insulin resistance to full-blown hyperglycemia (the high blood glucose level that is clinically diagnostic of type 2 diabetes) may take up to 10 years (see Fig. 7.2) (56). Unfortunately, the pathophysiology connected to the complications of hyperglycemia and inflammation may effect end-organ tissue prior to formal diagnosis.

Diagnostic Criteria for Prediabetes and type 2 diabetes (6)

Categories of Increased Risk (Prediabetes)
Impaired fasting* glucose: 100–125 mg/dl
Impaired glucose tolerance: 140–199 mg/dl (75 g oral glucose tolerance test)
Glycated hemoglobin: 5.7%–6.4%
Criteria for the Diagnosis of type 2 diabetes
Glycated hemoglobin: ≥6.5%
Fasting plasma glucose: ≥126 mg/dl (7.0 mmol/l)
2-hour plasma glucose: ≥200 mg/dl (11.1 mmol/l) during an oral glucose tolerance test

*Fasting is defined as no caloric intake for at least 8 hours.

A condition termed "prediabetes" (by the American Diabetes Association) is also prevalent among much of the population. The same pathophysiology underlies prediabetes—obesity, inflammation, insulin resistance, and hyperglycemia but at a level that does not cause overt symptoms. However, these individuals are characterized as having "impaired fasting glucose" or "impaired glucose tolerance" (3).

DIETARY PATTERN, TYPE 2 DIABETES, AND MetS

The pathophysiology of type 2 diabetes is tied closely to obesity (as stated above) and to physical inactivity (12,61). It is also strongly connected to dietary pattern, and in this section, we will discuss foods and nutrients related to the pathophysiology of MetS and type 2 diabetes, as well as what foods and nutrients are known to be preventive and may assist in correcting the underlying pathophysiology (21). An optimal prevention program includes optimal nutritional practices. A detailed discussion of dietary patterns and health can be found in Chapter 4. The American Diabetes Association in its Practice Guidelines makes specific recommendations about nutrition and energy balance (see Table 7.1 for these recommendations).

It is difficult to separate the implications of obesity and excess adipose tissue from those of diet and nutrition (see above, as well as Chapters 4 and 6). Indeed, one of the defining factors considered in the definition of MetS is waist circumference or abdominal obesity. Weight loss and/or maintenance of normal body weight are critical components of an optimal prevention program for either type 2 diabetes or MetS.

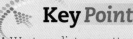

Key Point

A Western dietary pattern with a high intake of saturated fat, simple and refined carbohydrates, and processed meats is directly related to the pathophysiology and, therefore, the incidence of type 2 diabetes.

The impact of dietary pattern can be viewed from a number of different vantage points; we will discuss only those dietary influences that have been shown to be preventive or that are associated with increased risk and prevalence of type 2 diabetes and MetS. In addition, the dietary pattern that prevents or improves the pathophysiology (inflammation) that is associated with all four disorders—obesity, MetS, prediabetes, and type 2 diabetes—is of primary importance (see Fig. 7.3).

TABLE 7.1	American Diabetes Association Recommendations on Nutrition* and Diabetes (3)	

Category	Recommendations	Level of Evidence
Energy balance	• In overweight and obese insulin-resistant individuals, modest weight loss has been shown to improve insulin resistance. Thus, weight loss is recommended for all such individuals who have or are at risk for diabetes.	A
	• For weight loss, either low-carbohydrate or low-fat, calorie-restricted diets may be effective in the short term (up to 1 year)	A
	• For patients on low-carbohydrate diets, monitor lipid profiles, renal function, and protein intake (in those with nephropathy), and adjust hypoglycemic therapy as needed	E
	• Physical activity and behavior modification are important components of weight loss programs and are most helpful in maintenance of weight loss.	B
	• Weight loss medications may be considered in the treatment of overweight and obese individuals with type 2 diabetes and can help achieve a 5%–10% weight loss when combined with lifestyle modification	B
	• Bariatric surgery may be considered for some individuals with type 2 diabetes and BMI 35 kg/m^2 and can result in marked improvements in glycemia. The long-term benefits and risks of bariatric surgery in individuals with prediabetes or diabetes continue to be studied	B
Nutrition intervention	• Among individuals at high risk for developing type 2 diabetes, structured programs that emphasize lifestyle changes that include moderate weight loss (7% body weight) and regular physical activity (150 min/wk), with dietary strategies including reduced calories and reduced intake of dietary fat, can reduce the risk for developing diabetes and are therefore recommended	A
	• Individuals at high risk for type 2 diabetes should be encouraged to achieve the U.S. Department of Agriculture (USDA) recommendation for dietary fiber (14 g fiber per 1,000 kcal) and foods containing whole grains (one-half of grain intake)	B
	• There is not sufficient, consistent information to conclude that low–glycemic load diets reduce the risk for diabetes. Nevertheless, low–glycemic index foods that are rich in fiber and other important nutrients are to be encouraged	E

(continued)

TABLE 7.1	American Diabetes Association Recommendations on Nutrition* and Diabetes (3) (continued)	

Category	Recommendations	Level of Evidence
	• Observational studies report that moderate alcohol intake may reduce the risk for diabetes, but the data do not support recommending alcohol consumption to individuals at risk of diabetes	B
	• No nutrition recommendation can be made for preventing type 1 diabetes	E
	• Although there are insufficient data at present to warrant any specific recommendations for prevention of type 2 diabetes in youth, it is reasonable to apply approaches demonstrated to be effective in adults, as long as nutritional needs for normal growth and development are maintained	E
Secondary prevention	• A dietary pattern that includes carbohydrate from fruits, vegetables, whole grains, legumes, and low-fat milk is encouraged for good health	B
	• Monitoring carbohydrate, whether by carbohydrate counting, exchanges, or experienced-based estimation, remains a key strategy in achieving glycemic control	A
	• The use of glycemic index and load may provide a modest additional benefit over that observed when total carbohydrate is considered alone	B
	• Sucrose-containing foods can be substituted for other carbohydrates in the meal plan or, if added to the meal plan, covered with insulin or other glucose-lowering medications. Care should be taken to avoid excess energy intake	A
	• As for the general population, people with diabetes are encouraged to consume various fiber-containing foods. However, evidence is lacking to recommend a higher fiber intake for people with diabetes than for the population as a whole	B
	• Sugar alcohols and nonnutritive sweeteners are safe when consumed within the daily intake levels established by the Food and Drug Administration	A
Dietary fat and cholesterol	• Limit saturated fat to <7% of total calories	A
	• Intake of trans fat should be minimized	E
	• In individuals with diabetes, limit dietary cholesterol to <200 mg/day	E
	• Two or more servings of fish per week (with the exception of commercially fried fish filets) provide n-3 polyunsaturated fatty acids and are recommended	B

TABLE 7.1	American Diabetes Association Recommendations on Nutrition* and Diabetes (3) (continued)	
Category	**Recommendations**	**Level of Evidence**
Protein	• For individuals with diabetes and normal renal function, there is insufficient evidence to suggest that usual protein intake (15%–20% of energy) should be modified	E
	• In individuals with type 2 diabetes, ingested protein can increase insulin response without increasing plasma glucose concentrations. Therefore, protein should not be used to treat acute or prevent nighttime hypoglycemia	A
	• High-protein diets are not recommended as a method for weight loss at this time. The long-term effects of protein intake >20% of calories on diabetes management and its complications are unknown. Although such diets may produce short-term weight loss and improved glycemia, it has not been established that these benefits are maintained long term, and long-term effects on kidney function for persons with diabetes are unknown	E
Nutrition interventions for type 2 diabetes	• Individuals with type 2 diabetes are encouraged to implement lifestyle modifications that reduce intakes of energy, saturated and trans fatty acids, cholesterol, and sodium and to increase physical activity in an effort to improve glycemia, dyslipidemia, and blood pressure	E

*Plasma glucose monitoring can be used to determine whether adjustments in foods and meals will be sufficient to achieve blood glucose goals or if medication(s) needs to be combined with Medical Nutrition Therapy.

BMI, body mass index.

Reprinted with permission from American Diabetes Association, Bantle JP, Wylie-Rosett J, et al. Nutrition recommendations and interventions for diabetes: a position statement of the American Diabetes Association. Diabetes Care. 2008;31(Suppl 1):S61–S78.

Weight loss and a low-fat, low-refined-carbohydrate, and high-fiber diet with regular exercise are the primary components of the optimal lifestyle for preventing and managing prediabetes, type 2 diabetes, and MetS. Both are extremely effective in reversing the inflammation, insulin resistance, hyperglycemia, and/or lipid abnormalities that are all part of obesity and type 2 diabetes (6,26,40,53,59,69). In addition, it is clear that caloric restriction is extremely effective in modifying the pathophysiology of type 2 diabetes (25,65,66). It is difficult to separate the effects of the cutting back on calories from the effects of exercise, weight loss, and other nutritional changes. It is safe to conclude that exercise, weight loss, and cutting calories are all of great importance in overcoming the pathophysiology of type 2 diabetes (6,53).

Therefore, this discussion will not focus on the effectiveness of weight loss, coupled with caloric restriction and exercise, in preventing type 2 diabetes, MetS, and prediabetes as well as the underlying pathophysiology. Basic principles of weight-loss programs are discussed in Chapter 6 on Obesity.

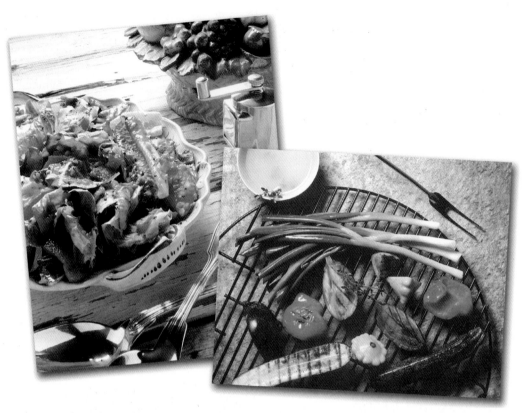

FIGURE 7.3 The Indo-Mediterranean dietary pattern has been shown to prevent type 2 diabetes as well as moderate the accompanying pathophysiology.

Energy Balance and Weight Loss

Weight loss and exercise are the primary considerations for lifestyle treatment of all three conditions. One important lifestyle consideration is to obtain and maintain an ideal body weight, through a low-fat, high-fiber diet and regular exercise and physical activity (PA) (see Fig. 7.4). Losing even a small amount of weight (5%–10% of body weight) is beneficial for insulin resistance, triglycerides, HDL, inflammation, and so forth (40,41,49,64,68).

The balance between caloric expenditure and caloric intake (energy balance) is the key to losing weight. Studies have demonstrated that groups of identical twins may respond differently to identical caloric intake, resulting in different amounts of weight gain or loss in among groups of twins (but not between identical twins) overfed by the same amount (see Fig. 7.5) (8). Therefore, the physiological response to caloric consumption may differ from person to person; thus, the old adage "a calorie is a calorie" may not be always true. It is clear that the daily balance of calorie intake and expenditure according to one's own physiology is the key.

Regardless of individual response, the long-term principle for successful weight loss remains caloric (energy) balance and energy flux. Increasing energy expenditure through increasing both regular exercise and overall daily activity levels is critical to successful weight loss and maintenance, thus to prevention of type 2 diabetes (19). Combining increased energy expenditure with decreased caloric intake are the key basic principles of effective weight loss programs.

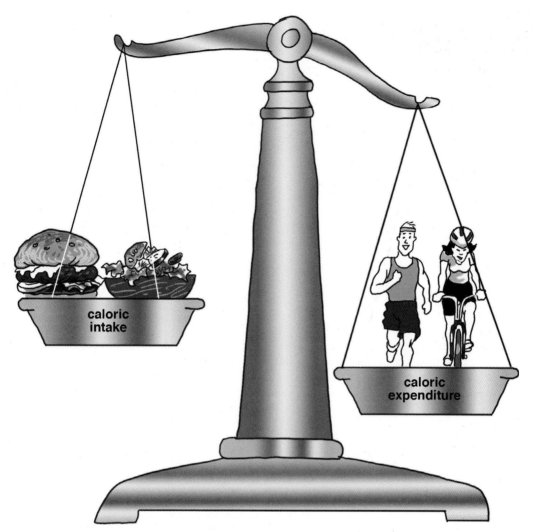

FIGURE 7.4 Establishing a "negative" balance between caloric expenditure and caloric intake on the side of increased caloric expenditure is one key to weight loss to prevent type 2 diabetes.

DIETARY CONTENT—CARBOHYDRATES AND GLYCEMIC LOAD

The effectiveness of decreasing the intake of simple and refined carbohydrates, as well as the effect of increasing the intake of complex carbohydrates (along with increased PA and weight loss), on preventing type 2 diabetes (both primary and secondary prevention) is supported by two studies: one called the "Finnish Diabetes Prevention Study" (46) and the other the US Diabetes Prevention Program (41). A low-fat, high-fiber diet coupled with exercise in persons with prediabetes was effective not only in reducing weight (5%–10%) but also in reducing the risk for diabetes compared with other diets that were either higher in fat or lower in fiber or both (46). Thus, high fruit and vegetable intake and high fiber and low fat (especially low saturated fat) intake are effective in preventing diabetes.

Consumption of large amounts of simple and processed carbohydrates, especially foods containing high amounts of sugar such as sweetened cereals, soft drinks sweetened with

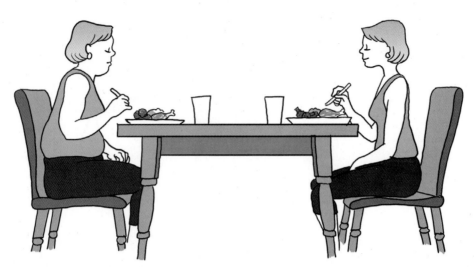

FIGURE 7.5 Some studies demonstrate the importance of genes in chronic disease. However, despite the genetic predisposition, the influence of the environment (health behaviors such as diet and exercise) is paramount in the development of type 2 diabetes.

high fructose corn syrup, or foods high in simple or refined carbohydrates (white bread, white rice, pasta, etc.), causes a large influx of glucose to the bloodstream almost immediately upon eating (13,21,32). In addition, increased blood glucose levels result in secretion of insulin from the pancreas in an attempt to reduce blood glucose levels by facilitating uptake in muscle, brain, and other cells (Fig. 7.6).

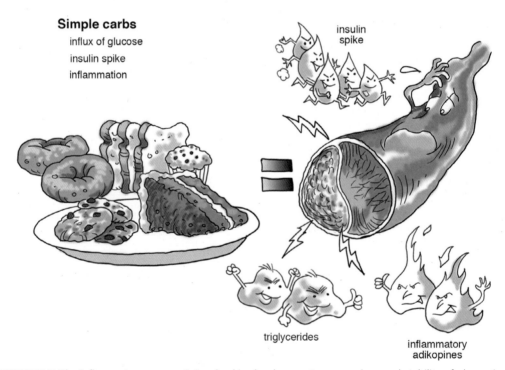

FIGURE 7.6 The inflammatory process is involved in development, progression, and stability of plaque in arteries.

A group of researchers at Harvard University has been following the health of more than 160,000 nurses in the United States for many years (Harvard Nurses Study) (47). They have demonstrated that a higher intake of whole grains is associated with decreased risk for type 2 diabetes in their population. A meta-analysis combined the Harvard nurses with 120,000 additional subjects (statistically) for a total population of more than 280,000. The group with the highest intake of whole grains (>40 g/day) had almost 25% less type 2 diabetes than the group with the lowest intake (<3 g/day) (25,47).

Another study (see Chapter 1) compared a well-known diabetes drug (metformin) to diet and exercise for prevention of diabetes. In this case, the lifestyle worked significantly better than the drug (41). The diet in this study consisted of a "healthy, low-fat, low-calorie diet and 150 minutes of exercise per week." The lifestyle group members lost 7% of their body weight (between 4 and 8 kg during 3 years of study), and the reduction in type 2 diabetes in the lifestyle group was 58% compared to 31% in the group on the drug (41).

In summary, two of the largest diabetes prevention studies ever performed (Finnish Diabetes Prevention study and US Diabetes Prevention Program) showed that diet and exercise are extremely effective in preventing type 2 diabetes in persons with prediabetes. The optimal diet is one consisting of high levels of complex carbohydrates such as fruits and vegetables, beans, whole grains, lean protein, low levels of saturated and trans fat, and increased levels of monounsaturated fatty acids (MUFA) and polyunsaturated fatty acids (PUFA). This high-fiber, low–saturated fat diet is effective in preventing type 2 diabetes, even in the absence of significant weight loss (16,64).

> **Optimize**
>
> ### Energy Balance
>
> Maintain optimal body weight based on body mass index (BMI), waist circumference, or waist-to-hip ratio (WHR).
>
> - Isocaloric diet if BMI is <25.0 or if
>   - ➤ Male with waist <40 or WHR <0.95
>   - ➤ Female with waist <35 or WHR <0.86
> - Hypocaloric diet if BMI is >25.0 or if
>   - ➤ Male with waist >40 or WHR >0.9
>   - ➤ Female with waist >35 or WHR >0.8

NUTRIENTS AND PATHOPHYSIOLOGY OF TYPE 2 DIABETES AND METS

The "postprandial state" describes the physiological state of the blood immediately after eating a meal. The postprandial state is important because the physiological changes that are related to the pathophysiology accompanying chronic diseases are often initiated by consumption of food. Figure 7.7 shows some of the effects of the postprandial state on the pathophysiology of type 2 diabetes, especially after a high-fat meal. More specifically, the amount of lipids in the blood (called "postprandial lipemia") is predictive of morbidity and mortality from heart attack (1). Postprandial lipemia is proinflammatory, increases insulin resistance, and decreases endothelial function. All are associated with the presence of type 2 diabetes as well as MetS.

Dietary composition is a driving force in the pathophysiology of inflammation and insulin resistance (4,32). Dietary composition can be subdivided by fat, carbohydrate, and protein, along with micronutrients and macronutrients (see Chapter 4). We will discuss the effects of various types of fat (e.g., monounsaturated and saturated) and carbohydrates, as well as some macronutrients, on the inflammatory state and insulin resistance.

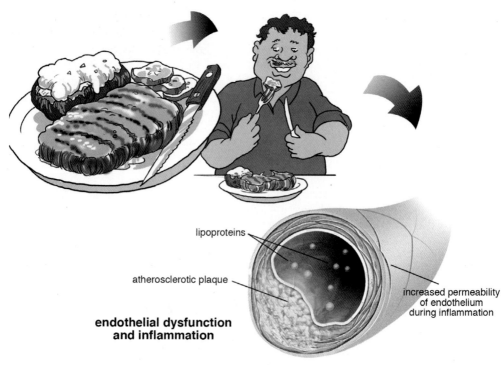

FIGURE 7.7 Postprandial lipemia results from consuming a high-fat meal and is characterized by the influx of lipids (lipoproteins and triglycerides) into the blood.

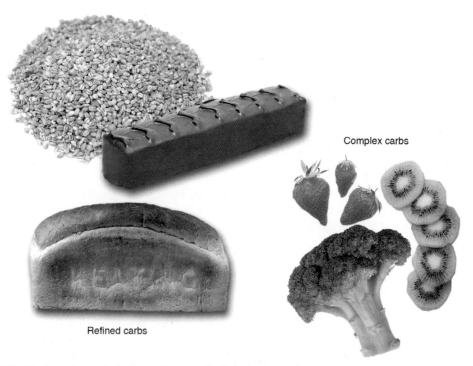

FIGURE 7.8 Complex carbohydrates increase the length of time for digestion to occur and moderate the influx of insulin. These are positive effects of decreasing refined carbohydrates and increasing complex in dietary pattern.

Glycemic Index and Glycemic Load

Glycemic Index: This measures how rapidly a food breaks down into glucose in the blood. The GI of glucose (e.g., white sugar) is 100; thus, this is the "reference" food. Foods with a GI of <60 are better choices because they do not break down as quickly and generally contain greater amounts of fiber and complex carbohydrates.

Glycemic Load: This measure is similar to GI, but it also attempts to add the extent to which a particular carbohydrate affects blood glucose. GL takes into account the GI, the type, and the serving size of the food.

Some common foods, along with their GI and GL (according to portion size), are listed in Table 7.2. An excellent and informative Web site is located at www.glycemicindex.com.

Simple and refined carbohydrates and saturated and trans fat are proinflammatory. Meals containing high amounts of these foods increase insulin secretion, insulin resistance, and fat mobilization into the blood while decreasing glucose utilization (see Fig. 7.8). In addition, these increase low-density lipoprotein levels, triglyceride levels, and inflammatory adipokines while lowering HDL levels. In short, these produce changes that make the low-level, systemic inflammation worse and are harmful to people who have or are susceptible to prediabetes, MetS, and type 2 diabetes (12,17,32). On the other hand, foods such as complex carbohydrates, high-fiber foods, MUFA, PUFA, omega-3 fats, and foods rich in polyphenols or flavonoids all promote vascular health and are anti-inflammatory (4,6,56,66).

Two measures often used to determine the influence of food, especially carbohydrates, on postprandial state are glycemic load (GL) and glycemic index (GI). GI is a number that reflects the action of a particular food on blood sugar. Refined sugar has a GI of 100. GL takes into account both the GI and the relative carbohydrate content of the food, and therefore may be a better measure of the effect of that food on blood glucose and metabolic status (see Chapter 4 for more information). Diets with high GL are proinflammatory, and decreasing the GL decreases or prevents the inflammatory response (see Fig. 7.9) (4,28,32). The box below and Table 7.2 further explain GI and GL as well as provide some examples of foods and their GI/GL.

Optimize

Carbohydrate Intake

	Daily calories (%)	Grams per day
Total carbohydrates	50–55 (95% complex)	200 (may be higher with regular, vigorous exercise) (190 complex)
Simple carbohydrates/ sugar	<5	20–25
Fiber		>30–45

Optimal Carbohydrate Intake

- Insoluble fiber from fruits, vegetables, beans, nuts, legumes, and whole grains is recommended as the primary source of this fiber.
- Weight-loss diets should utilize whole grains to replace most, if not all, of the carbohydrates from refined and processed grain carbohydrates.
- Simple sugars should be replaced either by eliminating sweeteners and foods and beverages sweetened by simple sugars or by using limited amounts of natural products such as honey (<5% of total calories).

TABLE 7.2	Glycemic Index and Glycemic Load of Common Foods (31,64)	
Food	**Glycemic Index**	**Glycemic Load**
Potatoes, baked	98	High
Carrots	85	Low
Corn	70	Low
Pot, red boiled	58	Medium
Green peas	51	Low
Sweet potatoes	50	Medium
Tomatoes	38	Low
Black beans	30	Low
Kidney beans	29	Low
Lentils	29	Low
Cantaloupe	65	Low
Banana	60	Medium
Kiwi	52	Low
Grapes	50	Low
Pears	45	Low
Orange	40	Low
Apple	40	Low
Strawberries	32	Low
Peaches	30	Low
Prunes	29	Low
Grapefruit	26	Low
Cherries	23	Low
Instant rice	87	High
Corn tortilla	72	Low
White rice	70	High
Corn meal	68	Low
Taco shells	68	Low
Refined pasta	65	High
Couscous	61	High
Brown rice	55	Medium
Air popped popcorn	55	Low
Whole wheat pasta	45	Medium

Source: Available from www.glycemicindex.com.

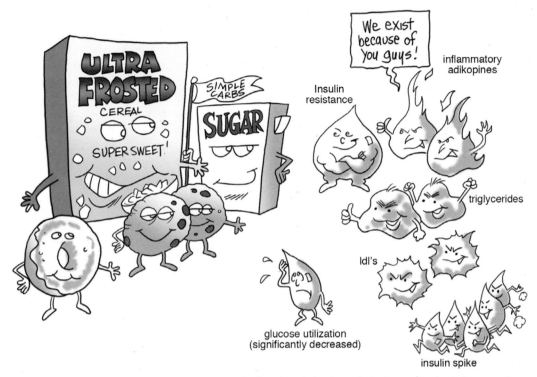

FIGURE 7.9 Consumption of large amounts of refined and simple carbohydrates results in increased insulin outflow, fat metabolism, adipokine production, and inflammation.

PREVENTING TYPE 2 DIABETES AND MᴇᴛS WITH DIET

Specific diet composition has been shown to prevent the pathophysiology associated with MetS, prediabetes, and type 2 diabetes independent of weight loss. Increasing amounts of MUFA, PUFA, omega-3 fats, complex carbohydrates, and fiber have all been shown to reverse inflammation, endothelial dysfunction, and insulin resistance. Dietary pattern is related to decreased death rate from heart disease and other chronic disease (11,21). Similar results have been reported for whole grain intake (47).

Chapter 4 contains more detail on diet, but the Mediterranean dietary pattern has been demonstrated to be effective in preventing chronic disease, including prediabetes, type 2 diabetes, and heart disease (71).

OPTIMAL EXERCISE FOR THOSE WITH TYPE 2 DIABETES AND MᴇᴛS

Exercise and prevention of the pathophysiology present in many chronic diseases was discussed in detail in Chapter 3. Whether the preventive benefits come from PA or cardiorespiratory fitness (CRF) is controversial, but in reality, both are necessary for optimal health. Review the "Digging Deeper" section in Chapter 3 for a detailed discussion of this controversy.

Optimize

Dietary Composition

The values below (portion of total calories) summarize specific optimal dietary pattern* recommendations for the prevention of type 2 diabetes (56).

Fat: 15%–25%
Saturated fat: ≤5%
Trans fat: <1%
MUFA: 5%–12%
PUFA: 5%–10% (omega-3 fatty acids)
Cholesterol: <150 mg/day
Fiber: 30–40 g/day total soluble and insoluble fiber
Omega-3: 1 g/day (EPA, eicosapentaenoic acid; DHA, docosahexaenoic acid) in addition to 1 g/day of ALA, alpha-linoleic acid

*Include functional foods (e.g., stanols, increased soluble fiber).

There is substantial information showing that higher levels of exercise, PA, and CRF are protective for MetS, prediabetes, and type 2 diabetes (4,6,46,57). Besides improving insulin resistance and endothelial function, PA and CRF are also related to lower levels of systemic inflammation and improved insulin sensitivity (decreased insulin resistance) and glucose metabolism (4,6,7,12,26,32,35,65,66). In addition, several large epidemiological studies (one with more than 200,000 subjects) have shown that increased PA and intensity of exercise reduces the incidence of type 2 diabetes among both men and women (36,38). In addition, PA reduces the death rate associated with heart disease among people with type 2 diabetes (36,38). It has also been shown that low CRF and PA (sedentary lifestyle) are related to increased prevalence of prediabetes, MetS, and type 2 diabetes (5,65).

Tanasescu et al., in a meta-analysis, concluded that body composition and "vigorous" activity are important in the pathophysiology of these diseases (60). In fact, the protective effect is most significant when exercise and weight loss or weight maintenance of ideal body weight are part of the lifestyle change. Thus, the optimal exercise program includes high amounts of daily activity, leisure-time PA, regular vigorous exercise, and a weight-loss program that includes exercise for those whose weight is above the ideal body weight. In another study, Boule et al. (9) concluded that vigorous exercise was more effective in increasing VO_2 max and in decreasing glycated hemoglobin (Hb A_{1c}). This and other research indicates that the exercise portion of the program should be relatively vigorous (>75% VO_2 reserve) and that losing body weight (5%–10% of total body weight) is helpful for improving insulin resistance and Hb A_{1c} (9,60).

Two important studies demonstrate the effectiveness of PA and CRF in decreasing mortality from heart disease and other chronic diseases among people with type 2 diabetes. Church et al. found that men who had a low fitness level and were not active had higher mortality than men in higher fitness categories (moderate and high) who were normal weight, overweight, or obese (12). This finding is important in that it demonstrates the contribution of PA and CRF in both normal and overweight populations. Regardless of weight, PA and CRF are protective (12).

Kokkinos et al. used the Aerobics Center database of men with estimated CRF levels to examine a similar question among African Americans and white men (42). This study demonstrates a dose–response effect of CRF. Each one metabolic-equivalent increment of increased CRF yielded 16% lower mortality for CVD in these men diagnosed with and treated for type 2 diabetes.

The relationship between obesity and type 2 diabetes, as well as the relationship with MetS and prediabetes, highlights another important factor. An exercise program should promote weight loss and, in particular, prevention of weight regain. Cardiovascular endurance exercise is the most efficient activity to both expend calories and increase fitness and to be effective for weight management. Higher CRF levels are associated with lower levels of insulin resistance (and impaired glucose tolerance) and type 2 diabetes (44). Interestingly, it has also been demonstrated that exercise in a weight-loss program, *even without weight loss*, decreases the risk for type 2 diabetes and insulin resistance

(43,64). Importantly, in this study, subjects who benefited from exercise without significant weight loss did approximately 4 hours/week of cardiovascular endurance exercise.

Optimal lifestyle for either the prevention or management of MetS, prediabetes, or type 2 diabetes includes exercise and weight loss. However, given the results stated in the Finnish study mentioned earlier, significant benefits can be obtained from about 45 to 60 minutes of moderate-intensity exercise at least 5 to 7 days per week. Some of the most beneficial effects of exercise in these diseases (MetS and type 2 diabetes) are the subacute effects that have been discussed in Chapter 3. Briefly, these effects occur subsequent to a single exercise session but are diminished or disappear within 6 to 24 hours after the exercise. Increased insulin sensitivity is one of these effects, as is enhanced glucose metabolism (37). The intensity of the exercise may also be a significant factor in promoting some of the important changes that prevent and moderate type 2 diabetes, thus supporting the Finnish conclusions that "moderate"-intensity PA (mostly walking in that study) is necessary to facilitate some of the beneficial changes (64).

Exercise increases insulin sensitivity. Both single exercise sessions and chronic exercise training are associated with the increase. Single exercise sessions cause temporary changes in insulin sensitivity related to the total energy expenditure of the exercise, rather than intensity (30). In addition, it is known that individuals with higher cardiovascular fitness have greater insulin sensitivity after a single session of exercise than do less fit individuals (8,30,37). Therefore, persons who exercise on a regular basis obtain the beneficial subacute effects of increased insulin sensitivity. This means that there is benefit to both single sessions of activity (being active and exercising on a daily basis) and increasing fitness levels through regular exercise.

We can, therefore, provide basic principles for an optimal exercise program for those with MetS, prediabetes, and type 2 diabetes. Sixty minutes of cardiovascular endurance exercise per day, coupled with lifestyle activity equivalent to 10,000 to 15,000 steps per day, is optimal (60). Thus, exercise is effective in reducing type 2 diabetes, decreasing insulin resistance and impaired glucose tolerance, and in reducing MetS.

Key Point

Diet and PA (exercise and leisure time PA) are intimately related to type 2 diabetes. A lifestyle that includes both increased levels of PA and CRF, along with a healthy dietary pattern, is required for optimal prevention.

Optimize

Exercise for Type 2 Diabetes and MetS

Frequency	6–7 Days Per Week
Intensity (include both high- and moderate-intensity exercise)	Moderate to vigorous: heart rate in the range of 40%–75% HRR (85%–90% of total weekly duration)
	High: heart rate in the range of 75%–85% HRR (10%–15% of total weekly duration)
Duration	60 minutes per day; may be divided into shorter sessions but not <15 minutes and preferably at least one session >30 minutes
Type	Walking or other weight-bearing exercise is preferred; swimming or aerobics may be substituted; resistance training can be used as an adjunct
Caloric expenditure	Caloric expenditure should equal >2,000 kcal/week outside of normal daily activities

HRR, heart rate reserve.

DIGGING DEEPER

Resistance Training in Diabetes

Resistance training (RT) has been shown to effectively enhance several fitness-related varia-bles. RT is effective for improving muscular strength and endurance. It has also been shown to be effective for changing the risk factors for CAD (10,22,48,58,62). Indeed, the health benefits from RT are similar to those from cardiovascular endurance, assuming the exercise prescription for RT is appropriate (Table 7.3) (10,22).

Moderate- to high-intensity RT, including circuit training (which is actually a combina-tion of RT and CV endurance training), is associated with increases in lean tissue (muscle), which, in turn, has effects on lipid and glucose metabolism, insulin resistance and insulin sensitivity, and metabolic control and Hb A_{1c} (22). All of these effects are beneficial for those with MetS, prediabetes, and type 2 diabetes and are preventive measures for type 2 diabetes, MetS, and CAD. Thus, prevention of type 2 diabetes and MetS is included in the effects of properly prescribed RT that is done on a regular basis to supplement a program of cardiovascular endurance training (22).

Optimize

Resistance Training for Those with Type 2 Diabetes and MetS

Frequency: 2–3 days per week
Intensity: 2–3 sets; 8–12 repetitions per set at 60%–80% 1 RM
Type: 8–10 multijoint exercises; all major muscle groups in same or split sessions; emphasize proper technique and caution against Val-salva maneuver to prevent exagger-ated blood pressure response

The recommendation of the American Col-lege of Sports Medicine for the RT exercise pre-scription is 60% to 80% one repetition maximum (RM) for resistance (62). One RM is the maxi-mum amount of resistance that can be lifted one time. A program that is inclusive of 60% to 80% is relatively high intensity. Table 7.4 presents a sample ("optimal") RT program appropriate for those with type 2 diabetes. This program should be combined with cardiovascular endurance training, preferably at a minimum of 3 days per week of RT combined with cardiovascular endur-ance and high levels of activity for best results.

Many of the complications of type 2 diabetes are vascular in nature. People with type 2 diabe-tes are at significantly increased risk of having CAD, and, in fact, the standard of care in lipid management is that people with type 2 diabetes be treated *as if they have CAD* (24,33). It is clear that appropriately prescribed and per-formed RT can modify many of the risk factors for CAD, as well as the pathophysiology that is associated with type 2 diabetes, obesity, MetS, and CAD (10,22,54).

Some of the changes include moderating the inflammation that is present in type 2 diabetes and obesity—improved glucose metabolism, improved endothelial function, weight loss, and positive changes in both HDL and low-density lipoprotein levels are pre-ventive for CAD (10,22,54). These changes seem to be associated mainly with circuit and moderately high intensity RT, rather than lighter intensity (muscular endurance training) or muscular strength training.

RT can be an excellent adjunct to a cardiovascular endurance program for people with prediabetes, MetS, and type 2 diabetes. We believe, however, that it should not be the sole method of exercise and that cardiovascular endurance exercise should be the centerpiece of such programs. The effects of cardiovascular endurance programs coupled with the simplicity and the ease of implementing in most populations make them more suited to facilitate the desired outcomes (Table 7.3).

TABLE 7.3	Benefits of Resistance Training on Various Physiological Variables (7,14,22,38,48,58)

Risk Factors	Effect of Risk Factor Apparently Healthy	Type 2 Diabetes	Notes
Glucose tolerance	NA	↑	Reduction of acute response to glucose tolerance test; decreased Hb A$_{1c}$; decreased use of insulin
Glycemic control, Hb A$_{1c}$	NA	↑, ±	Improved if hyperglycemia is present in one study
Insulin sensitivity	↑	↑	In hyperglycemia and glycemic clamps during hyperinsulinemia
Insulin dose	NA	↓	Improved in both type 1 diabetes studies
Hypertension	↓, ↑, ±	±	
Blood pressure	↓	±	Significant but small decrease caused by RT
Arterial stiffness	↓, ↑, ±	Unknown	Mixed results from research
Endothelial function	↑	↑	One controlled study demonstrates ↑ flow-mediated dilation in overweight women
Obesity prevention	±	↑	Rationale provides positive effects, but is not yet confirmed
Obesity	↓, ±	↓	Modest weight loss with increased muscle mass
Visceral adipose tissue	↓	↓	May be gender specific
Fat-free mass	±	↑	
High-density lipoprotein	±, ↑	↓, ±	Changes with circuit training or AT combined with RT
Low-density lipoprotein	↓, ±	Unknown	
Cardiovascular endurance fitness	↑	↑	Circuit training increases VO$_2$ significantly, but less than aerobic training

↓, decrease; ↑, increase or improved; ±, no effect.

AT, aerobic training; RT, resistance training.

Adapted from Braith RW, Stewart KJ. Resistance exercise training: its role in the prevention of cardiovascular disease. Circulation. 2006;113:2642–2650; Eves ND, Plotnikoff RC. Resistance training and type 2 diabetes: consideration for implementation at the population level. Diabetes Care. 2006;29(8):1933–1941.

TABLE 7.4 Sample Resistance Training Program for Type 2 Diabetes and Metabolic Syndrome

Period	Weeks	Reps (#/set)	Sets	Load (%1 RM)	Rest (seconds)	RPE (6–20 scale)	Speed (seconds)	Structure	Frequency (hours between)
One (linear)	0–6	11–15	1–3	50–70	60	11–14	3 sec Ecc 2 sec Con	Total body Workout Each session Super sets	Every 48 hours
Two (linear)	7–12	7–10	2–4	70–90	90	13–16 last set to fatigue	3 sec Ecc 2 sec Con	Total body Workout Each session Super sets	Every 48 hours
Three (linear)	13–18	3–6	3–5	80–100	90–120	16–19	3 sec Ecc 3–4 sec Con	Total body Workout Each session Do each exercise separately	Every 48 hours
Four (undulating)	19–24	Day 1–11–15 Day 2–6–10 Day 3–2–5	2–4 3–5 4–6	60–80 75–90 85–100	30–60 60–90 90–120	12–15 15–17 16–19	3 E/2 C 3 E/2 C 3 E/3–4 C	Total body Super set Super set Each separately	Every 48 hours

1 RM, maximum weight lifted for one repetition; Ecc or E, eccentric contraction; Con or C, concentric contraction; total body workout, all major upper, lower body, and trunk muscles worked in same session; super set, alternating push/pull (i.e., shoulder presses alternated with lat pull down behind neck) or agonist/antagonist pattern; each separately, all sets of one exercise followed by all sets of the antagonistic exercise (i.e., bench press then underhand chin sets). RPE, rating of perceived exertion.

RPE, rating of perceived exertion.

TABLE 7.5	Nutrient Effects on Postprandial State and Pathophysiology	
Nutrient	**Postprandial State**	**Pathophysiology**
Carbohydrates		
Refined and simple	➢ Increased ➢ Triglycerides ➢ Increased insulin secretion ➢ Increased insulin resistance ➢ Decreased glucose utilization ➢ Increased fat mobilization	➢ Increased inflammatory substances ➢ Increased adipokines ➢ Decreased endothelial function
Complex, fiber	➢ Increased HDL ➢ Decreased insulin secretion ➢ Increased insulin resistance	➢ Decreased inflammatory substances ➢ Improved endothelial function
Fats		
Saturated fat, trans fat	➢ Increased LDL, cholesterol ➢ Increased insulin resistance ➢ Increased oxidized LDL ➢ Increased fat mobilization	➢ Increased inflammatory substances ➢ Increased proinflammatory adipokines ➢ Decreased endothelial function
Monounsaturated fat, polyunsaturated fat	➢ Increased LDL, cholesterol ➢ Increased insulin resistance ➢ Increased oxidized LDL ➢ Increased fat mobilization	➢ Increased inflammatory substances ➢ Increased proinflammatory adipokines ➢ Decreased endothelial function
Omega-3	➢ Increased LDL, cholesterol ➢ Increased insulin resistance ➢ Increased oxidized LDL ➢ Increased fat mobilization	➢ Increased inflammatory substances ➢ Increased proinflammatory adipokines ➢ Decreased endothelial function

HDL, high-density lipoprotein; LDL, low-density lipoprotein.

Significant RESEARCH

Two articles fit this category for this chapter. The first is a straightforward account of the role of dietary carbohydrates in obesity, MetS, and type 2 diabetes by Griel and colleagues (32). The alarming increase in the rate of overweight and obesity during the past 25 years, as well as the increased interest in low-carbohydrate diets, merits some additional reading. Paired with this, we recommend an article by Basu and colleagues (4) that discusses the influence of diet on inflammation. These two articles provide professionals with high-quality, in-depth information for clients about nutrition, dietary pattern, and the pathophysiology of chronic disease.

(continued)

Dietary Carbohydrates

Griel AE, Ruder EH, Kris-Etherton PM. The changing roles of dietary carbohydrates: from simple to complex. Arterioscler Thromb Vasc Biol. 2006;26(9):1958–1965.

The "changing role" of carbohydrates is an important distinction provided up front (the title) by the authors. Initially, Griel et al. briefly review the history of dietary recommendations with respect to carbohydrates beginning with early recommendations to substitute carbohydrates for fat in the diet that date back to the 1970s. These recommendations were based on the relationship between dietary fat and heart disease and the evidence that increasing carbohydrates and decreasing total fat in the diet resulted in lower lipid levels. These recommendations have evolved with the recognition that "all carbohydrates are not equal." Griel discusses the relationships between the carbohydrate content of meals, postprandial insulin production, insulin resistance, lipid metabolism, and dyslipidemia. She correctly remarks that high-carbohydrate diets have been demonstrated to induce dyslipidemia, especially in people who are overweight and sedentary (i.e., type 2 diabetes!). She follows with a discussion of both simple and complex carbohydrates (all carbohydrates are not equal!) and closes the article with a very nice discussion on dietary carbohydrates and weight loss. Finally, the authors make some practical recommendations. This article is packed with information and is well worth reading.

Dietary Pattern and Inflammation

Basu A, Sridevi D, Ishwarlal J. Dietary factors that promote or retard inflammation. Arterioscler Thromb Vasc Biol. 2006;26(5):995–1001.

Basu and his colleagues provide an excellent summary of the literature on both the proinflammatory and the anti-inflammatory effects of foods and nutrients. He summarizes the effects of various types of dietary fats, including saturated, trans, polyunsaturated, monounsaturated, and omega-3s on inflammatory markers. Basu et al. discuss proteins, carbohydrates, dietary cholesterol, alcohol, and micronutrients with respect to their inflammatory effects and present a straightforward "nutritional" account of the literature without lots of biochemistry and pathophysiology intervening to bog down the reader unfamiliar with the pathophysiology. This article is simple, straightforward, and clear. An interested reader can follow the references to find more in-depth reading, but Basu et al. provide most of what the exercise professional needs to discuss this issue with clients and patients.

REFERENCES

1. Alberti KG, Eckel RH, Grundy SM, et al. Harmonizing the metabolic syndrome. A joint interim statement of the International Diabetes Federation Task Force on Epidemiology and Prevention. Circulation. 2009;120:1640–1645.
2. Altena TA, Michaelson JL, Ball SD, et al. Single sessions of intermittent and continuous exercise and postprandial lipemia. Med Sci Sports Exerc. 2004;36(8):1364–1371.
3. American Diabetes Association, Bantle JP, Wylie-Rosett J, et al. Nutrition recommendations and interventions for diabetes: a position statement of the American Diabetes Association. Diabetes Care. 2008;31(Suppl 1):S61–S78.
4. Basu A, Devaraj S, Jialal I, et al. Dietary factors that promote or retard inflammation. Arterioscler Thromb Vasc Biol. 2006;26(5):995–1001.
5. Batty GD, Kivimaki M, Smith GD, et al. Obesity and overweight in relation to mortality in men with and without type 2 diabetes/impaired glucose tolerance: the original Whitehall Study. Diabetes Care. 2007;30(9):2388–2391.
6. Bazzano LA, Serdula M, Liu S. Prevention of type 2 diabetes by diet and lifestyle modification. J Am Coll Nutr. 2005;24(5):310–319.
7. Borghouts LB, Keizer HA. Exercise and insulin sensitivity: a review. Int J Sports Med. 2000;21:1–12.
8. Bouchard C, Tremblay A, Despres JP, et al. The response to long-term overfeeding in identical twins. N Engl J Med. 1990;322(21):1477–1482.

9. Boule NG, Kenny GP, Haddad E, et al. Meta-analysis of the effect of structured exercise training on cardiorespiratory fitness in Type 2 diabetes mellitus. Diabetologia. 2003;46:1071–1081.

10. Braith RW, Stewart KJ. Resistance exercise training: its role in the prevention of cardiovascular disease. Circulation. 2006;113:2642–2650.

11. Brunner EJ, Mosdol A, Witte DR, et al. Dietary patterns and 15-y risks of major coronary events, diabetes, and mortality. Am J Clin Nutr. 2008;87: 1414–1421.

12. Church TS, LaMonte MJ, Barlow CE, et al. Cardiorespiratory fitness and body mass index as predictors of cardiovascular disease mortality among men with diabetes. Arch Intern Med. 2005;165: 2114–2120.

13. Dandona P, Aljada A, Bandyopadhyay A. Inflammation: the link between insulin resistance, obesity and diabetes. Trends Immunol. 2004;25(1):4–7.

14. Dandona P, Aljada A, Chaudhuri A, et al. Garg R. Metabolic syndrome: a comprehensive perspective based on interactions between obesity, diabetes, and inflammation. Circulation. 2005;111(11): 1448–1454.

15. Dekker JM, Girman C, Rhodes T, et al. Metabolic syndrome and 10-year cardiovascular disease risk in the Hoorn Study. Circulation. 2005;112(5):666–673.

16. de Munter JS, Hu FB, Spiegelman D, et al. Whole grain, bran, and germ intake and risk of type 2 diabetes: a prospective cohort study and systematic review. PLoS Med. 2007;4(8):e261.

17. Despres JP, Lemieux I. Abdominal obesity and metabolic syndrome [published online ahead of print December 13, 2006]. Nature. 2006;444:881–887. doi: 10.1038/nature05488.

18. Dobbelsteyn CJ, Joffres MR, MacLean DR. A comparative evaluation of waist circumference, waist-to-hip ratio and body mass index as indicators of cardiovascular risk factors. The Canadian Heart Health Surveys. Int J Obes Relat Metab Disord. 2001;25(5):652–661. doi: 10.2337/dc08-S061.

19. Donnelly J, Blair SN, Jakicic JM, et al. ACSM's Position Stand on appropriate physical activity intervention strategies for weight loss and prevention of weight regain for adults. Med Sci Sports Exerc. 2009;41(2):459–471.

20. Esposito K, Giugliano D. Diet and inflammation: a link to metabolic and cardiovascular diseases. Eur Heart J. 2006;27:15–20.

21. Esposito K, Nappo F, Marfella R, et al. Inflammatory cytokine concentrations are acutely increased by hyperglycemia in humans: role of oxidative stress. Circulation. 2002;106(16):2067–2072.

22. Eves ND, Plotnikoff RC. Resistance training and Type 2 diabetes: consideration for implementation at the population level. Diabetes Care. 2006;29(8):1933–1941.

23. Executive Summary: Standards of Medical Care in Diabetes—American Diabetes Association. Nutrition recommendations and interventions for diabetes. Diabetes Care. 2010;33:S1–S100. doi: 10.2337/dc10-S004.

24. Executive Summary: Third Report of the National Cholesterol Education Program Expert Panel on Detection, Evaluation, and Treatment of High Blood Cholesterol in Adults (Adult Treatment Panel III). JAMA. 2001;285:2486–2497.

25. Flight I, Clifton P. Cereal grains and legumes in the prevention of coronary heart disease and stroke: a review of the literature. Eur J Clin Nutr. 2006;60(10):1145–1159.

26. Fontana LA. Calorie restriction and cardiometabolic health. Eur J Cardiovasc Prev Rehabil. 2008;15(1):3–9.

27. Ford ES, Giles WH, Dietz WH. Prevalence of the metabolic syndrome among US adults: findings from the third National Health and Nutrition Examination Survey. JAMA. 2002;287(3):356–359.

28. Gastrich MD, Lasser NL, Wien M, et al. Dietary complex carbohydrates and low glycemic index/load decrease levels of specific metabolic syndrome/cardiovascular disease risk factors. Top Clin Nutr. 2008;23(1):76–96.

29. Giada F, Biffi A, Agostoni P, et al. Exercise prescription for the prevention and treatment of cardiovascular diseases: Part I. J Cardiovasc Med. 2008;9(5):529–544.

30. Gill JMR. Physical activity, cardiorespiratory fitness and insulin resistance: a short update. Curr Opin Lipidol. 2007;18:47–52.

31. Glycemic Index Web Site. Available at: www.glycemicindex.com. Accessed March 10, 2008.

32. Griel AE, Ruder EH, Kris-Etherton PM. The changing roles of dietary carbohydrates: from simple to complex. Arterioscler Thromb Vasc Biol. 2006;26(9):1958–1965.

33. Grundy SM, Cleeman JI, Merz C, et al; Coordinating Committee of the National Cholesterol Education Program. Implications of recent clinical trials for the National Cholesterol Education Program Adult Treatment Panel III guidelines. Arterioscler Thromb Vasc Biol. 2004;24(8):e149–e161.

34. Gustafson B, Hammarstedt A, Andersson CX, et al. Inflamed adipose tissue: a culprit underlying the metabolic syndrome and atherosclerosis. Arterioscler Thromb Vasc Biol. 2007;27(11):2276–2283.

35. Hamer M, Chida Y. Intake of fruit, vegetables, and antioxidants and risk of type 2 diabetes: systematic review and meta-analysis. J Hypertens. 2007;25(12):2361–2369.

36. Helmrich SP, Ragland DR, Paffenbarger RS Jr. Prevention of non-insulin-dependent diabetes mellitus with physical activity. Med Sci Sports Exerc. 1994;26(7):824–830.

37. Horowitz JR. Exercise-induced alterations in muscle lipid metabolism improve insulin sensitivity. Exerc Sports Sci Rev. 2007;35(4):192–196.

38. Jeon CY, Lokken RP, Hu FB, et al. Physical activity of moderate intensity and risk of type 2 diabetes: a systematic review. Diabetes Care. 2007;30(3):744–752.

39. Kahn R, Buse J, Ferrannini E, et al. The metabolic syndrome: time for a critical appraisal. Joint statement from the American Diabetes Association and the European Association for the Study of Diabetes. Diabetologia. 2005;48(9):1684–1699.

40. Klein S, Sheard NF, Pi-Sunyer X, et al. Weight management through lifestyle modification for the

prevention and management of type 2 diabetes: rationale and strategies: a statement of the American Diabetes Association, the North American Association for the Study of Obesity, and the American Society for Clinical Nutrition. Diabetes Care. 2004;27:2067–2073.

41. Knowler WC, Barrett-Connor E, Fowler SE, et al; Diabetes Prevention Program Research Group. Reduction in the incidence of type 2 diabetes with lifestyle intervention or metformin. N Engl J Med. 2002;346(6):393–403.

42. Kokkinos P, Myers J, Nylen E, et al. Exercise capacity and all-cause mortality in African American and Caucasian men with type 2 diabetes. Diabetes Care. 2009;32(4):623–628.

43. Laaksonen DE, Lindstrom J, Lakka TA, et al. Physical activity in the prevention of type 2 diabetes: the Finnish diabetes prevention study. Finnish diabetes prevention study. Diabetes. 2005;54(1):158–165.

44. LaMonte MJ, Blair SN, Church TS. Physical activity and diabetes prevention. J Appl Physiol. 2005;99:1205–1213.

45. Lee YH, Pratley RE. Abdominal obesity and cardiovascular disease risk: the emerging role of the adipocyte. J Cardiopulm Rehabil Prev. 2007;27(1):2–10.

46. Lindstrom J, Peltonen M, Eriksson JG, et al. High-fibre, low-fat diet predicts long-term weight loss and decreased type 2 diabetes risk: the Finnish Diabetes Prevention Study. Diabetologia. 2006;49:912–920.

47. Liu S, Stampfer MJ, Hu FB, et al. Whole-grain consumption and risk of coronary heart disease: results from the Nurses' Health Study. Am J Clin Nutr. 1999;70(3):412–419.

48. Marwick TH, Hordern MD, Miller T, et al. Exercise training for type 2-diabetes mellitus: impact on cardiovascular risk. A scientific statement from the American Heart Association. Circulation. 2009;119:3244–3262.

49. Mertens IL, Van Gaal LF. Overweight, obesity, and blood pressure: the effects of modest weight reduction. Obes Res. 2000;8(3):270–278.

50. National Diabetes Information Clearing House Web Site. Available at: http://diabetes.niddk.nih.gov/dm/pubs/pima/obesity/obesity.html. Accessed May 9, 2008.

51. National Institutes of Health Web Site. Available at: http://diabetes.niddk.nih.gov/dm/pubs/statistics/#allages. Accessed March 3, 2010.

52. National Institutes of Health Web Site. http://www.nhlbi.nih.gov/health/dci/Diseases/ms/ms_whatis.html. Accessed March 3, 2010.

53. Nicklas BJ, You T, Pahor M. Behavioural treatments for chronic systemic inflammation: effects of dietary weight loss and exercise training. CMAJ. 2005;172(9):1199–1209.

54. Olson TP, Dengel DR, Leon AS, et al. Moderate resistance training and vascular health in overweight women. Med Sci Sports Exerc. 2006;38(9):1558–1564.

55. Praet SFE, van Loon LJC. Optimizing the therapeutic benefits of exercise in Type 2 diabetes. J Appl Physiol. 2007;103:1113–1120.

56. Rizvi A. Type 2 diabetes: epidemiologic trends, evolving pathogenic concepts, and recent changes in therapeutic approach. South Med J. 2004;97(11):1079–1087.

57. Roitman JL, LaFontaine TP. Secondary prevention of coronary artery disease. In: AACVPR Resource Manual for the Guidelines for Cardiovascular Rehabilitation. Champaign, IL: Human Kinetics, 2005.

58. Sigal RJ, Kenny GP, Wasserman DH, et al. Physical activity/exercise and type 2 diabetes: a consensus statement from the American Diabetes Association. Diabetes Care. 2006;29:1433–1438.

59. Slentz CA, Tanner CJ, Bateman LA, et al. Effects of exercise training intensity on pancreatic beta-cell function. Diabetes Care. 2009;32:1807–1811.

60. Tanasescu M, Leitzmann MF, Rimm EB, et al. Physical activity in relation to cardiovascular disease and total mortality among men with type 2 diabetes. Circulation. 2003;107:2435–2439.

61. Thomas DE, Elliott EJ, Naughton GA. Exercise for type 2 diabetes mellitus. Cochrane Database Syst Rev. 2006;3:CD002968. doi: 10.1002/14651858.CD002968.pub2.

62. Thompson WA, ed. ACSM's Guidelines for Exercise Testing and Prescription. 8th Ed. Baltimore, MD: Lippincott Williams & Wilkins, 2010.

63. Tudor-Locke C, Hatano Y, Pangrazi RP, et al. Revisiting "how many steps are enough?" Med Sci Sports Exerc. 2008;40(7, Suppl):S537–S543.

64. Tuomilehto J, Lindstrom J, Eriksson JG, et al; Finnish Diabetes Prevention Study Group. Prevention of type 2 diabetes mellitus by changes in lifestyle among subjects with impaired glucose tolerance. N Engl J Med. 2001;344:1343–1350.

65. Unger RH. Weapons of lean body mass destruction: the role of ectopic lipids in the metabolic syndrome. Endocrinology. 2003;144(12):5159–5165.

66. Ungvari Z, Parrado-Fernandez C, Csiszar A, et al. Mechanisms underlying caloric restriction and lifespan regulation: implications for vascular aging. Circ Res. 2008;102(5):519–528.

67. USDA Agricultural Research Service, Fast Facts Web Site. Available at: http://www.ars.usda.gov/SP2UserFiles/Place/12355000/pdf/0304/Table_1_NIF.pdf. Accessed June 10, 2009.

68. Wei M, Gibbons LW, Kampert JB, et al. Low cardiorespiratory fitness and physical inactivity as predictors of mortality in men with type 2 diabetes. Ann Intern Med. 2000;132(8):605–611.

69. Weyer C, Hanson K, Bogardus C, et al. Long-term changes in insulin action and insulin secretion associated with gain, loss, regain and maintenance of body weight. Diabetologia. 2000;43:36–46.

70. Willett WC, Sacks F, Trichopoulou F, et al. Mediterranean diet pyramid: a cultural model for healthy eating. Am J Clin Nutr. 1995;61:1402S–1406S.

71. Wong ND, Pio JR, Franklin SS, et al. Preventing coronary events by optimal control of blood pressure and lipids in patients with the metabolic syndrome. Am J Cardiol. 2003;91:1421–1426.

CHAPTER 8

Hypertension

ABBREVIATIONS

ACE	Angiotensin-converting enzyme	LTPA	Leisure-time physical activity
BP	Blood pressure	PA	Physical activity
CAD	Coronary artery disease	PEH	Postexercise hypotension
CREF	Cardiorespiratory endurance fitness	RAAS	Renin–angiotensin–aldosterone system
DASH	Dietary Approaches to Stop Hypertension	ROS	Reactive oxygen species
HR	Heart rate	SNS	Sympathetic nervous system
JNC7	The Seventh Report of the Joint National Committee on Prevention, Detection, Evaluation, and Treatment of High Blood Pressure		

Hypertension is, perhaps, the second most prevalent chronic disease in the United States (obesity is the most prevalent). More than 30% of the population, about 73 million people aged 20 and older, have hypertension and almost 60% have either prehypertension or hypertension (2,45). According to the Centers for Disease Control and Prevention (31), only 70% of the people with hypertension are aware that they have it; approximately 60% are being treated and less than 35% of these are adequately controlled (31). Hypertension is generally asymptomatic; thus, many people are not aware of having it. Unfortunately, this lack of awareness, as with type 2 diabetes, leads to premature end-organ damage, such as heart and kidney diseases. It is also a disease that, though not difficult to control, requires compliance with exercise, a healthy diet, and medication. These types of behaviors are practices that most of our population is not compliant with; thus, a significant portion of people who are diagnosed are not adequately controlled.

The incidence of hypertension is higher in non-Hispanic blacks (42.6%) than in non-Hispanic whites (32.5%) and Mexican Americans (28.7%) (31). The incidence of hypertension rises proportionately (and almost linearly) with age. Figure 8.1 highlights the age-related incidence of hypertension. Moreover, death rates from hypertension are more than three times higher in black men (51%) than in white men (15.7%). It is likely that this is because of a combination of the increased incidence and ineffective treatment in black men. In 2008, direct and indirect costs of hypertension in the United States were almost $70 billion (2).

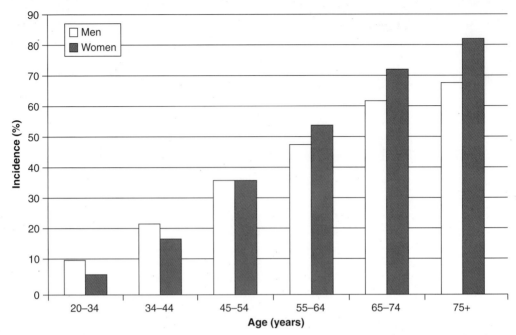

FIGURE 8.1 The incidence of hypertension by age group and sex in the U.S. population. Used with permission from Lloyd-Jones et al. (27).

HYPERTENSION AND RISK FACTORS

Hypertension not only comprises a distinct and unique chronic disease, it is (like many of the other chronic diseases discussed in this book) often present with coronary artery disease (CAD), metabolic syndrome, obesity, and type 2 diabetes. The American Heart Association considers hypertension to be a primary risk factor for CAD (2). Hypertension significantly increases the risk of death from CAD, stroke, diabetes, and renal (kidney) disease. In an important set of guidelines on hypertension from the Joint National Committee on Prevention, Detection, Evaluation, and Treatment of High Blood Pressure, it is reported that the "lifetime risk" of hypertension is more than 90% (32). This means that 90% of all adults, if they live long enough, will develop hypertension. In fact, this high degree of lifetime risk led to the formation of a new category called "prehypertension" in the most recent guidelines. This new category represents an effort to encourage early identification of individuals at risk for hypertension and to address that risk early in the disease process, thus avoiding some of the serious complications of long-standing hypertension, including heart and kidney diseases (32).

The risk of death from CAD and stroke increases almost linearly at systolic blood pressure (BP) levels beginning at 115 mm Hg and at diastolic BP levels beginning at 75 mm Hg. In these cases, the literature supports a twofold increase in mortality for every 20-mm Hg rise in systolic BP and for every 10-mm Hg rise in diastolic BP. The Framingham Heart Study as well as others show that the relative risk of cardiovascular disease is twice that in people with prehypertension (32,43).

Risk factors are characteristics that are "associated" with increased risk of a disease. In this case, hypertension is significantly associated with the prevalence of, incidence of, and mortality from CAD. The fact is that having hypertension or prehypertension increases

TABLE 8.1	Diet-Related Lifestyle Modifications That Effectively Lower Blood Pressure
Weight loss	For overweight or obese persons, lose weight, ideally obtaining a BMI of <25.0 kg/m^2; for non-overweight persons, maintain desirable BMI
Reduced salt intake	Lower salt (sodium chloride) intake as much as possible, ideally to 1.5 g sodium/d (or less)
DASH-type dietary pattern	Consume a diet rich in fruits and vegetables (8–10 servings/d), rich in low-fat dairy products (2–3 servings/d), and reduced in saturated fat and cholesterol
Increased potassium intake	Increase potassium intake to 4.7 g/d, which is also the level provided in the DASH diet
Moderation of alcohol intake	For those who drink alcohol, consume no more than two alcoholic drinks per day (men) and no more than one alcoholic drink per day (women)

Reproduced with permission from JNC (32)

BMI, body mass index; DASH, dietary approaches to stop hypertension.

the risk of heart attack, stroke, and death from either of these events (see Chapter 1 for a more detailed discussion of risk factors and chronic disease).

People with multiple risk factors have higher risk than those with one or no risk factors. The more risk factors present, the higher the risk for disease. For example, current guidelines for lipids recommend that people with type 2 diabetes be treated as if they have heart disease, even if they have no clinical diagnosis (17,19,32). In addition, guidelines for treatment of type 2 diabetes recommend that hypertension be aggressively treated to decrease risk (40). Thus, hypertension is not only a primary risk factor; it multiplies the risk of disease in the presence of other risk factors and must be treated as a significant disease entity by itself. Table 8.1 shows lifestyle and dietary pattern modifications that have been demonstrated to lower BP.

CLASSIFICATION OF BP

In 2004, the U.S. Department of Health and Human Services issued JNC7 (The Seventh Report of the Joint National Committee on Prevention, Detection, Evaluation, and Treatment of High Blood Pressure). This comprehensive report provides guidelines on BP diagnosis, prevention, and treatment (32). Table 8.2 shows the current classification of BP.

What is classified as "prehypertension" in this report would previously have been classified as "high normal" (32,43). Thus, it is recognized that there is no "threshold" for high versus normal BP, but rather there is an increasing risk with increasing BPs >115 mm Hg systolic and >75 mm Hg diastolic. This was demonstrated almost 10 years ago (43). In summary, hypertension is a chronic disease; hypertension is a risk factor for chronic disease; and hypertension magnifies risk when combined with other risk factors or in the presence of other chronic disease (43).

This chapter briefly discusses the pathophysiology of hypertension and prehypertension, some basic details of nutrition, diet and hypertension, prevention of hypertension,

TABLE 8.2	JNC7 Classification of Blood Pressure for Adults	
Blood Pressure Classification	**Systolic Blood Pressure (mm Hg)**	**Diastolic Blood Pressure (mm Hg)**
Normal	<120	and <80
Prehypertension	120–139	or 80–89
Stage 1 hypertension	140–159	or 90–99
Stage 2 hypertension	>160	or >100

JNC7, The Seventh Report of the Joint National Committee on Prevention, Detection, Evaluation, and Treatment of High Blood Pressure

and the optimal exercise program for preventing and managing hypertension. It is sufficient to say that, like most of the other risk factors and like most chronic diseases (certainly all of them in this book), hypertension can be prevented and/or effectively treated with lifestyle modifications, especially with exercise, diet, and weight-loss intervention.

PATHOPHYSIOLOGY OF HYPERTENSION

Although it may seem repetitive, hypertension is associated and coupled with low-grade, systemic inflammation (23,42). Another consequence of longer-standing hypertension is increased vascular stiffness (sometimes called "hardening" of the arteries or arteriosclerosis) that results from arterial remodeling (primarily in arterioles) to withstand the ongoing elevated internal pressure (52). Two primary physiological systems control BP: the sympathetic nervous system (SNS) and the renin–angiotensin–aldosterone system (RAAS). Both systems may be dysfunctional in hypertension. The origins of the inflammatory process in hypertension are not entirely clear, but the causes of vascular stiffness are thought to be the remodeling process in arterioles and other resistance vessels (52). It is clear that the low-grade, systemic inflammation that we have discussed throughout this book is present in and linked to the pathophysiology of hypertension and is an important pathophysiologic component of hypertension (23,42).

CONTROL OF BP

The SNS controls BP through a series of interactions between neurohormones and other substances and direct nervous system input from the vascular system, the kidneys, and adrenal glands (Fig. 8.2). The RAAS is a system through which interactions between various physiologically active substances (enzymes, neurohormones, etc.) result in increased BP. Most of these substances work through stimulating increased production and circulation of the primary components of the system—renin, angiotensin, and aldosterone. These substances act in the kidneys (on fluid and electrolyte balance) and also within the circulatory system. The RAAS and SNS are interconnected and act jointly to raise and lower BP in response to physiological and neural signals. The dysfunction of these systems is thought to be a primary component of hypertension. They are also primary targets for control, both with lifestyle modifications and with medication (1,20,23).

SYMPATHETIC NERVOUS SYSTEM

The SNS is the system often described as the "fight or flight" nervous system (see Fig. 8.3). Fight or flight refers to the response that Hans Selye originally described as the "stress" response (20). See the box titled "Fight or Flight" Physiological Responses" below for a more detailed discussion of "flight or fight."

Activating the SNS stimulates a general neurohormonal reaction with epinephrine (adrenaline) and norepinephrine (noradrenaline) and several other catecholamine and neurohormonal compounds that act primarily to increase BP, heart rate (HR) (thus cardiac output), peripheral resistance (through vasoconstriction), and metabolism (20). The end result of this activation is to prepare the body for fighting or for running

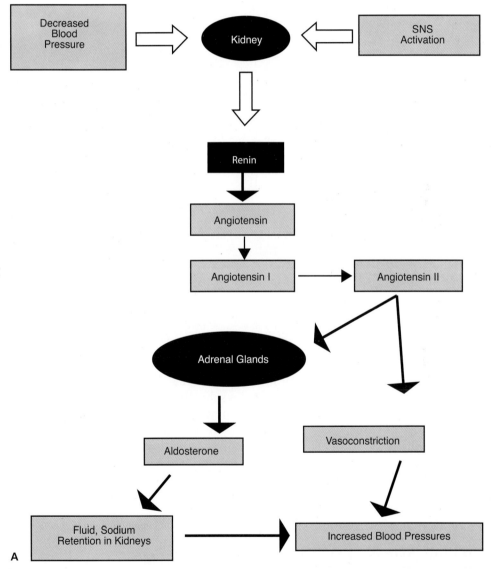

FIGURE 8.2 Primary control of blood pressure is balanced between the kidneys and the sympathetic nervous system. **A** shows a view of the whole system with interactions of the renin–angiotensin–aldosterone system (RAAS) and its influence on blood pressure. (*continued*)

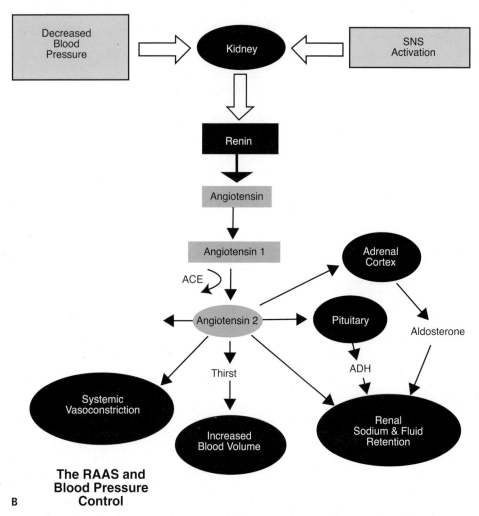

FIGURE 8.2 (*continued*) **B** illustrates the RAAS, a major control system for blood pressure. Renin and angiotensin are primary elements of this system that controls blood pressure through influencing kidney function, fluid regulation, vasoconstriction, and vasodilation, among other things.

away from danger. However, in our modern world, the SNS is often (now, in fact, almost always) activated for nonemergency situations that the body interprets as "emergencies," but that do not require drastic alteration in physiological function. These situations are often associated with "stress" or perceived stress and are usually accompanied by the pathophysiologic changes found in hypertension and other chronic diseases.

The components of fight or flight work in a feedback system that can be visualized in Figure 8.3 on page 187. Activation of the SNS also stimulates (separately from the mechanisms described below) the release of renin from the kidney. Thus, there is a direct link between the SNS and the RAAS.

THE RENIN–ANGIOTENSIN–ALDOSTERONE SYSTEM

The RAAS is similar to most physiological feedback systems. It is intended to control BP by altering renal function (kidneys) and increasing vascular resistance (through selective vasoconstriction and vasodilation). Renin, angiotensin, and aldosterone are

Fight or Flight Response

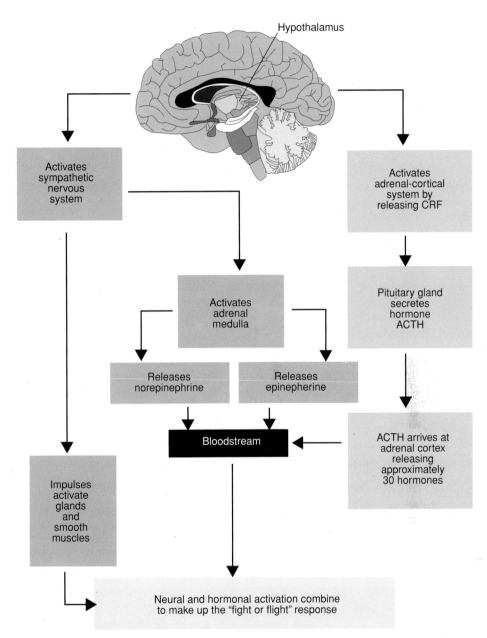

FIGURE 8.3 Fight or flight refers to a group of physiological responses to stress. It is controlled by both neurological and hormonal influences and can cause both short-term and long-term increases in blood pressure. (Courtesy of HowStuffWorks.com.)

the central active substances of the system. They are integrated into the regulation of BP through fluid volume, electrolyte reabsorption in the kidneys, and vasoreactivity (20).

Renin is released from the kidneys because of decreased BP. The sequence of this system is described in the box titled "RAAS Sequence of Action" below.

Renin acts as an enzyme that facilitates the formation of angiotensin I. The conversion of angiotensin I to angiotensin II is stimulated by angiotensin-converting enzyme (ACE).

DID YOU KNOW?

"Fight or Flight" Physiological Responses (20)

The SNS is the mediator of this response. It is a classic physiological feedback system first described by Hans Selye as a reaction to a stressor. The brain interprets external events in many different ways. In more primitive times (i.e., prehistoric), humans were primarily hunter/gatherers. The immediate prospect of danger in the form of life-threatening attacks resulted in the development of this system that prepares the body for very high levels of physical performance. The outcome of stimulating the fight or flight system is a set of physiological responses that

- increase the HR and BP;
- increase blood flow to active skeletal muscle and organs such as the heart;
- decrease blood flow to inactive skeletal muscle, the gastrointestinal system, and kidneys;
- increase cellular metabolism;
- increase blood glucose, mainly through glycolysis in the liver; and
- increase the rate of blood clotting.

These changes result in increased ability to move (flee or fight), as well as a physiology that is prepared to quickly repair itself in the case of injury (increased blood clotting). In this modern age, the importance of such a reaction is much diminished. We simply do not have many life-threatening circumstances. In fact, it seems fair to state that most people in the United States seldom encounter such circumstances. The fact is, however, that we still have the potential for this kind of reaction to stressful situations where we experience the response, but "fighting" or "fleeing" are not options. Thus, it does affect us negatively and the effect is often pathological in nature.

Angiotensin II has many actions, including stimulating the release of aldosterone by adrenal glands and causing general arteriolar vasoconstriction, which, in turn, increases BP rapidly (in seconds). Angiotensin II has several other physiological actions that contribute to increasing BP.

Activating the RAAS is also associated with increased SNS activity, since the release of renin is also stimulated by the SNS. Chronic activation of the SNS is one of the hallmarks of hypertension (20).

DID YOU KNOW?

RAAS Sequence of Action

Renin → Angiotensin I $\xrightarrow{\text{angiotensin-converting enzyme (ACE)}}$ Angiotensin II

One class of antihypertensive medications is called angiotensin-converting enzyme (ACE) inhibitors. They block the action of the enzyme (ACE) that converts angiotensin I to angiotensin II; thus, one of the primary points in the pathway of RAAS is blocked by this drug. In addition, there is a newer class of drugs called "angiotensin II receptor blockers" that block the cell membrane receptors where angiotensin II acts in the vascular system and the kidney.

Aldosterone is the final link in the RAAS. Increased aldosterone secretion causes increased water and sodium reabsorption in the kidneys, as well as release of potassium, and therefore increased BP. The RAAS is an example of a classic physiological feedback system. A physiological change (e.g., decreased BP) is recognized by sensors in various regions of the body and resolved by a sequence of physiological adjustments. When such systems go awry (e.g., the RAAS in the case of hypertension), the complex actions of the components can cause various outcomes, many of which often result in further disease-related pathophysiology (20).

THE RAAS AND HYPERTENSION

Dysfunction in the RAAS, which is meant to control BP, causes a cascade of physiological changes (actually "pathophysiologic" changes) that affect such wide-ranging processes as inflammation, vascular remodeling, BP, and other functions. The origin of this dysfunction is thought to be found in such "risk factors" as obesity, inflammation, insulin resistance, and hypertension itself (20).

In fact, the RAAS may be involved in a "positive feedback loop," in which increased BP resulting from increased RAAS activation results in more inflammation and vascular stiffening, resulting in further elevated BP (20,30). These positive feedback loops are consistently present in the pathophysiology of chronic disease. Inflammation, reactive oxygen species (ROS), oxidative stress, and SNS activation are some of them. They form a core of pathophysiologic conditions that are found in nearly every chronic disease discussed in this book.

HYPERTENSION AND INFLAMMATION

Hypertension is accompanied by the same low-level, systemic inflammation that is common to each of the chronic diseases discussed in this book (9,42). Whether the inflammation originates with the chronic hypertensive state or rather is part of associated changes and other risk factors is not clear. The fact is that inflammation is a product of the risk factors and the disease process. It is, therefore, inherent in hypertension and associated with most of the comorbid (risk) factors, such as obesity and endothelial dysfunction (20,30).

Whatever its origin, the inflammation is present from the earliest stages of hypertension (9). The mechanical stress of the pressure on the vessel wall may be one cause of the initial inflammation (30,42). But the problem may also be related to other factors such as increased angiotensin II levels (see Chapter 2 for a more detailed discussion of inflammation). In addition, obesity, insulin resistance, atherosclerosis, and other comorbid "risk" factors for hypertension and CAD are all accompanied by an inflammatory state (26). Regardless of the origin, hypertension is accompanied by a low-grade, systemic inflammation and the level of inflammatory markers is also reduced by reducing BP.

ARTERIAL STIFFENING

Evidence is accumulating that a missing piece of the pathophysiologic puzzle of hypertension is the stiffening or "remodeling" of arteries (primarily arterioles) as BP becomes chronically increased. Remodeling occurs as the amount and the structure of connective tissue in arterial sections of the vasculature increases (30,33,52). Connective tissue (composed of collagen and elastin) forms the primary *structural* component of vessel walls (52). Connective tissue provides support for arteries and allows them to withstand the daily demands of the elevated internal pressures associated with hypertension. The relative content of connective tissue in arterial walls increases in response to increased chronic intra-arterial pressure and the associated need to withstand the ongoing conditions that exist within a closed, pressurized vascular system. The progressive arterial stiffening may also result from the interactions that are associated with inflammation, angiotensin II, and from type 2 diabetes, insulin resistance, and obesity. The increased general vascular stiffening results in increased peripheral vascular resistance, which also chronically increases BP (52).

Pharmacological intervention to modify the physiological systems that are part of hypertension is difficult and complicated. Interrupting or changing one or more of the steps in some of these systems (as is done with almost all pharmacological attempts at medical therapy) may, indeed, modify BP, but the intervention does not affect the whole regulatory system. The intervention is likely to be partially effective or entirely ineffective in the long term because of the influence and complex nature of the interactions within these systems.

Later, we discuss the influence of exercise and diet in moderating hypertension. Many of the effective nutritional therapies were discussed in detail in Chapter 4. We believe it is safe to say that only exercise, diet, and weight loss can successfully intervene at several points along each of these physiological pathways; thus, lifestyle must be the primary focus of successful prevention of hypertension.

WHAT CAUSES HYPERTENSION?

The brief introduction (above) of the systems that control and change BP demonstrates the complexity of the issue. It is well known that, for example, chronic stimulation of the SNS results in increased BP. Indeed, many people perceive constant and ongoing "stress" in their life, which repeatedly activates this system. In fact, the system is chronically activated in many people with hypertension (20). However, this cannot be the sole reason for what amounts to the epidemic prevalence of hypertension in the United States—evidenced by 60% of the population that has hypertension or prehypertension and 90% of the population is at risk for developing hypertension during their lifetime (31). Thus, it would be beneficial to know the cause.

There are a number of hypotheses, although none of them is likely to provide a single acceptable answer. Collectively they are comprehensive enough to cover most of the likely causes. In most individuals, it is also likely that more than one of these mechanisms is involved.

First and foremost, the epidemic prevalence of obesity is one overriding reason for the epidemic of hypertension (see Chapter 6 for a detailed discussion of the pathophysiology of obesity). Obesity carries with it various inflammatory and SNS reactions that set up much of the pathophysiology common to hypertension and atherosclerosis. There are also physiological hypotheses that propose systemic and renal vasoconstriction, microvascular pathology, and an autoimmune response involving ROS and angiotensin II (23).

Hypertension most likely results from the physiological and biochemical interplay of risk factors, clinical pathophysiology, and interactions of the SNS, RAAS, and the feedback mechanisms that link these systems, as well as the clinical conditions associated with their function and dysfunction.

LIFESTYLE AND HYPERTENSION

JNC7 states that "the adoption of healthy lifestyles by all persons is critical for the prevention of high BP and is an indispensable part of the management of those with hypertension" (32). That, however, is essentially the extent of the support and information about lifestyle in JNC7, with the exception of a brief review of the literature and an affirmation of the efficacy of lifestyle intervention for the treatment of hypertension. We propose that lifestyle *must be the primary mode* of treatment if adequate control of BP is to be effective in the long term. Figure 8.4 illustrates the negative health behaviors that influence BP and contribute to hypertension.

In randomized trials, lifestyle modification has been shown to be effective in lowering BP in hypertensive persons (15). In an excellent meta-analysis of randomized trials of lifestyle intervention, the positive effects of exercise and diet were reported to be statistically significant. Other effective interventions include dietary alcohol and sodium restriction and omega-3 supplementation. Generally, these interventions result in a decrease of approximately 2.3- to 5.0-mm Hg in both systolic and diastolic BP (15). The trials reviewed by this meta-analysis lasted 6 months or less, so they are not long-term interventions, but they do show the effectiveness of lifestyle intervention for hypertension. A more recent study demonstrated a 16.9 mm Hg/9.9 mm Hg (systolic BP/diastolic BP) reduction in BP using the DASH (Dietary Approaches to Stop Hypertension) diet with exercise and weight loss (7). This and other studies demonstrate that more significant reductions in BP result from increased ("optimal") lifestyle intervention.

Randomized trials investigating the efficacy of exercise or diet for lowering BP verifies the effectiveness of exercise in both normotensive and hypertensive populations (18,37). The benefits of moderate-to-vigorous activity and increased CREF are confirmed by this research. Randomized trials satisfactorily account for some confounding variables. Fagard and Cornelissen (18) review these randomized trials and state that the changes in systolic BP and diastolic BP are consistent in these trials and that the

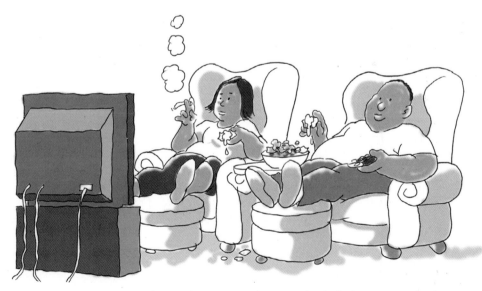

FIGURE 8.4 The environmental factors that promote hypertension include exposure to tobacco smoke, sedentary lifestyle, high saturated and trans fat foods, and food from refined grains. These are essentially the same factors that are pro-inflammatory and promote most chronic disease.

reduction in BP is greater in people with hypertension and prehypertension than in those with normal BP.

Other, large epidemiological, nonrandomized research supports the effectiveness of both increased physical activity (PA) and cardiorespiratory endurance fitness (CREF) with lower BP in men and women. Williams (47–51) has been one of the most active proponents of the benefits of exercise for preventing chronic disease. Both runners and walkers (in large, prospective cross-sectional studies) demonstrate that PA and CREF are associated with lower BP. Williams supports the effectiveness of intensity over duration and frequency, with respect to lowering BP. Interestingly, Williams also documents decreased use of antihypertensive medication (as well as cholesterol-lowering and antidiabetic medicines) in runners (47,49–51). The mechanisms for these changes appear to be decreased systemic vascular resistance (SNS) accompanied by positive changes in RAAS, as well as improved endothelial function (1,18,44).

DIET AND NUTRITION IN HYPERTENSION

This is a summary discussion of diet, nutrition, and BP. A detailed discussion of nutrition and chronic disease is given in Chapter 4. The connection between increased sodium intake and BP is well known and sufficiently documented to preclude extensive discussion here (3).

Dickinson's (15) review also verifies the effectiveness of healthy nutrition for preventing hypertension. Low-sodium diets have been documented to effectively lower BP in people with hypertension. The DASH diet (see discussion below and in Chapter 4) has been demonstrated to be effective in controlling BP (7,14,41). Many nutritional patterns have been found to lower BP in both people with and without hypertension. Common characteristics of these diets include daily intake of foods low in sodium; high in potassium and calcium; high in fiber, fruits, vegetables, and whole grains; and low in fat, particularly saturated fat (see Chapter 4 for a complete discussion of healthy dietary patterns). The DASH diet clearly demonstrates that sodium restriction is one part of a healthy nutritional pattern for management and prevention of hypertension. These studies, along with the epidemiological research on dietary patterns and chronic disease (as well as health), clearly demonstrate the effectiveness of a healthy diet in helping to prevent not only hypertension but also other chronic diseases (13,14,41). Table 8.3 shows some basic details of the DASH diet.

DIETARY CONTENT—THE DASH DIET

The DASH diet (see Fig. 8.5) can be found in detail online (see Chapter 4 for a detailed discussion of the DASH diet) (13). A recent study shows not only the positive effects of the DASH diet but the additive effects of exercise and weight loss as well. A group of researchers at Duke University studied the effects of the DASH diet alone, the DASH diet plus exercise and weight loss, and "usual diet control" (instructed to consume their usual diet and not to begin an exercise program) in a group of subjects with prehypertension or stage 1 hypertension and obesity. See the box titled "DASH Weight Loss Study Results" on page 193 for a summary of those results (7).

The differences between the DASH diet group and the DASH diet plus weight loss group (as well as the control group) were statistically significant in each of the areas shown in the box. The usual diet group demonstrated no significant change from baseline in any of the variables measured in the study. This study confirms the major theme of this book.

TABLE 8.3	DASH Diet Eating Plan	
Type of Food	Number of Servings for 1,600–3,100-cal Diets	Servings on a 2,000-cal Diet
Grains and grain products (include at least three whole-grain foods each day)	6–12	7–8
Fruits	4–6	4–5
Vegetables	4–6	4–5
Low fat or nonfat dairy foods	2–4	2–3
Lean meats, fish, and poultry	1.5–2.5	≤2
Nuts, seeds, and legumes	3–6/wk	4–5/wk
Fats and sweets	2–4	Limited

From DASH (13).
DASH, Dietary Approaches to Stop Hypertension.

"Optimal" lifestyle management of hypertension (and other chronic disease) cannot be dependent on a single mode of treatment, but in fact must be multifactorial. *Optimal treatment* means addressing all the lifestyle factors that increase risk for a particular chronic disease. In this case, hypertension is much more effectively treated using diet, exercise, and weight loss than diet alone (7).

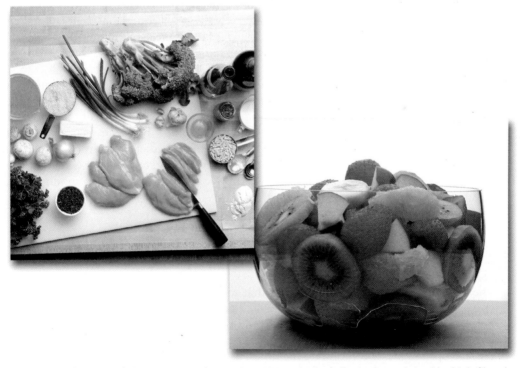

FIGURE 8.5 The DASH (Dietary Approaches to Stop Hypertension) diet is characterized by high fiber, low saturated and trans fat, and high amounts of fruits and vegetables.

DASH Weight Loss Study Results (7)

Variable	DASH + Exercise & Weight Loss	DASH Alone	Usual Diet
Systolic blood pressure decrease (mm Hg)	16.1	11.2	3.4
Diastolic blood pressure decrease (mm Hg)	9.9	7.5	3.8
Weight loss (kg)	−9.4	−0.1	+0.9
Aerobic fitness increase (%)	+19	−1.2	−3.2

DASH, Dietary Approaches to Stop Hypertension.

NUTRIENTS AND PATHOPHYSIOLOGY

The connection between nutrition, dietary pattern, and the pathophysiology of chronic disease, including inflammation and the other common pathophysiologic characteristics, is also well documented. The discussion in Chapter 2 is a more detailed discussion about this connection, but the current thinking is summarized below.

Food is a prime suspect in the inflammatory condition that is associated with chronic disease. A low-saturated-fat, high-fiber diet is preventive for those without clinical manifestation of disease and for new and recurrent events (secondary prevention) for those with documented chronic disease (3,4,7,12). Meals high in saturated fat and/or trans fat promote inflammation. High blood triglycerides after high-fat meals (called *postprandial lipemia*) also promotes inflammation. Conversely, high-fiber intake as well as intake of polyunsaturated, monounsaturated, and omega-3 fats in meals all inhibit inflammation. These nutrients, for the most part, also inhibit the formation of pro-inflammatory free radicals (ROS) (3,7,12,39).

Increased intake of vegetables and fruits is anti-inflammatory and is associated with lower prevalence of diabetes, heart disease, obesity, and other chronic diseases (4,12). In addition, high levels of blood triglycerides, high levels of low-density lipoproteins, low levels of high-density lipoproteins, overweight, and obesity are associated with increased inflammation even in youth (5,22,24). In fact, diet and physical inactivity may initiate the inflammatory process and certainly propagate it once it is present (26). Figure 8.6 illustrates many of the positive lifestyle behaviors known to modify hypertension.

EXERCISE AND HYPERTENSION

The epidemiological research concludes that increased PA and CREF are related to decreased BP (11,18,37,46,49). There is a well-documented inverse relationship between both PA and BP as well as between CREF and BP. In addition, the development of hypertension in later life is inversely related to both PA and CREF. Even after adjusting for other risk factors and lifestyle variables, the difference between the least and the most active is approximately 5 mm Hg (18). The risk factors become increasingly confounding because

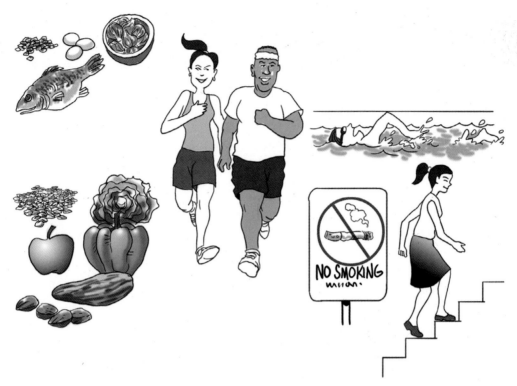

FIGURE 8.6 Positive health behaviors help to prevent hypertension and have been shown to lower blood pressure in those with hypertension.

of their pro-inflammatory nature and because of the continuing progression of the particular chronic disease. Regardless, it is clear that the lack of regular exercise and PA is directly related to both the development and the persistence of hypertension.

A large review of cardiorespiratory endurance exercise confirms the association of exercise with lower BP (46). The overall relationship documented in this study confirms a decrease of about 3 to 5 mm Hg in systolic BP and of 2 to 4 mm Hg in diastolic BP. The American College of Sports Medicine position stand on exercise and hypertension states that the reduction is 7.4/5.8 mm Hg after controlling for other risk factors (37). Although the influence of other risk factors could not be totally controlled, it was clear that even in the presence of other significant risk factors (e.g., obesity) this relationship is significant and persistent (46). Many others have confirmed this association (18,37).

The basis for the effect is likely to be multifactorial and includes both the anti-inflammatory effects of exercise and the improvement of endothelial function that is a subacute and a chronic effect of exercise (16,25,36). Positive effects on such diverse systems as vascular function, SNS, and RAAS all confirm that exercise has a positive effect on BP in both hypertensive and normotensive people (18).

The real question is what is the optimal exercise program? What defines the most effective intensity, duration, and frequency? Clear answers to this question are not currently known. Paul Williams (49–51) is a proponent of intensity as the important factor, and his prospective cross-sectional research from more than 100,000 runners confirms this. In his research, those runners with the fastest 10-K times had the least hypertension (as a group) and also used the least antihypertensive medication, and the relationship persisted even when body mass index was statistically controlled.

DID YOU KNOW?

Lifestyle Modifications to Manage Hypertension (32)

Modification	Recommendation	Approximate Systolic Blood Pressure Reduction Range (reference)
Weight reduction	Maintain or achieve normal body composition (body mass index 18.5–24.9 kg/m²)	5–20 mm Hg/10 kg of weight loss (37)
Adopt DASH eating plan	Consume a diet rich in fruits, vegetables, and low-fat dairy products, with a reduced content of saturated and total fat	8–14 mm Hg (41)
Dietary sodium reduction	Reduce dietary sodium intake to no more than 2.4 g sodium/d or 6 g sodium chloride/d	2–8 mm Hg (41)
Physical activity	Engage in regular aerobic physical activity such as brisk walking (at least 30 min/d, most days of the week)	4–9 mm Hg (37,49,51)
Moderation of alcohol consumption	Limit consumption to no more than two drinks (1–1.5 oz), e.g., 24 oz beer, 10 oz wine, or 3 oz of 80-proof whiskey) per day in most men and to no more than one drink per day in women and lighter-weight persons	2–4 mm Hg

DASH, Dietary Approaches to Stop Hypertension.

However, Robert Fagard, another accomplished and published author on this topic, finds no such relationship in his research, which has been confirmed by others (18,46). Despite finding no such relationship, they do report a "somewhat" more significant relationship between decreased BP and the magnitude of increased CREF (as measured by peak oxygen uptake). Thus, in studies where changes in fitness level were measured, the groups whose fitness level increased the most also had the greatest decreases in BP (18).

So, we have confusing and conflicting research results to deal with. One research group contends that increased CREF is related to decreased BP (49,51). Another group, in contrast, simply states that "exercise," regardless of the intensity, duration, or frequency, is related to decreased BP (18). Actually, the second approach has support from some recent studies by Blair et al. (6), as well as by Williams himself (47,48). The "Digging Deeper" section in Chapter 3 discusses the controversy between PA and CREF and their relative contribution to prevention of chronic disease. The conclusion is that the optimal exercise prescription would probably be the same—exercise and/or be physically active every day. Some of that exercise should be higher-intensity, fitness-related exercise, while some can (and should) be lower-intensity PA.

Longer-duration exercise has some clear advantages with respect to comfort, but some clear disadvantages with respect to time commitment. High-intensity exercise has advantages with respect to time but disadvantages in both comfort and in being associated with greater exercise-related risk of injury and other complications as well as noncompliance. Selecting a single intensity is not simple, but is perhaps unnecessary; it may be the mix of the two that is important in the exercise and PA prescription.

THE OPTIMAL EXERCISE PRESCRIPTION

The guidelines that we proposed earlier for the optimal exercise prescription for preventing hypertension are not significantly different from those proposed in Chapter 5 (and others). The box titled "Optimize: Exercise Prescription for Disease Prevention" below summarizes the optimal exercise and PA prescription. Exercise that targets increases in CREF as well as increased leisure-time physical activity (LTPA) (steps, movement, etc.) should be part of the optimal program. Although the improvement of CREF requires a higher intensity of exercise than LTPA, the end result is that people who want to prevent chronic disease in general or in intervening in a particular chronic disease—hypertension in this case—should endeavor to increase both CREF and PA for the most effective result (37).

_O_ptimize

CREF Exercise Prescription for Hypertension

Frequency	Cardiorespiratory endurance exercise: 3–4 d/wk
	Resistance exercise: 2–3 d/wk*
	LTPA: 3–4 d/wk (opposite cardiorespiratory endurance fitness exercise)
	Total: Exercise 7 d/wk
Intensity	Cardiorespiratory endurance exercise: 60%–75% VO_2R
	LMEx: 40%–60% VO_2R
Duration	Cardiorespiratory endurance exercise: 30 min of continuous exercise
	LMEx: 15–30 min
Mode	Cardiorespiratory endurance exercise: Repetitive, large muscle group exercise, e.g., walking, jogging, and swimming
	RT: A moderate program of RT should supplement CV endurance exercise
	LMEx: Any other activity including team sports, recreational activities, job-related, or household activities are in this category
Physical activity	See Lifestyle Modifications box, p. 196.

LTPA, leisure-time physical activity; LMEx, low-to-moderate exercise.

*For additional information about resistance training among patients with hypertension, see ACSM's Guidelines for Exercise Testing and Prescription, 8th Edition, and ACSM's Resource Manual for Guidelines for Exercise Testing and Prescription, 6th Edition.

DIGGING DEEPER

Hypotension after Exercise

The American College of Sports Medicine position stand on hypertension has an extensive and current discussion of postexercise hypotension (PEH). Others have noted PEH with interest and with speculation that it may well be relevant to the effects of exercise on hypertension (37,38).

PEH subsequent to individual bouts of exercise (a subacute effect) is well documented (21,28,37,38). PEH has been shown to occur after exercise of varying levels of intensity and duration. Although PEH has been demonstrated after both short and long bouts of exercise, the effect may be more pronounced after longer bouts and in individuals with hypertension. PEH may last 6 to 12 hours or more. Intermittent exercise has also been shown to be associated with PEH; in fact, the effect may be equally prevalent after shorter bouts (perhaps 5–10 minutes) of exercise (21,38).

Both aerobic and resistance exercise are associated with PEH (8,11,38). A few studies have demonstrated that longer durations are associated with a greater response, especially in persons with hypertension (29,37). However, PEH has been demonstrated with exercise durations ranging from 3 to 90 minutes and with intensities as low as 40% of VO_2max. In fact, PEH has been demonstrated after LTPA of very low intensities (34,37).

PEH has also been demonstrated in people with and without hypertension (37). The amount of the decrease may be dependent on pre-exercise BP; thus, those with the highest pre-exercise BP may have the greatest reduction postexercise (37).

PEH may be linked to the known chronic effects of exercise on BP, but the exact mechanism of PEH is not known. Some hypertensive medications facilitate the effects of PEH. A specific dose–response relationship with exercise has not been established. What is clear is that PEH may add to the therapeutic efficacy of exercise and should be considered in developing exercise programs for those with hypertension and prehypertension (34,37).

Some research suggests that "accumulating" bouts of exercise also results in PEH (35). This research tried to determine whether one long bout (40 min) or four short, interrupted bouts (10 min, each over 4 hours) resulted in different PEH responses. The short, interrupted bouts, spread out over 4 hours, resulted in increased length of PEH (11 vs. 7 hours). The intensity of both exercises was held at 50% VO_2peak (29,35).

Neurohormonal adaptations are among the most plausible explanations for PEH. The effects on SNS activity, including global reductions in sympathetic activity, decreased neural norepinephrine release, and effects on insulin sensitivity and insulin release (both related to BP and hypertension), are among the possibilities. Indications that a primary neurotransmitter substance in the brain may be involved have also been proposed (10). Changes in the RAAS are possible, but unconfirmed (37).

Changes in vascular function and vascular smooth muscle may contribute to the effect. As discussed previously, endothelial function is improved subacutely and chronically with exercise (25). Conversely, uncontrolled hypertension impairs endothelial function. Improved endothelial function may be related to the beneficial effect of exercise on hypertension (21).

Structural vascular changes and changes in gene expression secondary to the effects of environmental influences (such as diet or exercise) may also provide some clue to the basis for this benefit of regular exercise. Possible structural changes include vascular remodeling, increased vessel diameter, and the generation of new blood vessels. Genomic influences on BP and PEH have been observed in humans and that component, though small, appears to contribute (37).

What is known can be summarized as follows:

- Most of the time, exercise causes PEH.
- PEH is more pronounced in persons with hypertension than in those without.
- PEH is probably influenced by both intensity and duration of exercise, but duration (>30 minutes in most studies) may be equally effective, especially in patients who cannot tolerate higher intensity for longer duration.
- PEH is influenced by PA as well as structured exercise; thus, persons with hypertension and prehypertension should be encouraged to be as active as possible every day, throughout the day.
- PEH is a subacute response to exercise.

PEH is a subacute effect of exercise and thus merits some attention in the period after exercise, perhaps even precautions to persons with hypertension who are also medicated since it may interact with medication causing symptoms such as lightheadedness, weakness, dizziness, and near syncope. Precautions should include proper hydration and heat precautions (in the appropriate climate and season), appropriate precautions after exercising with respect to additional PA, diet, and fluid replacement, as well as symptom recognition.

Significant RESEARCH

The two articles selected for hypertension represent two very different content areas. The article by Johnson on the pathogenesis of hypertension is a review article that is comprehensive but challenging. The second article, by Blumenthal, is one of the most recent out of the DASH diet publishing group, demonstrating the effectiveness of the DASH diet coupled with exercise in treating hypertension.

Essential Hypertension

Johnson RJ, Feig DI, Nakagawa T, et al. Pathogenesis of essential hypertension: historical paradigms and modern insights. J Hypertens. 2008;26:381–391.

This article is an excellent review of the pathophysiology of hypertension integrated with some historical perspective of the theories along with current thinking. The article is relatively recent; thus, most of this information at a broad level remains accurate and valid. The historical discussion is interesting and also allows exercise professionals to put some of the myths and misunderstandings about BP and hypertension to rest. Johnson ties together the common pathophysiological paradigms of hypertension—connections between BP, arteriosclerosis, and kidney function—to the chronic disease of hypertension. He discusses the renal function pathways extensively and in detail, which contributes to the complexity of this article.

The article concludes with a section about the causes of the modern epidemic of hypertension. Obesity and diet are discussed here, but exercise and PA are largely ignored. The importance of this article is found in the nature of this review, with historical and current pathophysiological models explained and integrated with each other. The brief treatment of both diet and exercise is a bit disappointing, but the physiological detail is rewarding.

(continued)

Diet, Weight Loss, and BP Management

Blumenthal JA, Babyak MA, Hinderliter A, et al. Effects of the DASH diet alone and in combination with exercise and weight loss on blood pressure and cardiovascular biomarkers in men and women with high blood pressure. Arch Int Med. 2010;170(2):126–135.

The choice of Blumenthal's article really acknowledges the important roles of diet and exercise in controlling and moderating hypertension. Blumenthal has written about research demonstrating that the DASH diet plus what they call "weight management" (WM) was more effective than diet alone or than "usual care" in a control group. Although the research angle is important, the outcome of this study is what should be studied and put into perspective by the exercise professional.

The follow-up period for this study was 4 months. The three groups consisted of a control group, who were asked to maintain diet and exercise habits for the period of the study. The DASH diet and the DASH + WM groups had educational sessions about the DASH diet on a weekly basis throughout the study. Each group demonstrated compliance with the diet, as well as a significant difference between their group and the control group with respect to all factors of the diet. In addition, the DASH + WM group had supervised exercise sessions 3 d/wk, and the attendance to these sessions was documented at >90% as was compliance with the target HR range during exercise (>94%).

The DASH diet significantly reduced both diastolic and systolic BP (11.2/3.4 mm Hg) compared with controls. However, the combination of DASH + WM was more effective in reducing BP (16.1/9.9 mm Hg). The essential and only difference between DASH and DASH + WM was exercise. Thus, Blumenthal and his group demonstrate that the most effective treatment for hypertension is diet and exercise. These subjects were all diagnosed with hypertension, had obesity (body mass index ≥ 30.0 kg/m^2), and were not medicated for hypertension. The "Comment" section of this study provides an excellent discussion of the results along with some comparison to previous research. They also state that this study is part of an ongoing, larger, longer-term study. It is an excellent example of the use and efficacy of lifestyle in the moderation of chronic disease.

REFERENCES

1. Adams V, Linke A, Krankel N, et al. Impact of regular physical activity on NAD(P)H oxidase and angiotensin receptor system in patients with coronary artery disease. Circulation. 2005;111:555–562.

2. American Heart Association Web site: Publications and statistics. Available at: http://www.americanheart.org/presenter.jhtml?identifier=3055922.

3. Appel LH, Brands MW, Daniels SR, et al. Dietary approaches to prevent and treat hypertension: a scientific statement from the American Heart Association. Hypertension. 2006;47(2):296–308.

4. Bazzano LA, Serdula M, Liu S. Prevention of type 2 diabetes by diet and lifestyle modification. J Am Coll Nutr. 2005;24(5):310–319.

5. Berenson GS, Wattigney WA, Tracy RE, et al. Atherosclerosis of the aorta and coronary arteries and cardiovascular risk factors in persons aged 6 to 30 years and studied at necropsy (The Bogalusa Heart Study). Am J Cardiol. 1992;70:851–858.

6. Blair SN, Cheng Y, Holder JS. Is physical activity or physical fitness more important in defining health benefits? Med Sci Sports Exerc. 2001;33(6, Suppl):S379–S399.

7. Blumenthal JA, Babyak MA, Hinderliter A, et al. Effects of the DASH diet alone and in combination with exercise and weight loss on blood pressure and cardiovascular biomarkers in men and women with high blood pressure. Arch Intern Med. 2010;170(2):126–135.

8. Brashers VL. Alterations in cardiovascular function. In: Huether SE, McCance KL, eds. Understanding Pathophysiology. St. Louis, MO: Mosby-Elsevier, 2008, pp. 608–613.

9. Chae CU, Lee RT, Rifai N, et al. Blood pressure and inflammation in apparently healthy men. Hypertension. 2001;38:399–403.

10. Chen C-Y, Bechtold AG, Tabor J, et al. Exercise reduces GABA synaptic input to nucleus tractus solitarii baroreceptor second-order neurons via NK1 receptor internalization in spontaneously hypertensive rats. J Neurosci. 2009;29:2754–2761.

11. Cornelissen VA, Fagard RH. Effect of resistance training on resting blood pressure: a meta-analysis of randomized controlled trials. J Hypertens. 2005;23:251–259.

12. Dandona P, Aljada A, Chadhuri A, et al. Metabolic syndrome: a comprehensive perspective based on interactions between obesity, diabetes and inflammation. Circulation. 2005;111:1448–1454.

13. DASH Diet Eating Plan Web site: http://dashdiet.org/. Accessed December 29, 2008.

14. Dauchet L, Kesse-Guyot E, Czernichow E, et al. Dietary patterns and blood pressure change over 5-y follow-up in the SU.VI.MAX cohort. Am J Clin Nutr. 2007;85(6):1650–1656.

15. Dickinson HO, Mason JM, Nicolson DJ, et al. Lifestyle interventions to reduce raised blood pressure: a systematic review of randomized controlled trials. J Hypertens. 2006;24:215–233.

16. Edwards KM, Ziegler MG, Mills PJ. The potential anti-inflammatory benefits of improving physical fitness in hypertension. J Hypertens. 2007;25: 1533–1542.

17. National Cholesterol Education Program. Executive Summary of the Third Report of the National Cholesterol Education Program (NCEP) Expert Panel on Detection, Evaluation, and Treatment of High Blood Cholesterol in Adults (Adult Treatment Panel III). JAMA. 2001;285:2486–2497.

18. Fagard RH, Cornelissen VA. Effect of exercise on blood pressure control in hypertensive patients. Eur J Cardiovasc Prev Rehabil. 2007;14:12–17.

19. Grundy SM, Cleeman JI, Merz C, et al, for the Coordinating Committee of the National Cholesterol Education Program. Implications of recent clinical trials for the National Cholesterol Education Program Adult Treatment Panel III guidelines. Arterioscler Thromb Vasc Biol. 2004;24(8):e149–e161.

20. Guyton AC, Hall JE. Textbook of Medical Physiology. 10th ed. Saunders Publishing Co., Philadelphia, PA. 2007.

21. Halliwill JR. Mechanisms and clinical implications of post-exercise hypotension in humans. Exerc Sport Sci Rev. 2001;29(2):65–70.

22. Jarvisalo MJ, Harmoinen A, Hakanen M, et al. Elevated serum C-reactive protein levels and early arterial changes in healthy children. Arterioscler Thromb Vasc Biol. 2002;22:1323–1328.

23. Johnson RJ, Feig DI, Nakagawa T, et al. Pathogenesis of essential hypertension: historical paradigms and modern insights. J Hypertens. 2008;26:381–391.

24. Kapiotis S, Holzer G, Schaller G, et al. A proinflammatory state is detectable in obese children and is accompanied by functional and morphological vascular changes. Arterioscler Thromb Vasc Biol. 2006;26:2541–2546.

25. Laughlin HM. Physical activity in prevention and treatment of coronary disease: the battle line is in exercise vascular cell biology. Med Sci Sports Exerc. 2004;36(3):352–362.

26. Libby P. Atherosclerosis: the new view. Sci Am. 2002;286:47–53.

27. Lloyd-Jones D, Adams RJ, Brown TM, et al. Heart disease and stroke statistics—2010 update: a report from the American Heart Association. Circulation. 2010;121:e46–e215.

28. MacDonald JR, MacDougall JD, Hogben CD. The effects of exercise intensity on post exercise hypotension. J Hum Hypertens. 1999;13:527–531.

29. Mach C, Foster C, Brice G, et al. Effect of exercise duration on post-exercise hypotension. J Cardiopulm Rehabil. 2005;25:366–369.

30. Matfin G. Disorders of blood flow and blood pressure. In: Porth CM, ed. Essentials of Pathophysiology: Concepts of Altered Health States. Baltimore, MD: Lippincott, Williams & Wilkins, 2007:360–374.

31. National Health and Nutrition Examination Survey Web site: http://www. cdc.gov/nchs/nhanes.htm. Accessed December 17, 2008.

32. National High Blood Pressure Education Program. The Seventh Report of the Joint Commission on Prevention, Detection, Evaluation and Treatment of High Blood Pressure. Hypertension. 2003;42:1206–1252.

33. O'Rourke MF, Hashimoto J. Arterial stiffness: a modifiable cardiovascular risk factor? J Cardiopulm Rehabil Prev. 2008;28(4):225–237.

34. Padilla J, Wallace JP, Park S. Accumulation of physical activity reduces blood pressure in pre- and hypertension. Med Sci Sports Exerc. 2005;37: 1264–1275.

35. Park S, Rink LD, Wallace JP. Accumulation of physical activity leads to a greater blood pressure reduction than a single continuous session, in prehypertension. J Hypertens. 2006;24(9): 1761–1770.

36. Penco M, Petroni R, Pastori F, et al. Should sports activity be encouraged or contraindicated in hypertensive subjects? J Cardiovasc Med. 2006;7: 288–295.

37. Pescatello LS, Franklin BA, Fagard R, et al. American College of Sports Medicine position stand: exercise and hypertension. Med Sci Sports Exerc. 2004;36(3):533–553.

38. Pescatello LS, Kulikowich JM. The aftereffects of dynamic exercise on ambulatory blood pressure. Med Sci Sports Exerc. 2001;33:1855–1861.

39. Qi L, Hu FB. Dietary glycemic load, whole grains, and systemic inflammation in diabetes: the epidemiological evidence. Curr Opin Lipidol. 2007;18(1):3–8.

40. Rosenzweig JL, Ferrannini E, Grundy SM, et al. Primary prevention of cardiovascular disease and type 2 diabetes in patients at metabolic risk: an Endocrine Society clinical practice guideline. J Clin Endocrinol Metab. 2008;93(10):3671–3689.

41. Sacks FM, Svetkey LP, Vollmer WM, et al, for the DASH-Sodium Collaborative Research Group. Effects on blood pressure of reduced dietary sodium and the Dietary Approaches to Stop Hypertension (DASH) diet. N Engl J Med. 2001;4; 344(1):3–10.

42. Savoia C, Schiffrin E. Inflammation in hypertension. Curr Opin Nephrol Hypertens. 2006;15: 152–158.

43. Vasan RS, Larson MG, Leip EP, et al. Impact of high-normal blood pressure on the risk of cardiovascular disease. N Engl J Med. 2001;345:1291–1297.

44. Wan WH, Powers AS, Li J, et al. Effect of post-myocardial infarction exercise training on the renin–angiotensin–aldosterone system and cardiac function. Am J Med Sci. 2007;334:265–273.

45. Wang Y, Wang QJ. The prevalence of prehypertension and hypertension among US adults according to the new joint national committee guidelines: new challenges of the old problem. Arch Intern Med. 2004;164:2126–2134.

46. Whelton SP, Chin A, Xin X, et al. Effect of aerobic exercise on blood pressure: a meta-analysis of randomized, controlled trials. Ann Intern Med. 2002;136(7):493–503.

47. Williams PT. Physical fitness and activity as separate heart disease risk factors: a meta-analysis. Med Sci Sports Exerc. 2001;33(5):754–761.

48. Williams PT. The illusion of improved physical fitness and reduced mortality. Med Sci Sports Exerc. 2003;35(5):736–740.

49. Williams PT. A cohort study of incident hypertension in relation to changes in vigorous physical activity in men and women. J Hypertens. 2008;26(6):1085–1093.

50. Williams PT. Reduced diabetic, hypertensive, and cholesterol medication use with walking. Med Sci Sports Exerc. 2008;40(3):433–443.

51. Williams PT. Relationship of running intensity to hypertension, hypercholesterolemia, and diabetes. Med Sci Sports Exerc. 2008;40(10):1740–1748.

52. Zieman SJ, Melenovsky V, Kass DA. Mechanisms, pathophysiology and therapy of arterial stiffness. Arterioscler Thromb Vasc Biol. 2005;25:932–943.

9

Prevention and Management of Dyslipidemia with Lifestyle: Diet, Exercise, and Weight Loss

ABBREVIATIONS

Apo	Apoprotein	LDL-C	Low-density lipoprotein
CAD	Coronary artery disease		cholesterol
CREF	Cardiorespiratory endurance	LPL	Lipoprotein lipase
	fitness	PPL	Postprandial lipemia
CVD	Cardiovascular disease	RM	Repetition maximum
HDL	High-density lipoprotein	RT	Resistance training
HDL-C	High-density lipoprotein	STRRIDE	Studies of Targeted Risk
	cholesterol		Reduction Intervention through
IDL	Intermediate-density lipoprotein		Defined Exercise
LDL	Low-density lipoprotein	VLDL	Very low–density lipoproteins

This chapter will address a key cardiovascular disease (CVD) risk factor—dyslipidemia—and its role in the development and progression of atherosclerosis. The primary goal of this chapter is to describe the pathophysiology of dyslipidemia and the effectiveness of lifestyle interventions, specifically exercise to prevent (primary prevention) and reverse dyslipidemia (secondary prevention), thus reducing the risk for events caused by CVD.

EPIDEMIOLOGY OF DYSLIPIDEMIA

Dyslipidemia (abnormal blood lipids) represents a significant health problem in the United States. Dyslipidemia is a primary risk factor for atherosclerosis. Excess cholesterol, particularly oxidized low-density lipoprotein (LDL), is deposited within the intima of arteries, which can eventually cause arterial narrowing and obstruction of blood flow. See Chapter 5 for a detailed description of the development and progression of atherosclerosis. Table 9.1 presents guidelines for blood lipids levels of the National Cholesterol Education Program as well as the authors' opinion for optimal levels for the prevention of atherosclerosis development and progression.

Nearly 107 million U.S. citizens aged 20 years and older (50 million women and 55 million men) have total blood cholesterol levels of ≥200 (36); 37.2 million have levels of ≥240 mg/dl. Figure 9.1 presents data about the percentages of non-Hispanic white, non-Hispanic black, and Mexican Americans who have high LDL levels (>130 mg/dl) and low high-density lipoprotein (HDL) levels (<40 mg/dl).

TABLE 9.1	Guidelines for Blood Lipoprotein Levels Based on the National Cholesterol Education Program (www.nhlbi.nih.gov), ACSM's (American College of Sports Medicine) Guidelines for Exercise Testing and Prescription and the Authors' Opinions for Optimal Atherosclerosis Prevention (2)				
	Optimal	**Desirable**	**Borderline**	**High Risk**	**Very High Risk**
Total cholesterol (mg/dl)	<160	<200	200–239	240–299	300+
LDL-C (mg/dl)	<100	100–129	130–159	160–189	190+
HDL-C (mg/dl)	>60	50–59	40–49	30–39	<30
Triglycerides (mg/dl)	<100	100–149	150–199	200–249	250+
TC/HDL Ratio	<3.0	3.0–3.99	4.0–4.99	5.0–5.99	6.0+

LDL-C, low-density lipoprotein cholesterol; HDL-C, high-density lipoprotein cholesterol; TC, total cholesterol.

Among Americans 20 years of age and older, more non-Hispanic white men and women have a high-density lipoprotein cholesterol (HDL-C) lower than 40 mg/dl than do non-Hispanic black men and women or Mexican-American men, but not women (7,10). During a recent 10-year period of the Framingham Heart Study, HDL-C levels increased from a mean of 44.6 mg/dl to 46.6 mg/dl in men and 56.9 mg/dl to 60.1 mg/dl in women (20).

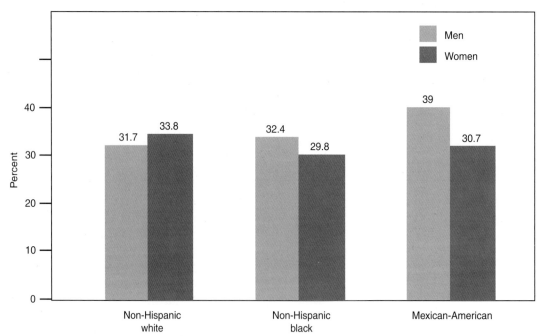

FIGURE 9.1 Prevalence of high low-density lipoprotein cholesterol (LDL-C) (>130) and low high-density lipoprotein cholesterol (HDL-C) (<40) in American adults of differing ethnicities.
Source: From American Heart Association heart facts and statistics: update 2010. Circulation 2010;121:46–215.

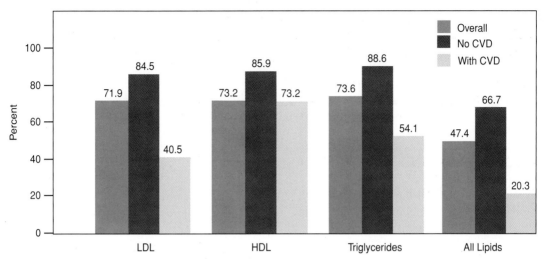

FIGURE 9.2 Percent of Americans at recommended lipid levels according to NHANES data. LDL, low-density lipoprotein; HDL, high-density lipoprotein.
Source: From American Heart Association heart facts and statistics: Update 2010. Circulation 2010;121:46–215.

Triglycerides decreased from a mean of 144.5 mg/dl to 134.1 mg/dl in men and 122.3 mg/dl to 112.4 mg/dl in women. Total cholesterol levels did not change in either men or women and persons with the least increase in body mass index had the most favorable improvements in HDL-C and triglycerides.

Recent studies also show that abnormal levels of postprandial lipids (the level of lipids in the blood after a meal is called "postprandial lipemia," or PPL), particularly triglycerides, are a strong predictor of risk for coronary artery disease (CAD) (4,31). Figure 9.2 presents data on the number of U.S. adults whose lipids are at the recommended levels (12). PPL level in response to a typical Western dietary pattern is of significant interest and concern (see Chapter 4 for a description of the Western dietary vs. the Prudent dietary pattern).

PATHOPHYSIOLOGY OF DYSLIPIDEMIA

PLAQUE FORMATION IN ATHEROSCLEROSIS

The formation of lipid-filled plaque is the underlying process in atherosclerosis. The pathophysiology of atherosclerosis is described in detail in Chapter 5. The initiating event in this process appears to be an "injury" to the endothelium, which causes inflammation and/or endothelial dysfunction. The original injury may be associated with lifestyle behaviors linked to risk factors for atherosclerosis such as diet, sedentary lifestyle, or smoking (29). As a result, lipids, particularly oxidized low-density lipoprotein-cholesterol (LDL-C), along with other cells such as white blood cells, blood platelets, and smooth muscle cells from the arterial media accumulate within the lining of the vessel (the endothelium) to form plaque (blockage). The plaque is deposited under the endothelium, and it progresses at varied rates, depending largely on the presence of risk factors (29). Figure 2.10 in Chapter 2 provides an illustration of some of the events involved atherogenesis.

Dyslipidemia plays a major role in the development and progression of atherosclerotic plaque, but other major risk factors also contribute to the pathophysiology and the process. Fat and cholesterol are not soluble in plasma; thus, they must be transported by circulating molecules, which are called "lipoproteins." Elevated fasting levels of LDL-C, triglycerides, and postprandial levels of triglycerides (PPL), as well as low levels of HDL-C, are strongly associated with increased risk for atherosclerosis. High levels of HDL (>60 mg/dl) are protective and decrease the risk for atherosclerosis.

LIPOPROTEINS AND HEART DISEASE

One example of the potential of LDL-C to cause atherosclerosis is an inherited condition called "familial hypercholesterolemia" in which liver LDL-C receptors are not present in sufficient amounts for LDL-C to be effectively removed from plasma. Individuals with familial hypercholesterolemia who inherit a single defective gene have blood cholesterol levels between 300 and 400 mg/dl. They develop premature atherosclerosis and often experience angina pectoris and myocardial infarction before 40 years of age. In a more rare form of familial hypercholesterolemia, individuals who inherit 2 defective genes from parents have cholesterol levels >600 mg/dl; atherosclerosis usually occurs at a very early age, sometimes before the age of 6 (41).

Research consistently demonstrates a direct relationship between levels of LDL-C and triglycerides and CAD, cerebrovascular disease, and peripheral vascular disease (11,27,44). Other well-controlled studies demonstrate an inverse relationship between HDL and the development and progression CAD, although the mechanisms for this benefit are not clear (11,53).

Numerous other studies demonstrate that lowering LDL-C, non-HDL-C, and triglycerides and/or raising HDL-C levels results in a reduced risk for atherosclerosis and the prevalence of heart attacks and strokes (14,15,17,19,35,50). Figure 9.3 shows some of the lipoprotein types and basic structure.

Recently, studies have suggested a causal link between lipoprotein(a) and ischemic heart disease, although definitive results from randomized clinical trials are lacking (22).

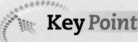 **Key Point**

The scientific evidence clearly implicates LDL-C, particularly the small dense particles and triglycerides as atherogenic. HDL-C is antiatherogenic.

LIPOPROTEIN BASICS

Lipoproteins are primarily composed of lipids (fat), protein, and cholesterol. There are five major types of lipoprotein, and each has several subclasses. For example, there are seven types of LDL-C, based on particle size and density (9,47). Research shows that the smaller, denser LDL-C particles are more atherogenic, whereas larger, less dense particles are protective or neutral (47). The following box provides a basic description of each of the major classes of lipoproteins and their basic biological functions.

There are two sources of cholesterol:

1. Digestion of food containing cholesterol (exogenous)
2. Synthesis of cholesterol, predominantly by the liver (endogenous)

Even though excessive cholesterol is atherogenic, it is an essential substance that is used throughout the body for many biological functions (see the following box). Figure 9.4 illustrates both pathways.

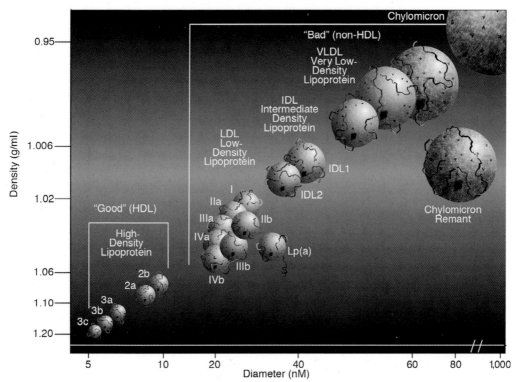

FIGURE 9.3 Lipoproteins come is a variety of types and sizes. Each has specific functional and biological qualities. There is a wide range of particle size and density relating to the specific types of lipoproteins and their atherogenicity. HDL, high-density lipoprotein; IDL, intermediate-density lipoprotein; LDL, low-density lipoproteins; VLDL, very low–density lipoprotein.

DID YOU KNOW?
Major Categories of Lipoproteins

Category	Biological Function(s)
VLDL	Major transporter of triglycerides in blood
LDL	Major transporter of free cholesterol in blood, most atherogenic of lipoproteins
IDL	Transitional lipoprotein in the metabolism of LDL, highly related to the progression of atherosclerosis
Triglycerides	Storage form of fat; provides energy when fatty acids are degraded by the enzyme lipoprotein lipase and released in to working muscle; an atherogenic lipoprotein, particularly those present in postprandial blood
HDL	Transports cholesterol to the liver from peripheral arterial sites where it is used to form bile acids; HDL is considered anti-atherogenic and partly through the mechanism of "reverse cholesterol transport"; HDL is also anti-inflammatory.
Chylomicrons	Digested form of lipoprotein which is converted to VLDLs in the liver

VLDL, Very low–density Lipoprotein; LDL, low-density lipoprotein; IDL, intermediate-density lipoprotein; HDL, high-density lipoprotein.

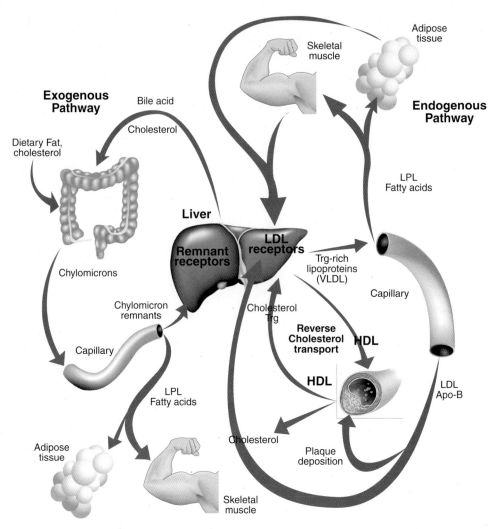

FIGURE 9.4 Exogenous and endogenous cholesterol transport pathways. In the exogenous pathway, cholesterol and fatty acids from food are absorbed through the GI tract. Triglycerides and cholesterol are packaged into chylomicrons, and lipids are bound to proteins to form lipoproteins. In fat or muscle tissue the triglyceride is removed from the very low–density lipoprotein (VLDL) with the aid of lipoprotein lipase (LPL). High-density lipoproteins (HDLs) take up cholesterol from cells. In the endogenous pathway, the liver synthesizes cholesterol from macronutrient materials.
Source: From Rubin R, Strayer DS. Rubin's Pathology: Clinicopathologic Foundations of Medicine, 5th ed. Philadelphia: Lippincott Williams & Wilkins, 2008.

DID YOU KNOW?
Key Biological Functions of Cholesterol

- Component of cell membranes
- Backbone structure of sex hormones, including testosterone and estrogen
- Backbone structure of vitamin D
- Component of bile acids

PROTEIN CONTENT OF LIPOPROTEINS

There are several major proteins associated with lipoproteins, called "apoproteins" (apo). ApoB-100 is the primary protein of LDL, and B-48 is the main protein component of chylomicrons (transport form of triglycerides from the gut to the liver) and very low–density lipoproteins (VLDLs). ApoB proteins bind to LDL receptors, resulting in uptake and activation of cellular metabolism. ApoE protein is involved in the recognition of HDL-C by cells and also in clearing other lipoproteins (such as VLDLs) from the liver. ApoA-1 is a major constituent of chylomicrons. Apo(a) is strongly associated with CVD risk. LDL and Apo(a) combine to form lipoprotein(a), a highly atherogenic lipoprotein (22). These Apos serve several functions, including recognition of cell membrane receptors for lipoproteins and acting as cofactors in lipoprotein metabolic reactions.

ENZYMES INVOLVED IN LIPOPROTEIN METABOLISM

Several enzymes are involved in the biochemistry of lipoproteins. Lecithin cholesterol acyltransferase facilitates "reverse cholesterol transport" through HDL-C. This is a process that allows cholesterol to be transported from arteries to the liver, where it is taken up and used to synthesize bile acids and is eliminated. Two other proteins, Apo CI and CII (components of both HDL and VLDL), activate lecithin cholesterol acyl transferase and lipoprotein lipase (LPL), both of which are antiatherogenic. Finally, ApoE

DID YOU KNOW?

Key Enzymes Involved in Lipid Metabolism

Enzyme	Function(s)
HMG Co-A reductase	Rate-limiting enzyme in synthesis of cholesterol in the liver; also the target of "statin" medications that lower LDL-C.
Hepatic lipase	Converts HDL_2 to HDL_3. HDL_3 decreases cholesterol in foam cells, thus may be anti-atherogenic. Together with another enzyme—cholesterol ester transfer protein—hepatic lipase is believed to interact with HDL_2 to reduce the risk for atherosclerosis.
Lecithin cholesterol acyltransferase	Responsible for facilitating reverse cholesterol transport.
Lipoprotein lipase	An enzyme that breaks down fat; located on the surface of vascular endothelial cells and on macrophages. It is responsible for the breakdown of triglycerides; low levels of lipoprotein lipase are associated with high triglycerides and low HDLs; exercise and weight loss increase LPL activity and result in lower triglycerides and may also result in a substantial increase in HDL-C.

HMG Co-A reductase, 3-hydroxy-3-methyl-glutaryl-CoA reductase, or HMGCR; LDL-C, low-density lipoprotein cholesterol; HDL-C, high-density lipoprotein cholesterol.

facilitates cholesterol uptake and elimination. Some of the key enzymes involved in lipid metabolism are summarized in the box titled "Key Enzymes Involved in Lipid Metabolism."

EXERCISE AND PREVENTION OF DYSLIPIDEMIA

Exercise, diet, and weight loss are powerful tools in the prevention and management of dyslipidemia. Among the most consistent and reliable benefits of regular cardiorespiratory endurance fitness (CREF) exercise are its effects on blood levels of lipoproteins and the chronic adaptations in lipoprotein metabolism. CREF exercise training, along with a low-saturated fat, low-trans fat, and high-fiber diet and decreased body fat has been documented to decrease triglycerides and LDL-C and increase HDL-C (28,42,45,46,55,58,60,62,63). A single session of CREF exercise for 30 to 45 minutes at 60% to 85% of VO_{2max} lowers triglycerides and raises HDL-C (5,18,37). This beneficial, subacute effect of exercise on plasma lipoproteins may be sustained for 24 to 96 hours.

> ### Key Point
> A CREF exercise training session of 30 to 45 minutes at 60% to 85% of VO_{2max} results in a subacute lowering of triglycerides and an increase in HDL-C that may be sustained for 24 to 96 hours or longer.

Cross-sectional studies demonstrate an inverse relationship between weekly amount of CREF exercise and levels of triglycerides and LDL-C (23,24,25,26,55,57,59). In contrast, there is a positive relationship between levels of HDL-C and the weekly amount of CREF exercise (23,55,57). Williams et al. (57,58) reported a strong, consistent, and beneficial relationship between weekly running distance and all major lipoproteins among more than 10,000 runners. More recently, Williams et al (56) demonstrates an inverse relationship between weekly running volume and the use of lipid-lowering medications. These studies clearly demonstrate a positive and beneficial relationship between volume of running per week (physical activity) and levels of blood lipoproteins.

Although the effects of resistance training (RT) on lipid metabolism are less well defined, several recent studies suggest a beneficial effect of RT alone or in combination with aerobic exercise training (21,33,39,49,54). In addition, the American Heart Association recently updated their position statement on RT and cardiovascular disease prevention and rehabilitation (56). In this statement the authors conclude that

1. a modest benefit on lipoproteins can be anticipated following a consistent and properly designed RT program, and
2. RT combined with CREF exercise may be more effective than either alone.

> ### Key Point
> Aerobic exercise is of primary importance in planning exercise for dyslipidemia. However, RT, particularly when combined with aerobic exercise, may be as beneficial.

They also conclude though that RT should be viewed as a compliment to rather than a replacement for CREF endurance exercise.

Several randomized longitudinal studies show that chronic CREF exercise with a weekly calorie expenditure ≥1200 results in decreased triglycerides and increased HDL-C (28,43,45,59,62). However, the response among individuals is variable, suggesting a genetic influence on the response of lipids to CREF exercise training (58,60). Wood and his colleagues published several randomized studies showing that a 12-month CREF exercise program (equivalent of 18 miles per week of jogging/walking) significantly improves lipoprotein metabolism and blood levels (62,63). The benefit is enhanced when weight and body-fat loss occurred simultaneously with the CREF exercise program (45,62). These findings support the conclusion that that the benefits of CREF exercise training on lipoproteins are enhanced when combined with a healthy low-fat, high-fiber diet and weight loss (43,46).

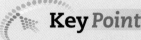

Key Point

Early randomized trials support the conclusion that the benefits of CREF exercise training on lipid metabolism and lipid levels are enhanced when combined with a healthy diet and weight loss.

Recently, Kraus and colleagues (28) published the results of the "STRRIDE" project. STRRIDE stands for "Studies of Targeted Risk Reduction Intervention through Defined Exercise." This study examined several lipoprotein risk factors using three different combinations of intensity and duration in the exercise prescriptions (28,42). Kraus divided participants into four groups, including a control group and three exercise groups: (1) high-duration/high-intensity exercise group (the caloric equivalent of 18 miles of jogging/week at 60%–85% of peak VO_{2max}), (2) low-duration/high-intensity group (caloric equivalent of 12 miles of jogging per week at 60%–85% of peak VO_{2max}), and (3) low-duration/moderate-intensity group (caloric equivalent of 12 miles per week at 40%–55% of peak VO_{2max}) (28).

After an initial 2-month period of progression to the prescribed exercise program, participants trained for 8 months. Exercising participants were asked to maintain their bodyweight, and 84 of the 111 participants were successful. The improvement of lipoproteins was significantly better in the high-duration/high-intensity group than the other exercise groups on all but one of the 11 lipoprotein variables. Improvement in lipoproteins did not seem to be associated with intensity. A serious limitation of this otherwise well-controlled study was the lack of a high-duration/moderate-intensity group.

A follow-up report from the STRRIDE study demonstrated that just 5 days of inactivity after the 8 months of training resulted in significant increases in total LDL-C and other atherogenic LDL-C subparticles (42). In the high-duration/high-intensity group, improvements in HDL-C, HDL-C particle size, and levels of large HDL-C were maintained after 15 days of inactivity. Both of these studies will be discussed in more detail in the "Digging Deeper" section later in this chapter.

The beneficial effects of exercise on PPL are well documented. In cross-sectional studies, higher levels of CREF are associated with improved PPL, and, in randomized trials, CREF exercise has been shown to improve PPL (13,16,43,46). The improvement in PPL seems to be related to increased LPL activity after a 30- to 45-minute CREF exercise session (13,43,46,48,65,66). The breakdown of blood triglycerides is increased during and for a prolonged period after exercise (5,18,37). This represents another subacute effect that supports the importance of daily exercise (see Chapter 3 for a discussion of the subacute effects of exercise). Figure 9.5 represents the effects of exercise on PPL.

In addition, 30 minutes of brisk walking has been shown to offset the increase in postprandial triglycerides associated with a diet in which carbohydrates are substituted for fat (6,13). The effects of RT on PPL in general are not well defined; thus, conclusions are unclear right now (40,64). Finally, as indicated earlier, PPL may be a more significant risk factor for atherosclerosis and endothelial dysfunction than fasting lipids. A recent study reported that high-intensity aerobic interval training completely attenuated the endothelial dysfunction induced by PPL (52).

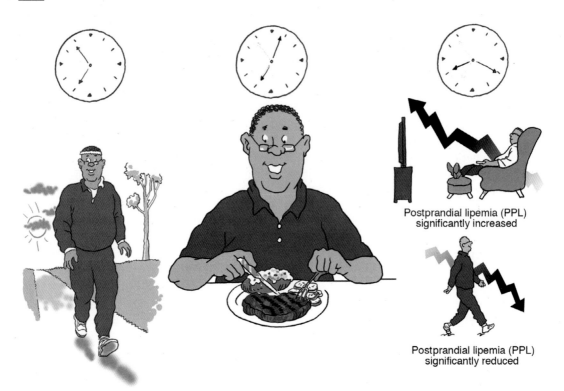

FIGURE 9.5 A high-fat meal is followed by a significant increase of fats (triglycerides) in the blood. That phenomenon is called "postprandial lipemia" (PPL). PPL is significantly reduced by moderate CREF exercise performed about 12 hours prior to the food intake.

As we stated previously, the favorable effect of exercise training on PPL is most apparent when the exercise is performed 8 to 12 hours before consuming a high-fat meal (43,46,48). The mechanism for this phenomenon is thought to be the increased activity of LPL in response to a single exercise session. LPL appears to peak between 8 and 12 hours after a moderate-to-vigorous session of exercise (43,46,48,66). This finding is thought to be related to the time necessary for protein synthesis and LPL gene expression to be induced and again illustrates the importance of daily physical activity (46). The peak in LPL activity after exercise generally corresponds to the time frame of the subacute, exercise-induced lowering of triglycerides. The increased LPL activity facilitates increased breakdown of VLDL-triglycerides and, thus, increased availability of triglycerides for energy production within the exercising muscle cell. The subsequent increased availability of VLDL-remnant molecules may, in turn, be related to the observed increase in HDL-C synthesis after an aerobic session of exercise.

Other studies have reported similar effects on PPL after accumulated exercise sessions. For example, the effects on PPL of three 10-minute sessions of exercise interrupted by 20 minutes of recovery versus one continuous session of 30 minutes, once per day at equivalent intensities, were similar (1,30). Though the evidence is not conclusive, it seems that if caloric expenditure is

> **Key Point**
>
> An exercise session of 30 to 45 minutes' duration at a moderate to high intensity attenuates PPL and seems to be most effective when the exercise occurs 8 to 12 hours before a meal, when LPL activity is greatest.

equal, triglycerides and HDL-C may be improved to the same degree after a 4- to 12-week period of either accumulated or continuous exercise sessions. Thus, persons with dyslipidemia may achieve similar benefits from performing a minimum of three 10-minute sessions or one 30-minute session of exercise per day. One significant issue with the generalization of this recommendation, however, is that, because of the intermittent exercise, it requires more than an hour to perform 30 minutes of exercise. This approach may not be practical for most busy people. Thus, the authors believe that it is premature to suggest that intermittent exercise is as effective as 30 to 60 minutes of continuous exercise for optimizing blood lipids and lipoproteins.

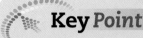

Key Point

Although intermittent exercise in 10 to 15 minutes per session may be as effective as a continuous 30- to 45-minute session of exercise in attenuating PPL, the evidence remains equivocal, and, thus, continuous exercise at moderate to high intensity is preferred.

GUIDELINES FOR EXERCISE AND LIFESTYLE

The literature clearly supports the effectiveness of exercise for improving lipoprotein profile. Both higher-intensity exercise (e.g., for HDL-C) and lower-intensity exercise (for triglycerides) have been shown to be effective for specific lipoproteins. Increased

DID YOU KNOW?

General Nutrition Tips for Improving Blood Lipids

- Lose weight and body fat if necessary to achieve ideal body composition
- Consume <7% of daily calories from saturated fat
- Consume little or no trans-fat
- 20% to 30% of daily calories may come from fat sources, but 13% to 23% should be mono- or poly-unsaturated
- Consume <150 milligrams of cholesterol per day
- Consume a ¼ cup of berries every day
- Consume 2 to 3 fish meals (salmon, tuna, mackerel, sardines, trout) per week
- Consume 25 mg of soy protein per day
- Consume ¼ cup of nuts (walnuts, almonds, pecans, pistachios) per day
- Consume ½ to 1 cup of cooked beans and legumes (black, pinto, garbanzo, lima, navy, etc.)
- Consume 15 to 20 g of soluble fiber per day, along with 35 to 45 g of total fiber per day
- Consume only whole grains (oats, barley, brown rice, quinoa, bulgur, other)
- Limit simple sugars to no >5% of calories per day
- Limit all processed foods
- Limit alcohol to 1 or 2 drinks for men and 1 drink for women per day

TABLE 9.2	Optimal Guidelines for Exercise Management of Dyslipidemia*			
Program Component	**Frequency (d/wk)**	**Intensity (%HRR/%1RM)**	**Duration (min/session/d)**	**Mode**
CREF training	4–7 (optimally aim for >5 d/wk.)	40%–85% 12–16 RPE	15–60 min, 1–4 sessions/d (2–4 to equal 60 min per day– optimal), 300 min/week ≥2,000 kcal/wk	Large muscle, rhythmic, for example, walk, jog, bike, swim, elliptical, and so on.
Resistance training	2–3	60%–80% 1RM 12–16 RPE Stop 2–3 reps from volitional fatigue	30–45 minutes per session 2–3 sets, 8–15 repetitions	8–12 large-muscle exercises preferable

HRR, heart rate reserve; 1RM, One repetition-maximum; CREF, cardiorespiratory endurance fitness; RPE, ratings of perceived exertion.

*Moderation of postprandial lipemia (PPL) is best accomplished by exercise 12 hours prior to the high-fat meal.

CREF and individual exercise sessions, including both aerobic, cardiovascular endurance exercise and RT, have been shown to improve dyslipidemia. For more information on RT, see ACSM's statement entitled "Progression Models in Resistance Training" (34). This leads to the logical conclusion that an exercise program combining vigorous/moderate exercise with periodic longer-duration exercise is most beneficial for mitigating this risk factor. Table 9.2 summarizes guidelines for exercise management of dyslipidemia. The following box provides some general nutrition tips that may favorably affect blood lipids. Additional information on diet and lipoproteins (lipids) may be found in Chapter 4 on Nutrition.

DID YOU KNOW?
What Are Processed Foods?

"Processed foods" have been somehow altered from their natural state. Generally, we are referring to processed grains that have had the germ and other nutrient components removed. Many of these grains, for example, white (refined) flour, are further processed by adding vitamins and other nutrients that were previously removed during the initial processing. Processed meat carries significant risk for cancer and heart disease and should be avoided. These meats are preserved by smoking, curing, or salting, and/or have added chemicals, namely, "nitrites" as preservatives. Sausages, bacon, hot dogs, and deli or luncheon meats are examples of processed meat.

DIGGING DEEPER

Exercise and Lipoproteins

In previous chapters, as well as earlier in this chapter, we have discussed the evidence that regular physical activity and/or structured exercise is associated with a significantly reduced risk for cardiovascular disease morbidity and mortality. One of the mechanisms for this frequently observed relationship is the beneficial effects of exercise on plasma lipoproteins. However, the optimal intensity and/or frequency of exercise for improving lipoproteins is not clearly established. In this section we will discuss the effects of exercise on lipoproteins and the optimal exercise prescription.

It has long been accepted that exercise has an overall beneficial effect on lipids and lipoproteins. Some of the earlier studies focused on total cholesterol, triglycerides primarily because that was the state of the knowledge (46). Regardless, this body of research did establish this important relationship.

There remains, however, information about exercise and lipoproteins that is unclear. The biological complexity of lipoprotein metabolism contributes to the difficulty of designing adequately controlled research to address the issue. The impact of macronutrient ingestion before and after exercise contributes to the problems with research design and interpretation. In addition, changes in body composition add to the difficulty of interpretation. The literature on this subject is very complicated. We will discuss a few studies that address lipoproteins and exercise, leaving the resolution of research design to the experts doing this research.

In this chapter we discussed several cross-sectional and randomized studies that suggest that a minimum calorie expenditure of approximately 1200 kcal/week of aerobic exercise is required for some benefit, but that additional benefit may be derived from additional weekly calorie expenditure from exercise. Recently, Kraus and colleagues published the results of the STRRIDE and the effects on plasma lipoproteins (28). Although this study is not definitive, there are a few important conclusions that may be derived from the results.

This study was a randomized trial with a cohort of 111 sedentary, overweight men and women, aged 40 to 65 years, with mild-to-moderate dyslipidemia. Participants were randomized to a control group (n = 26), a low-amount/moderate-intensity (n = 19), a low-amount/high-intensity (n = 17), or a high-amount/high-intensity group (n = 22). The study lasted 6 months; Table 9.3 summarizes the intensity and volume of exercise each group sustained throughout the study.

(continued)

TABLE 9.3	Intensity and Volume of Exercise by Group in the STRRIDE Study (42)			
	Amount of Exercise (miles/wk)	Intensity of Exercise (% VO_{2max})	Exercise Cal/Expend (cal/wk)	Frequency (d/wk)
Low amount/moderate intensity	10.5	40–55	1075	3.5
Low amount/high intensity	11.0	65–80	1104	2.9
High amount/high intensity	16.7	65–80	1681	3.6

TABLE 9.4	Changes in Selected Lipoproteins by Exercise Group in the STRRIDE Study (28,42)		
	LDL-C* (mg/dl)	**HDL-C* (md/dl)**	**Triglycerides* (mg/dl)**
Low amount/ moderate intensity	+3.7	+0.7	−49.6
Low amount/ high intensity	+3.6	+0.3	−13.1
High amount/ high intensity	−1.9	+4.6	−28.6

LDL-C, low-density lipoprotein cholesterol, HDL-C, high-density lipoprotein cholesterol.
*No significant differences among groups.

The low-amount/moderate-intensity group averaged 176 minutes per week, whereas the low-amount/high-intensity and high-amount/high-intensity groups averaged 117 and 174 minutes per week, respectively. Table 9.4 shows the changes in lipoproteins by exercise group. Although the results of this and subsequent STRRIDE research is complicated, Kraus and colleagues (28) summarize the findings by stating that exercise caused many beneficial changes in lipoproteins. They further state that a high amount (greater weekly caloric expenditure) appeared to be the critical factor rather than the intensity of the exercise. Though this is correct, we should point out that Kraus and colleagues (28) did not include "high amount/moderate intensity" in their research design. Thus, it remains unknown whether a high-amount/moderate-intensity group would have also improved the lipoprotein profile to a similar degree as the high-amount/high-intensity group (28).

The results also demonstrate that the high-intensity/high-amount group had significantly decreased concentrations of small LDL-C and total LDL-C particles as well as increased average size of LDL-C particles. The high-intensity/high-amount group also had a significantly greater increase in large HDL-C particles. The size and density of lipoprotein particles are significant with respect to their atherogenic effects. Small, dense LDL-C particles are more atherogenic than large, less dense particles. Likewise, HDL-C particle size and density also effect atherogenicity, with larger particles being more protective than smaller, denser particles (47).

These findings, therefore, are associated with an expected lower risk of CVD. It is also important to note that Kraus and colleagues (28) found that exercise, in any of these combinations of intensity and duration, was more effective than not exercising (the control group) with respect to the effects on lipoproteins.

Slentz et al. (42) published a second study from STRRIDE several years later. This study was significant because it included detraining data on all groups. Thus, the effects of exercise and detraining were documented as well as the persistence of the effects in a posttraining period with no exercise. The subacute and the chronic effects of exercise become more apparent in this research design. Three major findings from this study are summarized as follows:

1. HDL-C was most improved in the high-amount/high-intensity exercise group, and these effects were sustained up to 2 weeks posttraining with no exercise. HDL-C was significantly increased within 24 hours after a single exercise session. The size of the

HDL-C particles also increased significantly. These changes support the beneficial effects of high-amount/high-intensity exercise on HDL-C as opposed to moderate-intensity or high-intensity/low-volume exercise. Finally, this is a subacute effect that occurs with daily exercise, even though the changes were sustained over 2 weeks after the last exercise session. The length of the effect after exercise requires further study.

2. Triglycerides are most affected by low-amount/moderate-intensity exercise. The decrease in triglycerides in this group was double the size of the decrease in the other two groups. In this low-intensity group, this change was maintained over 15 days (as the triglycerides were), but in the two higher-intensity groups the change was maintained for 5 days and then were diminished at 15 days (the magnitude of change was less, thus accounting for the earlier loss of the benefit on triglycerides).

3. Sustained physical inactivity is associated with increased LDL-C particle number and density (these changes are associated with increased atherogenicity). The control group also demonstrated increased weight, waist circumference, and visceral fat—again, all changes that increase risk of disease and event (42).

We would like to discuss one additional significant finding in the STRRIDE study. Slentz and his colleagues (42) found that the moderate-intensity/moderate-amount exercise was associated with greater decreases in triglycerides than higher-intensity exercise in either the high-amount or low-amount group. The fact is that HDL-C (low-amount/high-intensity and high-amount/high-intensity) and VLDL triglycerides (all three groups) were both significantly changed 24 hours after an exercise session. In addition, LDL-C particle size and density both increased (positive changes) at 24 hours after exercise. Slentz et al. (42) (and Kraus et al. (28)) thus demonstrated that these beneficial effects of exercise occur consistently in the period immediately after exercise. These are subacute effects, and, as long as training (exercise) continues, the changes are likely to be sustained (28,42).

Clearly, anyone attempting to improve lipoprotein profile with exercise is not (hopefully) going to train for 9 months, then quit for 2 weeks, just because some of the benefits are sustained for that short period of time. The benefits are subacute benefits that will certainly disappear after some undetermined time of detraining. In fact, the benefits of the exercise training program were disappearing at the time of the last blood samples according to the results of this study.

One additional study merits attention in this discussion. Recently, Tsekouras and colleagues (51) studied the effects of a single session of resistance exercise on the removal of VLDL triacylglycerol (triglycerides) from the blood.

They closely controlled the exercise and nutrient intake after exercise by feeding the participants a specified meal after the exercise session and before sampling blood the next day. The blood samples were taken 14 hours after the exercise and the meal. The RT session was a low-intensity (HR = 125, VO_2 = 10.9 ml/kg-min, 80% peak torque) "aerobic" session but may be classified as a moderate-intensity session of RT exercise. The duration (90 minutes) is classified as "long" in comparison to the STRRIDE study.

Tsekouras et al. (51) found that VLDL triglyceride levels were significantly reduced (by approximately 30%) after a single session of resistance exercise. Interestingly, they also demonstrated a significant decrease in a lipoprotein called "ApoB100," which is a primary component of LDL-C. Coupled with the decreased triglycerides, this is clearly a beneficial, subacute effect of exercise.

What does all of this mean? Perhaps, it means that this confusing picture of the research on lipids, lipoproteins, and exercise is beginning to be sorted out. The older, long-term

(continued)

studies of exercise and lipoproteins examined changes subsequent to 12- to 52-week training programs and sampled participants only before and after exercise. In order to discern the subacute nature of these changes, they would have to sample participants sometime between 24 and 72 hours after exercise, and they did not do this.

From these studies, it can be concluded that many of the beneficial exercise-related changes in lipoprotein are subacute and that they occur in the period of 24 to 96 hours postexercise. Some of these changes persist with no subsequent exercise for a short period (e.g., 5–15 days in the Slentz study), but others do not. Thus, although the complete beneficial effects of exercise on lipoproteins have yet to be elucidated, what is known clearly demonstrates that regular exercise training is beneficial and that many of the benefits occur in the period shortly after exercise and may subside sometime between 24 hours and 2 weeks. The lesson to be learned from all of this is that compliance to a regular, daily program of varying-intensity exercise coupled with high amounts of physical activity is critical to improving this risk factor.

Significant RESEARCH

We have selected two studies that investigate exercise and PPL, because this topic is important for assessing cardiovascular risk and is underappreciated. Lipoprotein profile and PPL are amenable to improvement with exercise. The criteria for the effective dose of exercise also are relatively specific to PPL. The exercise required to modify PPL is most effective if it occurs about 8 to 12 hours before a (high-fat) meal. The two studies discussed here address the topic of PPL from two different approaches. Summarizing these results is relatively simple—exercise attenuates increased blood levels of triglycerides during the postprandial period. Continuous and intermittent exercise, as well as RT, seem to have similar effects.

Exercise and Postprandial Triglycerides

Burns SF, Hardman AE, Stensel D. Brisk walking offsets the increase in postprandial TAG concentration found when changing to a diet with increased carbohydrate. Br J Nutr. 2009;101(12):1787–1796.

Dr. Burns and colleagues performed some interesting research on walking and PPL after consumption of a high-carbohydrate meal. The point of their study was to determine whether the addition of a "brisk walk" would attenuate the increased triglycerides often experienced following a meal that is high in carbohydrates. The higher-carbohydrate meal was compared to the "standard United Kingdom" diet, in which the macronutrient mix is as follows: 40% fat, 45% carbohydrates, and 15% protein. The "recommended" diet aims for 30% fat, 55% carbohydrates, and 15% protein; this is a dietary pattern lower in fat and higher in carbohydrates. The research question is whether exercise can offset the increased PPL after the higher-carbohydrate meal compared to a meal that adheres to the United Kingdom's "usual" dietary pattern.

Unfortunately, the study was designed in a manner that did not measure triglycerides long enough into the postexercise period to assess the effects of the walk on PPL. Regardless, the authors point out that the research confirms that increasing dietary carbohydrates is associated with increased postprandial triglycerides and they did, in fact, demonstrate this in their control group.

The authors closely controlled dietary intake over 4 days, including the measurement day, under three different conditions—(1) a "typical U.K. diet"; (2) a "recommended" diet (presumably a healthier alternative to the typical U.K. diet); and (3) a "recommended diet with walk." All testing for each trial was done on day 4, in a laboratory where all participants were fed three meals on the prescribed diet and monitored at rest and during exercise for the entire day. The brisk walk was performed in the laboratory on a treadmill before the breakfast meal. Blood samples were taken at various intervals throughout the day following the walk (each hour at a minimum), resting metabolic rate was measured early in the morning before breakfast and walking, and exercise energy expenditure was measured.

The results are presented in a rather complex format, but the major finding and primary outcome is that walking when coupled with the higher-carbohydrate diet offsets the increase in triglycerides that has been demonstrated in this and other studies.

The walking exercise in this study can be considered a "moderate- intensity" session. The participants self-selected an average pace of 4.0 mph on the treadmill and exercise-related oxygen uptake was measured at 17.6 ml/kg-minute (about 4 METs after correcting for the resting energy expenditure). This was 53% of their estimated peak VO_2 from the exercise test performed during before testing. The mean total calorie expenditure during 30 minutes of walking was measured at 207 calories. Thus, in this study a brief session of "brisk" walking after consumption of a meal higher in carbohydrates resulted in lower triglycerides after exercise than in the event of consuming the same meal without walking. Exercise, then, produces a beneficial effect on triglycerides in the postprandial period.

Resistance Exercise and PPL

Zafeiridis A, Goloi E, Petridou A. Effects of low- and high-volume resistance exercise on postprandial lipaemia. Br J Nutr. 2007;97:471–477.

Dr. Zafeiridis and colleagues designed this study to determine whether PPL could be modified by a high-volume or a low-volume RT session. The researchers controlled the energy expenditure and the intensity of RT as well as the content of a high-fat meal fed to participants 16 hours after the RT trials. Two RT trials were performed in random order. One trial used a "low-volume" RT protocol (2 sets of 8 exercises at 12 repetitions maximum (RM) completed in 39 minutes), and the second used a "high-volume" RT protocol (4 sets of 8 exercises at 12 RM completed in 79 minutes). The low-volume RT resulted in an average calorie expenditure of approximately 215 calories for the entire session, and the high-volume calorie expenditure was approximately 400 calories.

The results demonstrate that both a high-volume and a low-volume RT program result in moderating PPL after a high-fat meal. In addition, and interestingly, neither RT protocol changed insulin sensitivity or blood glucose in the period after exercise. The authors suggest that calorie expenditure during exercise may not be the only variable that determines the postprandial effects of RT. PPL was attenuated after both high- and low-volume RT exercise sessions. Thus, the effect occurred despite the differences in energy expenditure of the two RT exercise sessions. They further speculate that perhaps RT presents a greater "metabolic stress" than aerobic exercise. In addition, the authors state that the intermittent nature of the RT may further contribute to the effect. They cite Altena et al. (1) (see discussion under "Exercise and Lipoproteins") whose study demonstrated that intermittent aerobic exercise (three 10-minute sessions at 60% VO_{2max}, separated by 20 minutes of rest) attenuates PPL as effectively as 30 minutes of continuous aerobic exercise for 30 minutes at 60% VO_{2max}.

REFERENCES

1. Altena TS, Michaelson JL, Ball JD, et al. Single sessions of intermittent and continuous exercise and postprandial lipemia. Med Sci Sports Exerc. 2004; 36:1364–1371.

2. American Heart Association Heart Facts and Statistics: Update 2010. Circulation. 2010;121: e46–e215.

3. Bansai S, Buring JE, Rifal N. Fasting compared with nonfasting triglycerides and risk of cardiovascular events. JAMA. 2007;298:309–316.

4. Berg A, Johns J, Baumstark M, et al. Changes in HDL subfractions after a single, extended episode of physical exercise. Atherosclerosis. 1983; 47:231–240.

5. Burns SF, Hardman AE, Stensel D. Brisk walking offsets the increase in postprandial TAG concentration found when changing to a diet with increased carbohydrate. Br J Nutr. 2009;101(12): 1787–1796.

6. Carroll MD, Lacher DA, Sorlie PD. Trends in serum lipids and lipoproteins of adults, 1960–2002. JAMA. 2005;294:1773–1781.

7. Crouse SF, O'Brien BC, Rohack JJ. Changes in serum lipids and apolipoproteins after exercise in men with high cholesterol: influence of intensity. J Appl Physiol. 1995;79:279–286.

8. Ellington AA, Kullo IJ. Atherogenic lipoprotein profiling. Adv Clin Chem. 2008;46:295–317.

9. Ford ES, Chaoyang L, Zhao G. Hypertriglyceridemia and its pharmacologic treatment among US adults. Arch Intern Med. 2009;169:572–578.

10. Framingham Heart Study Web Site [Internet]. Available at: www.nhlbi.nih.gov/about/framingham/. Accessed April 9, 2010.

11. Ghandehari HS, Kamai-Bahi S, Wong ND. Prevalence and extent of dyslipidemia and recommended lipid levels in US adults with and without cardiovascular comorbidities: the National Health and Nutrition Examination Survey 2003–2004. Am Heart J. 2008;156:112–119.

12. Gill JM, Hardman AE. Exercise and postprandial lipid metabolism: an update on potential mechanisms and interactions with high carbohydrate diets (review). J Nutr Biochem. 2003;14: 122–132.

13. Gordon NF, LaFontaine TP. Comprehensive cardiovascular risk reduction in patients with coronary artery disease. In: Roitman JL, ed. ACSM's Resource Manual for Guidelines for Exercise Testing and Prescription. 4th Ed . Baltimore, MD: Williams and Wilkins, 2003, pp. 254–266.

14. Gould AL, Davies GM, Alemao E. Cholesterol reduction yields clinical benefits: meta-analysis including recent trials. Clin Ther. 2007;29: 778–794.

15. Hardman AE. The influence of exercise on postprandial triacylglycerol metabolism. Atherosclerosis. 1998;131(Suppl 1):593–600.

16. Hausenloy DJ, Yellon DM. Targeting residual cardiovascular risk: raising high-density lipoprotein cholesterol levels. Heart. 2008;94:706–714.

17. Henderson GC, Krauss RM, Fattor JM. Plasma triglyceride concentrations are rapidly reduced following individual bouts of endurance exercise in women. Eur J Appl Physiol. doi: 10.1007/s00421-010-1409-7.

18. Houslay ES, Sarma J, Uren NG. The effect of intensive lipid lowering on coronary atheroma and clinical outcome. Heart. 2007;93:149–151.

19. Ingelsson E, Massaro JM, Sutherland P. Contemporary trends in dyslipidemia in the Framingham Heart Study. Arch Intern Med. 2009;169: 279–286.

20. Kamstrup PR. Lipoprotein(a) and ischemic heart disease—a causal association: a review. Atherosclerosis. 2010. doi: 10.1016/j.atherosclerosis.2009. 12.036.

21. Kelley GA, Kelley KS. Aerobic exercise and lipids and lipoproteins in men: a meta-analysis of randomized controlled trials. J Mens Health Gend. 2006;3:61–70.

22. Kelley GA, Kelley KS. Impact of progressive resistance training on lipids and lipoproteins in adults: another look at a meta-analysis using prediction intervals. Prev Med. 2009;49:473–475.

23. Kelley GA, Kelley KS, Franklin B. Aerobic exercise and lipids and lipoproteins in patients with cardiovascular disease: a meta-analysis of randomized controlled trials. J Cardiopulm Rehabil. 2006;26:131–139.

24. Kelley GA, Kelley KS, Tran ZV. Aerobic exercise and lipids and lipoproteins in women: a meta-analysis of randomized controlled trials. J Womens Health. 2004;11:46–64.

25. Kelley GA, Kelley KS, Tran ZV. Exercise, lipids, and lipoproteins in older adults: a meta-analysis. Prev Cardiol. 2005;8:206–214.

26. Keys A. Coronary heart disease in seven countries. Nutrition. 1997;13:250–252.

27. Kraus WE, Houmard JA, Duscha BD. Effect of amount and intensity of exercise on plasma lipoproteins. N Engl J Med. 2002;347:1483–1492.

28. Libby P, Theroux P. Pathophysiology of coronary artery disease. Circulation. 2005;111:3481–3488.

29. Miyashita M, Bruns SF, Stensel DJ. Accumulating short bouts of brisk walking reduces postprandial plasma triacylglycerol concentrations and resting blood pressure. Am J Clin Nutr. 2008; 88:1225–1231.

30. Nordestgaard BG, Benn M, Schnohr P. Nonfasting triglycerides and risk of myocardial infarction, ischemic heart disease, and death in men and women. JAMA. 2007;298:299–308.

31. Petitt DS, Amgrimsson SA, Cureton KJ. Effect of resistance exercise on postprandial lipemia. J Appl Physiol. 2003;94:694–700.

32. Pitsavos C, Panagiotakos DB, Timbalis KD. Resistance exercise plus aerobic activities is associated with better lipids' profile among healthy individuals in the ATTICA study. QJM. 2009; 102:609–616. doi: 10.1093/qjmed/hcp083.

33. Ratamess NA, Alvar BA, Evetoch TK, et al. American College of Sports Medicine position stand on progression models in resistance training for healthy adults. Med Sci Sports Exerc. 2009;41(3):687–708.

34. Robinson JG, Wang S, Smith BJ, et al. Meta-analysis of the relationship between non-high-density lipoprotein cholesterol reduction and coronary heart disease risk. J Am Coll Cardiol. 2009;53:316–322.

35. Schober SE, Carroll MD, Lacher DA, et al. High Serum Total Cholesterol: An Indicator for Monitoring Cholesterol Lowering Efforts in US Adults, 2005–2006. NCHS data brief no 2. Hyattsville, MD: National Center for Health Statistics, 2007.

36. Sgouraki E, Tsopanakis A, Tsopanakis C. Acute exercise: response of HDL-C, LDL-C lipoprotein and HDL-C subfraction levels in selected sport disciplines. J Sports Med Phys Fitness. 2001; 41:386–391.

37. Shannon KA, Shannon RM, Clore JN. Resistance exercise and postprandial lipemia: the dose effect of differing volumes of acute resistance exercise bouts. Metabolism. 2005;54:756–763.

38. Shaw I, Shaw BS, Kraslishchikov O. Comparison of aerobic and combined aerobic and resistance training on low-density lipoprotein cholesterol concentrations in men. Cardiovasc J Afr. 2009; 20:290–295.

39. Singhai A, Trilk JL, Jenkins NT. Effects of intensity of resistance exercise on postprandial lipemia. J Appl Physiol. 2009;6:823–829.

40. Slack J. Risks of ischaemic heart-disease in familial hyperlipoproteinaemic states. Lancet. 1969; 294(7635):1380–1382.

41. Slentz CA, Houmard JA, Johnson JL. Inactivity, exercise training and detraining, and plasma lipoproteins: STRRIDE: a randomized, controlled study of exercise intensity and amount. J Appl Physiol. 2007;103:432–442.

42. Sorace P, LaFontaine TP, Thomas TR. Know the risks: lifestyle management of dyslipidemia. Health Fit J. 2006;10:18–25.

43. Stamler J, Neaton JD. The multiple risk factor intervention trial (MRFIT)—importance then and now. JAMA. 2008;300:1343–1345.

44. Stefanick ML, Mackey S, Sheehan M. Effects of diet and exercise in men and postmenopausal women with low levels of HDL cholesterol and high levels of LDL cholesterol. N Engl J Med. 1998;339:12–20.

45. Superko HR, Gadesam RR. Is it LDL particle size or number that correlates with risk for cardiovascular disease? Curr Atheroscler Rep. 2008;10:377–385.

46. Thomas TR, LaFontaine TP. Exercise, nutritional strategies, and lipoproteins. In: Roitman JL, ed. Resource Manual for Guidelines for Exercise Testing and Prescription. Baltimore, MD: Lippincott Williams & Wilkins, 2003, pp. 294–301.

47. Thomas TR, Liu Y, Linden MA, et al. Interaction of exercise training and n-3 fatty acid supplementation on postprandial lipemia. Appl Physiol Nutr Metab. 2007;32:473–480.

48. Thompson WR, ed. ACSM's Guidelines for Exercise Testing and Prescription. 8th Ed. Baltimore, MD: American College of Sports Medicine. Lippincott Williams & Wilkins, 2010.

49. Timbalis K, Panagiotakos DB, Kavouras SA, et al. Responses of blood lipids to aerobic, resistance, and combined aerobic with resistance training: a systematic review of current evidence. Angiology. 2009;60:614–632.

50. Toth PP. When high is low: raising low levels of high-density lipoprotein cholesterol. Curr Cardiol Rep. 2008;10:488–496.

51. Tsekouras YE, Magkos F, Prentzas KI, et al. A single bout of whole-body resistance exercise augments basal VLDL-triacylglycerol removal from plasma in health untrained men. Clin Sci. 2009;116:147–156.

52. Tyldum GA, Schjerve IE, Tjonna AE. Endothelial dysfunction induced by post-prandial lipemia: complete protection afforded by high-intensity interval exercise. J Am Coll Cardiol. 2009;13: 200–206.

53. Vargeer M, Holleboom AG, Hastelein JJ, et al. The HDL-hypothesis—does high-density lipoprotein protect from atherosclerosis? J Lipid Res. 2010. doi:10.1194/jlrR001610.

54. Warner SO, Linden MA, Harvey BR. The effects of resistance training on metabolic health with weight regain. J Clin Hypertens. 2010;12:6–72.

55. Williams MA, Haskell WL, Ades PA, et al; American Heart Association Council on Clinical Cardiology; American Heart Association Council on Nutrition, Physical Activity, and Metabolism. Resistance exercise in individuals with and without cardiovascular disease: 2007 update: a scientific statement from the American Heart Association Council on Clinical Cardiology and Council on Nutrition, Physical Activity, and Metabolism. Circulation. 2007;116:572–584.

56. Williams PT. High-density lipoprotein cholesterol and other risk factors for coronary artery disease in female runners. N Engl J Med. 1996; 334:1298–1303.

57. Williams PT. Incident hypercholesterolemia in relation to changes in vigorous physical activity. Med Sci Sports Exerc. 2009;41:73–80.

58. Williams PT. Relationship of distance run per week to coronary heart disease risk factors in 9,920 male runners. The National Runners' Health Study. Arch Intern Med. 1997;157:191–198.

59. Williams PT, Blanche PJ, Kraus RM. Behavioral versus genetic correlates of lipoproteins and

adiposity in identical twins discordant for exercise. Circulation. 2007;112:350–356.

60. Williams PT, Blanche PJ, Rawlings R, et al. Concordant lipoprotein and weight responses to dietary fat change in identical twins with divergent exercise levels. Am J Clin Nutr. 2005;82:181–187.

61. Williams PT, Stefanick ML, Vranizan KM, et al. The effects of weight loss by exercise or dieting on high-density lipoprotein (HDL) levels in men with low, intermediate, and normal-to-high HDL at baseline. Metabolism. 1994;43:917–924.

62. Wood PD, Stefanick ML, Dreon DM. Changes in plasma lipids and lipoproteins in overweight men and women during weight loss through dieting as compared with exercise. N Engl J Med. 1988;319:1173–1179.

63. Wood PD, Stefanick ML, Williams PT, et al. The effects on plasma lipoproteins of a prudent weight-reducing diet, with or without exercise, in overweight men and women. N Engl J Med. 1991;325:461–466.

64. Zafeiridis A, Goloi E, Petridou A. Effects of low- and high-volume resistance exercise on postprandial lipaemia. Br J Nutr. 2007;97:471–477.

65. Zhang JQ, Ji LL, Nunez G. Effect of exercise timing on postprandial lipemia in hypertriglyceridemic men. Can J Appl Physiol. 2004;29:590–603.

66. Zhang JQ, Thomas TR, Ball SD. Effect of exercise timing on postprandial lipemia and HDL cholesterol subfractions. J Appl Physiol. 1998;85:1516–1522.

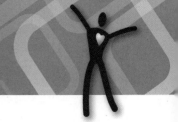

10

Changing Health Behaviors

ABBREVIATIONS

RC   Readiness for change
SCT   Social Cognitive Theory

SOC   Stages of change
TTM   Transtheoretical model

Changing habitual behavior is, perhaps, one of the most difficult challenges that a person can undertake. For the Exercise Professional who is working with individuals who are trying to change one or more lifestyle behaviors, it is also a daunting and difficult challenge. Negative health habits are reinforced by years of engaging in the behavior, by emotional currents that may originate far in the past, by a negatively reinforcing social support system, and by the cultural and societal environments in which individuals reside. Without great commitment on the part of the client and some knowledge of and capacity to implement the principles of behavior change, these negative health behaviors can be very difficult to overcome.

The behavior change process is the subject of volumes of research, which we will only cover superficially. Figure 10.1 summarizes some of the important parts of that process. This model does not describe all of the components that have been outlined in the literature, but centers on those we believe to be the most critical to the process. They are also the components that can be positively influenced by a knowledgeable Exercise Professional.

Stages of change (SOC), decision making, self-efficacy, and relapse prevention are the theoretical cornerstones to a successful behavior change program (see Fig. 10.1). These

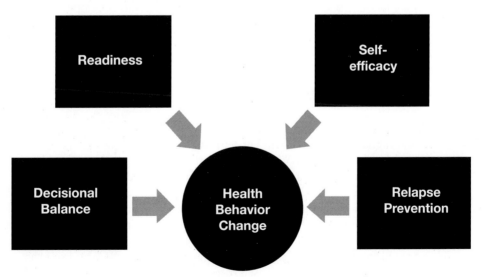

FIGURE 10.1 Health behavior change can be extremely challenging. These four factors are important considerations in the process.

What Is "Coaching"?

A more detailed description of the coaching process will be presented below, but a brief description may be helpful at this point. The traditional method for behavior change evolved from an approach that assumed the presentation of information ("education") that supported a specific change (increased level of physical activity, for example) would result in someone actually changing behavior. This approach was typical in the early days of Cardiac Rehabilitation programs, for example, where it was simply assumed that "patient education" about the positive effects of exercise or the negative effects of smoking would result in patients adopting a new, healthy lifestyle that included not smoking and regular exercise. Clearly, this was not the common outcome. Coaching theory evolved from several other methods that promote lifestyle behavior change and is based in "motivational interviewing." The basis of coaching lies in exploring a client's value systems, barriers to behavior, and it addresses the individual's strengths. Coaches focus on positives and on using energy in individuals to facilitate success. Coaching is based on asking questions that promote introspection and insight into personal behaviors. Coaching is not using the traditional "expert" method for changing behavior, though "expert advice" is certainly part of the coaching process.

components form the most logical parts of this difficult process of implementing and sustaining health behavior change. They are also critical considerations for the Exercise Professional focused on assisting the client in making successful change. The Exercise Professional will benefit from knowing the basic principles of the processes of change and their components in order to assist clients with progression through these SOC on the way to adopting new, healthy lifestyle behaviors permanently.

In this chapter, we will introduce the coaching process as a primary tool for fostering successful change. Coaching is a client-centered approach to developing behavior change that focuses on the individual's goals and perceptions of the need and importance for change (see the box titled "What Is 'Coaching'?").

THE TRANSTHEORETICAL MODEL (STAGES OF CHANGE)

The Transtheoretical Model (TTM) of behavior change was originally conceived by Dr. James Prochaska and Dr. Carlo DiClemente in the early 1980s (22). A key component of this model is the SOC (17). We will refer to this model using the terminology "readiness for change" (RC) in the remainder of this chapter. We will discuss the entire TTM, including the SOC, processes of change, decisional balance, and self-efficacy (17). The integration of all four components into a comprehensive behavioral change program allows the best chance for successful lifestyle changes to become internalized and permanent.

Over the years, the TTM has stood the test of time with respect to its validity and is well accepted by those knowledgeable in behavior change. RC, by itself, has become a useful and important tool for Exercise Professionals who are working with clients who are trying to change negative health behaviors such as lack of exercise and poor dietary patterns. We will provide some practical application and tools for using SOC as well as the entire TTM in this chapter.

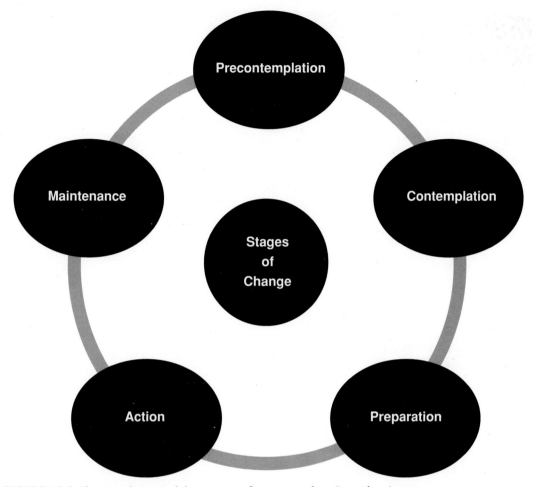

FIGURE 10.2 The transtheoretical theory states five stages of readiness for change.

STAGES OF CHANGE

There are five stages in the SOC model that are summarized and defined in Table 10.1 and illustrated in Figure 10.2. Those stages are as follows:

1. Precontemplation
2. Contemplation
3. Preparation
4. Action
5. Maintenance

With respect to the "permanency" of the change, it is important to remember that old habits, especially those such as smoking, a chemically addictive, as well as behaviorally addictive habit, are at some risk for relapse for a number of years after a change.

Stage of readiness can be easily assessed by asking simple questions about the health behavior and its place in the individual's life. (See the box titled "Survey to Assess SOC for physical activity" for an SOC questionnaire specifically related to physical activity.) SOC is important, not only with respect to whether a person will be able to successfully initiate an exercise program or other behavior change, but also whether that individual will be able to

TABLE 10.1	Stages of Change
Stage	**Characteristics**
Precontemplation	Individual is not thinking about changing behavior
Contemplation	Individual is thinking about changing behavior, but has not initiated any changes in behavior
Preparation	Individual has initiated changes in behavior, but is not at recommended or optimal levels of new behavior.
Action	Individual has initiated change, is at the recommended or optimal level, but has not maintained this level consistently for 6 months or more.
Maintenance	Individual has initiated change, is at the recommended or optimal level, and has maintained this level consistently for more than 6 months.

DID YOU KNOW?

Survey to Assess SOC for Physical Activity (12)

Answer the following questions by checking the appropriate box on the right.

1. I am not currently physically active and have no intention to become physically active.* ☐ Agree ☐ Disagree
2. I intend to become more physically active in the next 6 months. ☐ Agree ☐ Disagree
3. I currently engage in limited regular physical activity (not as defined below) but have done so for less than 6 months. ☐ Agree ☐ Disagree
4. I have been physically active regularly for less than 6 months. ☐ Agree ☐ Disagree
5. I have been physically active regularly for more than 6 months. ☐ Agree ☐ Disagree

*Physical activity is defined as a total of 30 minutes or more per day, 5 days or more every week or 150 minutes per week.

Scoring Stage of Readiness Classification

Precontemplation: Answers question 1 "Agree" and questions 2 through 5 "Disagree".
Contemplation: Answers question 1 with the response, "Disagree," and question 2 with, "Agree."
Preparation: Answers question 3 with the response, "Agree," but may not meet the precise definition of "Physical Activity" provided.
Action: Answers question 4, with the response, "Agree."
Maintenance: Answers question 5 with the response, "Agree."

Note: This survey can be adapted to assess SOC for any lifestyle behavior by changing the topic of the questions.

sustain it (get to the "maintenance" stage) over the long term. In addition, individuals generally move back and forth between stages as they progress. The change process is rarely linear and rarely proceeds without interruption (17).

The SOC survey is an important concept for a number of reasons. "Readiness" to change is one of the most important considerations with respect to the potential for achieving successful behavior change. The willingness to undertake and make a specific behavior change is a staged phenomenon. That is, unless one thinks about the change ("contemplation"), the pros and cons of the change (processes important to and part of the behavior change will be discussed later), as well as other important behavior-related variables, they generally are not willing to undertake and sustain the necessary processes to successfully and permanently adopt the new behavior. In fact, undertaking the change process at a time when readiness is low almost always results in a failure to achieve the desired behavior change.

CYCLING THROUGH STAGES

Individuals usually don't progress through these stages in a "linear" and orderly fashion. It is common for people to spend variable amounts of time at each stage as they progress in making the behavior part of a new healthy lifestyle. Cycling back and forth between stages as the change process moves forward is a fact of life (26). People often cycle back and forth between preparation and action or between precontemplation and contemplation (see Fig. 10.3). They may decide to start a lifestyle behavior change and even take

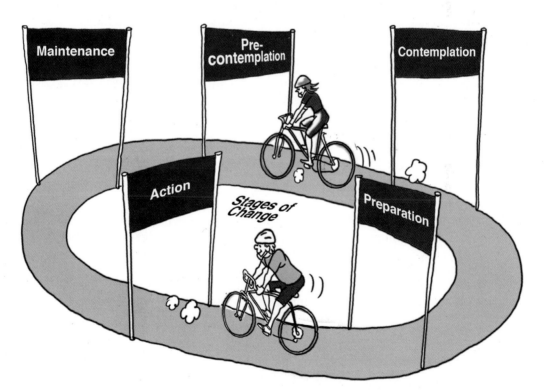

FIGURE 10.3 People rarely progress through the stages of change (SOC) in a linear fashion. It is normal to cycle back and forth between stages during the health behavior change process.

steps to make the change (preparation), then just as quickly cycle back to thinking about it (contemplation), but not actually doing it.

Contemplating change often involves experimentation with the change (this, in fact, may be the process of cycling in and out of various stages). For example, it is common for individuals who are considering initiating a structured exercise program and who are in the contemplation or preparation stages to actually increase their level of physical activity (though not to recommended levels), before they take action to implement any exercise program (15). Thus, shifting between the contemplation and preparation may help a person to experiment with the behavior.

STRATEGIES, PROCESSES, AND SOC

There are behavioral strategies and processes that seem to work well with specific SOC categories. Table 10.2 provides a brief outline of those strategies and stages. For example, providing someone who is in the precontemplation stage of beginning an exercise program with basic, simple information about the pros and cons of making the change can be helpful with respect to facilitating their thinking in some organized and positive way about the change they might consider. In fact, research demonstrates that the pros of making a particular change are significantly more important during the precontemplation and contemplation stages than at other stages in the change process (21). Thus, what better time to provide and discuss this information?

However, it is important to allow the client to discuss cons. This discussion can further the functional relationship between the coach/trainer and the client by allowing a discussion of how different the new behavior is from the old. In fact, the process of successful behavior change *requires* that it be different. Understanding this can promote the new behavior. Dwelling on cons is not helpful, and at some point the discussion should be refocused on the benefits of changing the behavior in question.

Understanding and discussing the barriers to starting an exercise program can also be helpful. Exercise Professionals will encounter clients who are in either the contemplation stage or especially the preparation stage because it is in these stages that people experiment with the new behavior. For these individuals, assessing SOC becomes important for helping Exercise Professionals understand where the client is cognitively and what may help reinforce the change process. The assessment can also help individuals begin the change process, understand where they are, why change is important, and what they need to do to successfully change.

Processes and Strategies

Processes and strategies related to SOC can be divided into domains such as experiential, behavioral, and cognitive. Since our concern is the practical implications and not research, we will not discuss these processes as part of any particular domain, but rather as practices that are helpful in increasing the success of the change process.

Below is a brief description of these processes and their meaning. We will provide practical hints and guidelines for implementing these in Table 10.2. These are given from the perspective of the practitioner and what they might provide or help the client consider, think about, and do.

Information Gathering

Collect information about the new behavior. Find simple and appropriate literature, especially literature discussing the benefits of the lifestyle change under consideration. The pros are twice as important as the cons at this point, though certainly cons that clients express

TABLE 10.2	Stages of Change: Goals, Processes, and Strategies	
Stage of Change	**Goals**	**Useful Behavioral Strategies and Tools**
Precontemplation	Begin to think about initiating the change List pros and cons of the change to be made	Think about appropriate and reasonable goals Provide list of benefits of change, discuss benefits, think about pros and cons
Contemplation	Weigh pro's and con's Set realistic goals about steps to take to implement change Implement the intended change in some form	Implement some kind of reinforcement program for achieving goals Identify a support system— one or more people who will provide helpful support
Preparation	Gradually increase the desired behavior to recommended levels	Implement reinforcement program for the behavioral change Identify barriers and obstacles as change occurs
Action	Fully achieve the intended behavior at recommended levels	Anticipate high-risk situations and formulate a relapse prevention strategy Find a method to add variety to the behavior change
Maintenance	Behavior change has been maintained at the recommended level for >6 months	Prepare for relapse prevention Increase enjoyment of new habit(s) Continue to review and consider positive benefits of the change

should be discussed (preferably using a "coaching" approach that allows the client to generate their own rebuttal for those cons (see the box above and the section below on "Coaching" for a more detailed explanation) (21).

Reward and Reinforcement

Reward for successful behavior is extremely important (12). The reward should be something that the individual enjoys, that supports the new behavior, and that is not "contrary" to the behavior being changed; for example, if exercise and weight loss are goals, do not reward with a trip to the Sunday all-you-can-eat buffet brunch!

Realistic and Specific Goals

Goals must be quantifiable and as objective as possible (12,17). "Walking on weekends" is not a measurable goal. Walking for 30 minutes on Saturday and Sunday is quantifiable, specific, and measurable. If the goal is too vague, the behavior has little chance of

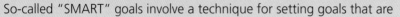

SMART Goals

So-called "SMART" goals involve a technique for setting goals that are

- Specific
- Measurable
- Attainable
- Realistic
- Timely

Briefly, by applying each of the words above to the goal allows the coach and the client to determine whether the goal is something that fits the conditions, the plan, and the individual at that time. Individualizing goals in this manner improves the likelihood that outcomes will be positive. Coaching can assist individuals to assure that goals fit the "SMART" acronym.

occurring regularly. Both short-term and long-term goals should be discussed and established and must be quantifiable and objective as well. In addition, serious consideration of a gradual progression toward the optimal physical activity and physical fitness goals should be part of the goal-setting process. Goal "ownership" is critically important to success in achieving goals. It has been demonstrated that a person with self-set goals (goals that are "owned") is almost twice as likely to achieve the goal as someone who has goals set for them (19). Coaching can assist clients to increase goal ownership. Finally, using the "SMART" goal technique (see the box titled "Smart Goals") can help make the goals clear and achievable (4).

Substitute Alternatives

Substituting positive alternatives for established negative behaviors are important tools for an individual in the process of changing health behaviors (17). Find something that will take the place of a totally sedentary weekend afternoon, or the traditional Saturday-night endless-shrimp meal. If your client is going to have a chance at success, these alternative behaviors are extremely important.

Modeling

The importance of exposing a client to others who have made a similar change and exhibit the behavior on a *regular* basis, under circumstances similar to theirs is critical (Fig. 10.4) (13). If possible, continuing exposure to this behavior is part of modeling. Observing others who are "similar" to the client is an effective example of modeling the correct behavior. This is also the appropriate time to add that we consider role modeling by Exercise Professionals to be of extreme importance and critical to the success and self-efficacy of the client and the change process itself.

Commitment

The individual must make the commitment to change. A personal contract stating the intended behavior in quantifiable and measurable terms can be very effective, especially if signed and witnessed by someone significant in the individual's life (e.g., spouse, child, or best friend) (2). Short of that, a clear verbal commitment (to the same individuals) in objective terms may also be effective.

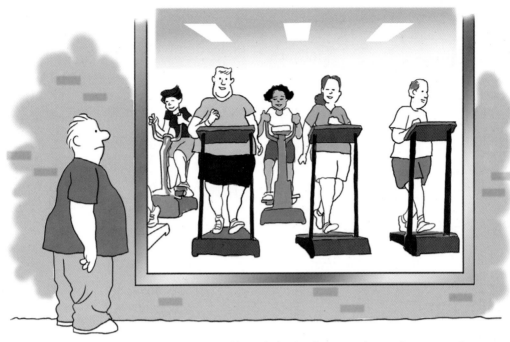

FIGURE 10.4 People who are attempting to change behavior, for example, starting an exercise program, can benefit from watching others (who are similar to themselves) model exercise behavior in an environment similar to their own intended exercise environment.

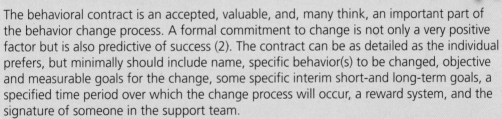

DID YOU KNOW?

Sample Behavior Change Contract

The behavioral contract is an accepted, valuable, and, many think, an important part of the behavior change process. A formal commitment to change is not only a very positive factor but is also predictive of success (2). The contract can be as detailed as the individual prefers, but minimally should include name, specific behavior(s) to be changed, objective and measurable goals for the change, some specific interim short-and long-term goals, a specified time period over which the change process will occur, a reward system, and the signature of someone in the support team.

In addition, the contract could specify tools and methods to measure progress, relapse prevention strategies, and SOC assessment, and perhaps a statement of the current behavior prior to initiating the change process and an ongoing personal journal of the change process.

Finally, if the individual resists or is reluctant to sign a contract, they should be encouraged to verbally commit to the change process to someone close, a friend, a spouse, or another significant person in their life. Formal commitment, as in such a statement or a signed contract is (as stated above) not only important but also predictive of success. Alternatively, this reluctance may be a sign that "readiness" for change is not sufficient to succeed at this time. Figure 10.5 is a sample of a contract that may be used for a client in the process of a health behavior change.

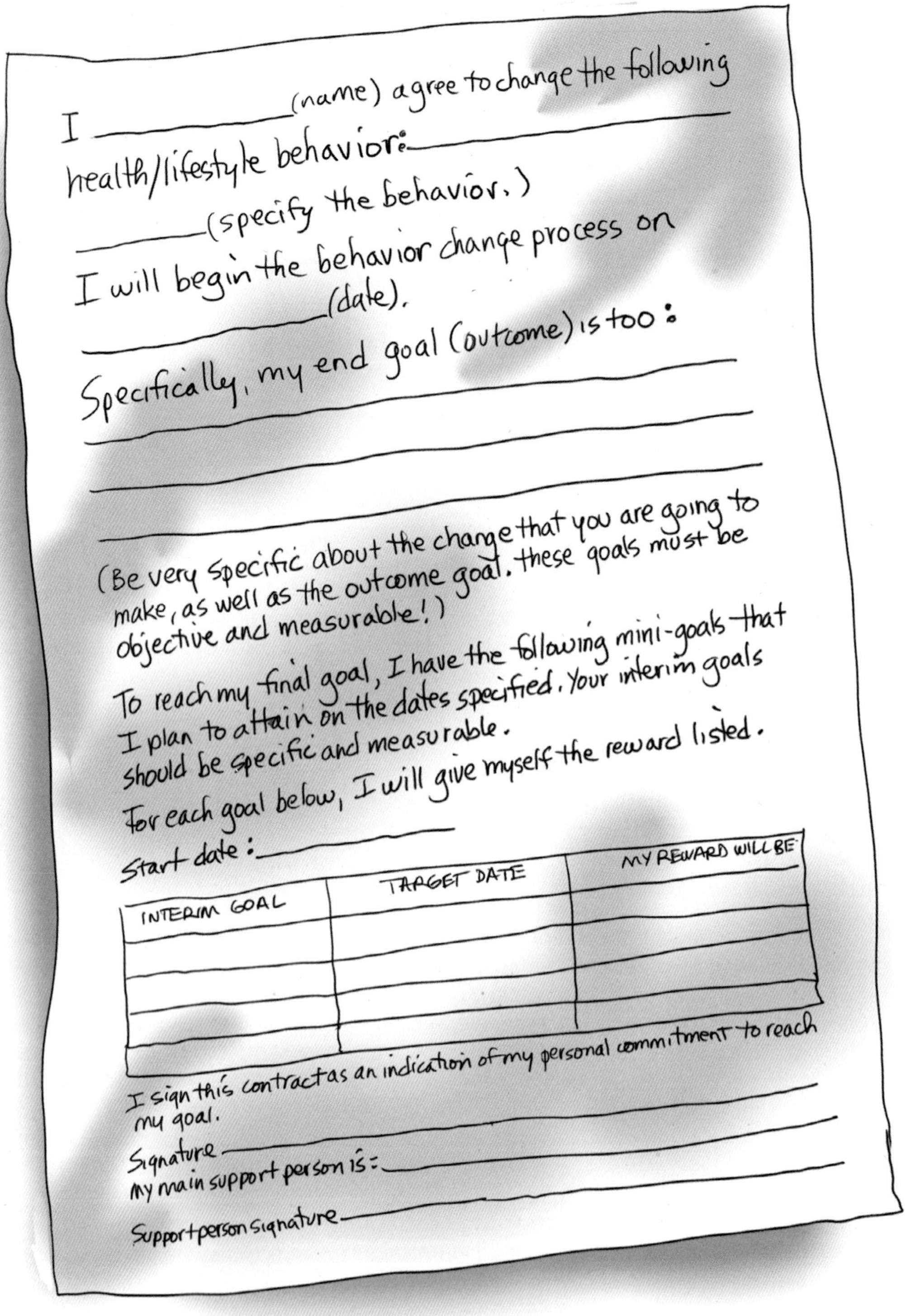

I _____(name) agree to change the following
health/lifestyle behavior: _____
_____(specify the behavior.)
I will begin the behavior change process on _____
_____(date).

Specifically, my end goal (outcome) is too: _____
_____
_____
_____

(Be very specific about the change that you are going to
make, as well as the outcome goal. these goals must be
objective and measurable!)

To reach my final goal, I have the following mini-goals that
I plan to attain on the dates specified. Your interim goals
should be specific and measurable.
For each goal below, I will give myself the reward listed.

Start date: _____

INTERIM GOAL	TARGET DATE	MY REWARD WILL BE

I sign this contract as an indication of my personal commitment to reach
my goal.
Signature _____
my main support person is: _____
Support person signature _____

FIGURE 10.5 This is a sample personal contract that can be modified for use with clients to accompany behavior change programs.

Sample Reminder Systems

Web sites:

- www.memotome.com
- www.thesitetoremember.com
- www.bigdates.com
- www.reminders.com

Electronic devices

- Almost all phones, especially any brand of "smartphone" will have the ability to provide you with reminders of many different kinds, including text to your phone, e-mail, and just a basic sound or vibrating reminder of events that you have put on your calendar that day.
- All computers with calendar capabilities have similar systems that can be used as reminders.

Reminders

Most individuals need to be reminded, but this is especially true of new routines, changing schedules, or new plans. Finding a reminder that is personal enough and reliable enough is important. In this time of electronic devices, cell phones, computers, texting, tweeting, Web sites like Facebook (and other social networking sites and tools), and e-mail can be sources for implementing an effective reminder system (7).

Support Systems

Helpful and positive support systems are at the core of successful behavior change. Having one or more persons who provide encouragement and verbal, mental, emotional, and physical support (especially in difficult times) is critical to the success of the behavior change process. People in the support system must be carefully selected. A spouse or a child may not always be the best choice, simply because of the closeness of the relationship. An excellent choice is someone who is positive and supportive without badgering and who is honest without being rude or insensitive.

Know the Pros and Cons

Knowing why a behavior change is important, what the expected benefits are, and how to facilitate and succeed are critical points of information for someone attempting to change a health behavior. Provide lists, literature, and any kind of information that is tailored to the individual. Do not provide scientific literature to someone who knows little about science or who is not interested. Likewise, do not provide lists or reasons for exercise and weight control for someone who has no intention (and, perhaps, no need) to lose weight. Remember that early in the change process (precontemplation and contemplation) pros are twice as important as cons (21).

Increase Opportunity

Help the client find ways to increase the opportunity to perform the behavior. Finding ways to generalize the new behavior to different situations is critical to long-term success. Being able to be active while traveling or in bad weather situations is a key to being successful in changing physical activity or exercise in particular (13). A different route home from work may require passing by a fitness center. Changing a lunch routine might allow a chance to eat healthy food. Planning and sticking to a plan are key factors in successful change.

DID YOU KNOW?

List of Samples of Pros and Cons to Changing Physical Activity Level

Pros

- Increased capacity to carry out daily activities without undue fatigue.
- Increased ability to engage in recreational activity.
- Increased feelings of mental and physical self-efficacy.
- Decreased risk for many chronic diseases.

Cons

- Regular exercise takes blocks of time that I don't have.
- Regular exercise requires some kind of facility or health club membership.
- Increasing physical activity requires that I leave my desk, and my boss will not allow that.
- Increasing physical activity takes too much time from my family.
- Increasing physical activity requires too much planning, and I cannot always plan my day.

Care about Consequences

Knowing the consequences of one's behavior on others, especially significant others, can be powerful (17). Knowing that second-hand smoke affects others in the family, the workplace, or even the environment itself (toxic chemicals, dirty ashtrays, smelly curtains, cars, and/or furniture) can be effective for reinforcing the desired behavior. These consequences are true for physical inactivity, eating behaviors, being overweight, and other unhealthy behavior. It is also true that the consequences of healthier choices can positively impact others. This, too, should be pointed out and discussed with clients.

Environmental Influences (Stimuli/Cues)

Search for, find, and note stimuli that facilitate the behavior that the person is changing. Many, in fact most behaviors, are a matter of habit (thus the term "behavior"). Habitual behavior may be stimulated by place, circumstance, people, even by factors that seem unimportant, such as social setting. Smoking is often a function of meals, social environments, and even friends who smoke. Finding those things that stimulate the new, positive habitual behavior and help your client find ways to extinguish the old, negative behavior and establish the new behavior are also critical factors that may facilitate success. Both negative and positive stimuli generally operate in an individual's environment. Leaving exercise equipment or clothing where it is immediately visible upon waking is a positive cue that "exercise should occur next!" On the other hand, being tempted by a breakfast meeting with a business associate rather than completing a morning exercise session is a negative cue or stimulus. Clients must be equipped to deal with the negative by placing many positive stimuli into their new environment.

Self-Monitoring and Tracking

Even for people who are notoriously unable (maybe unwilling) to write down and keep track of things like behavior, this is an extremely important task. One recent meta-analysis reports that self-monitoring was the most important variable when explaining successful behavior change. However, even though it is the strongest predictor, it accounts for less than 15% of the total picture; thus, there are many other variables to consider (15). In order to change, clients must know the what, why, where, and when associated with the old, negative behavior (13). They must find the negative influences, stimuli, and obstacles,

DID YOU KNOW?

Example of a Log of Behavior Change

Month/Day/Year	Type of Exercise	Duration	Ratings of Perceived Exertion*	Problems	If Not, Why Not?
10/10/2010	Walk	23 min	10	None	NA
10/12/2010	Walk	35 min	11	None	NA
10/14/2010	None	NA	NA	Weather (snow)	Snow
10/17/2010	Stat cycle	20 min	10	None	NA
10/19/2010	Walk	25 min	11	None	NA
10/22/2010	Stat cycle	15 min	10	Tired	Stop d/t bored
10/25/2010	None	NA	NA	Still tired, no time	No time
10/28/2010	Walk	35 min	11	Had to do it	NA

*How hard is the exercise?

as well as opportunities to establish and practice the new behavior. Although it is unnecessary to track behaviors forever, it is important to begin the process with a mechanism for tracking the established habits and the new behavior to see how it fits into daily life. Note that the sample log is a pencil-and-paper method for tracking behavior. Individualizing the method to the individual is most effective, and there are many other available means, including those available on computer, phone, and other hand-held devices.

These are processes that individuals may use as they progress through the stages to facilitate and assist with the behavior change process (they are divided into behavioral and cognitive processes). The box below defines these processes. These behavioral and cognitive processes are part of the behavior change process and may occur, in some form, in all stages, though some are more common and useful with specific stages (8).

DECISION MAKING

Part of the SOC model involves making decisions during the change process. The most powerful component of this decision-making process is, according to the research, the "pros and cons" of making the change. These are potent operators for making (or not making) most health behavior changes (18,21). Pros and cons appear to be common to many different types of health behavior change as well as to many of the stages. Pros are twice as important as cons for individuals progressing from the precontemplation to the contemplation stage (21). In fact, cons become increasingly less important as one progresses through the stages from contemplation to maintenance, whereas pros become increasingly more important from precontemplation through action stages (21).

DID YOU KNOW?

Processes of Behavior Change (12)

Behavioral Processes

1. **Reward:** provide yourself with tangible rewards for achieving behavior change goals.
2. **Substitution:** substitute new, healthier behaviors for the old, unhealthy behavior.
3. **Commitment:** make a strong commitment to the new behavior, preferably in the form of a behavioral contract.
4. **Reminders:** initiate a system for reminding yourself of the new behavior, for example, notes, alarms, and so on.
5. **Support:** find a helping network of support for your new behavior, for example, friends, colleagues, family, and so on.

Cognitive processes

1. **Understand the risks:** know the risks and understand the actual likelihood of their occurrence.
2. **Increase your knowledge:** read and think about the behavior change you want to make.
3. **Know the benefits:** be aware of, understand, and think about the benefits of the change.
4. **Increase opportunity:** find ways to increase your opportunities to do the new behavior.
5. **Care about consequences to others:** think about and understand how your current behavior and the new behavior affect others, that is, especially family and friends.

Decisional Balance

Decisional balance is part of the decision-making process. Decisional balance means balancing the pros and cons of making the change. The information above discusses where this strategy can be most important and effective. Many people benefit from actually listing the pros and cons. Over and above that, thinking about the pros and cons as the change process advances is important. Help clients be mindful of the pros. Talk about the pros and provide a list to clients in the appropriate stages—precontemplation, contemplation, and preparation are appropriate stages.

SOCIAL COGNITIVE THEORY AND SELF-EFFICACY

A second theory of behavior change is called "Social Cognitive Theory" (SCT). Dr. Albert Bandura developed this theory of behavior change. Indeed, from the early 1960s, Dr. Bandura studied, refined, and evolved SCT (3,17). Bandura stated that behavior change is a function of the interaction between the environment, the individual, and the behavior. There are personal, environmental, and behavioral factors that act together in varying proportions to control and direct behavior, including presumably health behavior (3).

One of the most important parts of SCT is "self-efficacy." Self-efficacy refers to the individual's beliefs about his or her ability to successfully make and sustain a behavior change (17). Some individuals believe they cannot control certain parts of their life and certainly some behaviors. For example, some people believe that they have no control over their time; thus, they "don't have time" to exercise. One strategy to address this is a "time inventory." Many individuals do not really know what they do with the time they have, particularly the discretionary time. Thus, tracking (making a time inventory) will illustrate where that time is used and, more important, where there may be room for additional activities, such as exercise.

For example, many persons unfortunately believe that having diabetes or heart disease is genetic and, thus, control over the disease process is not possible. Clearly, these are false beliefs, but without the self-efficacy to reinforce the lifestyle change, individuals are rarely able to make permanent changes in negative health behaviors. A recent review of correlates of physical activity states that of psychological factors, self-efficacy is the "most consistent positive correlate of physical activity behavior" in the literature (24).

An extremely important element of self-efficacy is the belief that success in achieving the desired outcome is possible. Without that belief, people are reluctant to even attempt a particular change. Few people contemplate attempting a behavior change that they perceive as impossible. People tend to try behaviors and physical tasks that they believe they can accomplish. In addition, failure to achieve change (relapse) after previous attempts detracts from self-efficacy (12). Someone who has tried to lose weight or quit smoking 2 or 3 or more times in the past may have difficulty believing they can succeed in another attempt. However, many people continue trying to change health-adverse behaviors such as smoking even in the face of repeated failed attempts.

DID YOU KNOW?
Influences on Self-Efficacy (3)

Bandura outlined four important influences on self-efficacy that can have practical impact on the Exercise Professional's practice with clients:

1. **Success at performing the lifestyle change or behavior:** The individual changing behavior must have some successes during the early parts of the process.
2. **Modeling of others:** The individual must see models for the change they are making. It is best if these models are "like them"; the best models are those in which the client sees themselves.
3. **Verbal persuasion:** Coaching, and persuading the client to be successful and to incorporate the change, is very helpful to the success of lifestyle change.
4. **Positive physiological and affective outcomes:** Clients should be part of this process by participating in goal setting as well as taking part in assessment that shows progress and change.

On a practical level, Exercise Professionals can implement many day-to-day practices that enhance each of these influences on lifestyle change with clients who are attempting to initiate a regular exercise program. For example, allowing a client to observe others who are successfully and, more importantly, "regularly" exercising is one such action. Introducing the client to different settings and situations where similar individuals exercise and are physically active is another. Providing them with information about the benefits and positive effects of exercise is another. Actually assessing and reassessing physical fitness and physical activity to provide both physiological and behavioral correlates of the exercise is vital to allowing the client to see and, more important, "feel" the results of regular exercise. Documenting this progress is an essential factor in permanent change. Similarly, starting the client at a level where exercise is neither tedious nor painful, while also providing for small successes, can confer reinforcement for further attempts to exercise and also show that exercise does not have to be painful to be beneficial.

Another important part of self-efficacy is perceived barriers to change (17,24). Barriers such as time, fatigue, weather, facilities, or lack of exercise partners are strong influences on self-efficacy for exercise behavior. Interestingly, these barriers cross other important cognitive and behavioral processes that support and facilitate behavior change, but, again, these are primarily of research interest and have little practical implication other than the fact that they are similar and confirm each other.

People must address barriers, both perceived and real, to a particular lifestyle change they are trying to make. These barriers are often integral parts of the old behavior, and not addressing them ignores the reality of the present. Time limitations are consistently perceived as a barrier by people who are attempting to change PA. Addressing schedules, responsibilities, and even circadian preferences (time of day for exercise), is critical to success for most sedentary individuals.

Self-efficacy translates to critical work for the Exercise Professional if clients are to be successful in achieving and maintaining permanent health behavior change. Role models of the desired behavior are important. For example, encouraging exercise or activity with someone with similar characteristics with respect to job, family life, and even body type may be very helpful. Observing others who are successfully carrying out regular exercise behavior can be supportive of the new behavior. Finding people who work in the same (busy and stressful) environment, and who exercise, clearly illustrates the possibility of successfully making change.

In addition, we continue to maintain that Exercise Professionals should be lifestyle role models for clients. "Walking the walk" is very reinforcing and, in fact, should be an expectation of Exercise Professionals.

LAPSE AND RELAPSE PREVENTION

Lapse and relapse are defined in the box below. These are terms applied to behavioral "slips" or return to previous behaviors. Planning for relapse prevention is important to success with the change process.

Relapse prevention involves anticipating barriers, obstacles, and high-risk situations that might be related to lapse or relapse from the planned behavior change. Developing strategies for addressing those situations in advance is an excellent way to plan for them and to feel more positive about addressing them. Success in avoiding lapse or in restarting after lapse or relapse may increase self-efficacy.

For example, your client might perceive that finding time for exercise (the planned behavior change) and the perceived discomfort of exercise are obstacles to starting and

DID YOU KNOW?
Lapse and Relapse

Lapse: A temporary or small "slip" in the intended behavior. An example is missing a week of exercise and then restarting successfully during a planned attempt to implement a regular exercise program.

Relapse: A full return to former behavior patterns. An example is missing 2 or 3 weeks of exercise, which is a return to former, sedentary habits after attempting to implement a regular, structured exercise program.

DID YOU KNOW?

Examples of Barriers and Strategies to Address

Barrier: time constraints

"I don't have time to add another activity to my day." "I'm so busy at work, that when I get home, I'm too tired and exhausted and don't want to exercise." "I have to get my children back and forth to their activities, to school and take care of my husband at the same time, when am I going to find time to exercise?"

Strategy to address this barrier: A time inventory is usually helpful, particularly to identify discretionary time. It does not need to be extremely detailed, but it should address time use during major portions of the day and suggest other times when exercise, activity, or whatever the behavior change is, could be fit in.

Barrier: distractions and environmental obstacles

"People around me smoke." "There is always snack food in the refrigerator and out on the counter in the kitchen." "My friends are always going out Friday and Saturday night, and I can't go with them because I don't want to eat." "No one I know leaves his desk for 5 minutes every hour just to walk around—it's not productive."

Strategy to address this barrier: These and similar statements are really statements of distraction. People who are trying to change often find environmental obstacles (distractions) surrounding them in many circumstances. It is likely that they did not recognize these distractions before they tried to change the behavior, but suddenly when food (or exercise) becomes a major focus, they appear and impede the change process. Each of the obstacles needs to individualized and managed in a way that either minimizes or completely eliminates it from the environment. For example, unwanted food in the house can either be put out of sight, or more preferably eliminated. "Out" with the unhealthy and "in" with the healthy food! The Exercise professional should help find ways to manage all of these distractions.

maintaining a regular exercise program. Time is, in fact, one of the most common barriers and reasons not to exercise. Finding time can be a significant challenge to a new exerciser. Attempting exercise at different times of the day to see what works can be helpful. Using many short bouts of activity in a day can demonstrate how effective an overall increase in physical activity can be. It may help to determine what *does not* work by attempting many different solutions and eliminating those that clearly don't work. Recording these journal entries often helps clients see "why" things aren't working and may lead them to solutions for these problems. Time logs (as suggested earlier) and planned scheduling of exercise are often effective methods to find time for exercise.

Discomfort is easy to resolve—the initial exercise prescription should be at a rating of perceived exertion that is not only tolerable, but in some cases "easy" (11–13 on the rating of perceived exertion scale; Fig. 10.6) (1). Demonstrating that exercise can be both comfortable and beneficial is an important component of "learning" to exercise.

Relapse prevention also requires a vision of the behavior change process as a whole. The road to change is not a "superhighway." Rather it is most often a twisty, curvy, hilly road with lots of yellow caution lights, "yield" signs, and detours. The list of "Lessons from Relapse" below has several pertinent points. One of the most applicable is number 7. It is critical to remember that a lapse (see definition above) is *not* failure. To set up a situation where one (or even two) slips is equated with failure is a sure setup for relapse. The inevitable lapses simply must be viewed as temporary detours from the path. They must be treated as temporary or occasional lapses in behavior that can be corrected. Clients should

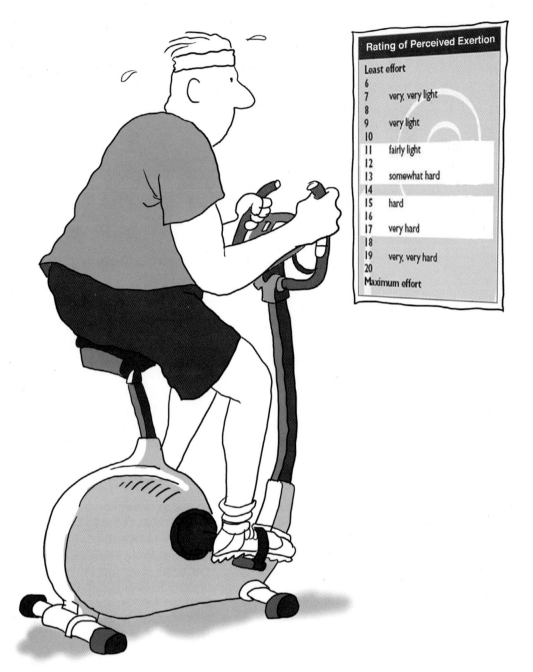

FIGURE 10.6 Regulating exercise intensity using rating of perceived exertion is one way to resolve issues with discomfort during exercise.

be clearly coached to arrive at methods for dealing with lapse. These methods are often appropriate for inclusion into the behavioral contract.

Missing a single exercise session, or even two in a row, does not mean that "all is lost." It simply means that one (or two) exercise sessions have been missed. Restarting the program at that point is easy, is relatively painless, and is very important to the overall behavior change process. In fact, one of the important components to relapse prevention is learning to restart the behavior after these temporary interruptions. Have a plan for restarting in

Lessons from Relapse (23)

1. **The first attempt at behavior change is rarely successful:** It is rare that individuals make successful, major behavior change successfully in the first attempt. Professional assistance is often helpful.
2. **Goals for change help promote specific change; attempting a nonspecific change is not an efficient way to facilitate successful behavior change:** The use of "trial and error" in discovering obstacles and successes during the change process is not efficient. Learn about why lapses, as well as successes occur.
3. **Change always requires more than you think it will:** Time, effort, and even financial commitments are commonly underestimated by individuals who are attempting behavior change.
4. **Use the correct processes at the correct time:** Many of the cognitive and behavioral processes that are associated with successful change are more effective when applied at specific points during the change process—use them appropriately.
5. **Complications always arise:** Unforeseen circumstances almost always intervene in behavior change; be aware and proceed logically.
6. **Making change is rarely a straight line from zero to 100:** Be aware of the twists and turns in your behavior change process and adapt accordingly.
7. **A lapse is not failure:** One slip or one fall "off the wagon" does not mean failure and certainly doesn't mean that you should just give up.
8. **Apparently inconsequential decisions often lead to major consequences:** Decisions, which at the time seem minor, often invoke unforeseen and unintended consequences, so stay on the path.
9. **Stress, distress, and social pressure all set up conditions for lapse and relapse:** Times of stress and distress are the most common causes of lapse and relapse, so be especially vigilant and aware of your own behavior during those times.
10. **Learning promotes success:** Learn from your mistakes and lapses; even more important, learn from your successes how to continue being successful.

case of full-blown relapse. Restarting is, in fact, an appropriate and helpful part of the change process if it is managed closely and carefully.

Situations that are perceived as risky, such as vacations, illness, family, or changes in work hours should be considered and discussed, then strategies should be devised and ready for use in these situations. There should also be a "tool kit" for unanticipated situations and lapses. Reminders, support systems, and reinforcement of the positive behaviors are all appropriate for such situations. They strengthen the chances that the behavior will occur regularly and be internalized as well as increase self-efficacy for positively and successfully dealing with lapses!

RELAPSE PREVENTION AND PROBLEM SOLVING

As summarized earlier, there are numerous relapse prevention techniques that can be applied to assist with a behavior change program. In addition, "problem-solving therapy" may be helpful (20). Using active problem-solving techniques to address the barriers and obstacles along with relapse prevention techniques adds additional tools to the client's repertoire that address the problems of lapse and relapse. A five-stage model has been described and is summarized in the box below (20). This problem-solving technique is particularly suited to coaching because the client can be coached toward recognizing the issues and ways to address them.

PRACTICAL SOLUTIONS TO BEHAVIOR CHANGE PROBLEMS

The practical issues related to behavior change are too numerous and complex to sort out and include in a single section of a chapter. Most Exercise Professionals are challenged by time, knowledge, and individual client differences while attempting to provide personal training and also deal with issues of behavior change. We will try to address some of the typical issues, offer practical solutions to often-encountered problems and provide some forms, surveys, and questionnaires that may be helpful. In the end, both Exercise Professionals and clients need to be acutely aware that (as stated previously) the process is neither easy, nor linear. Preparation for the curves and bumps in the road, as well as the inevitable lapse (and sometimes relapse) is part of an effective disease prevention process.

STAGE OF CHANGE

Assessment of SOC

Assessing SOC is usually the first practical step. Though it seems unlikely that most people who approach Exercise Professionals for assistance would be in the precontemplation stage, it is not necessarily a foregone conclusion. Some people who attempt change are "pushed" into it by others in their life (family, spouse, friends, coworkers, physicians), but are clearly neither ready, nor interested in changing. The box entitled "Stages of Change Questionnaire" is for assessing RC. Simply give the questionnaire to the client and ask for an honest answer to the questions. Individuals who admit to being precontemplative are

---

DID YOU KNOW?
Problem-Solving Therapy

The five recommended steps to this technique are as follows:

1. Develop a realistic perspective that acknowledges that difficulties with compliance and behavior change are normal and expected as "bumps in the road" along the way.
2. Define the specific problem and the goal behavior associated with that problem. "What is the problem? What can you do about that particular problem?"
3. Describe alternative solutions to address the barrier/obstacle. A greater number of solutions allow a broader approach to solving the problem.
4. What are the likely consequences and outcomes of particular (or different) decisions that a client might make in a given circumstance?
5. What decision will be implemented at this time and what is the likely outcome of that particular decision?

not good candidates for initiating an exercise (or any other) program that involves changing lifestyle. Give them written information and offer to help when they feel they are ready. Trying to persuade or coach someone who is not ready for the behavior change process is a waste of professional time and energy.

However, most clients who are initiating an exercise program (either for the first time or after relapse) are likely to be in either the contemplation, preparation, or the action stage. As such, the processes and strategies are different than for earlier stage clients.

Application of Appropriate Strategies to SOC

The next step is to attempt to help clients progress through one stage to the next. Table 10.2 addresses strategies appropriate to specific stages. In the previous example, getting someone in the precontemplation stage to begin thinking about the change is the first step. In addition, remember that in these first two stages, the pros are twice as important as the cons (21). Providing some kind of list as well as having the person write their own list of pros and cons can be very helpful and positive.

It is also an important time to remember that you (the Exercise Professional) are the expert, and though you cannot tell someone what is best for them, you can certainly give expert advice on appropriate and inappropriate goals and reasonable outcomes. Allowing a client to set goals that cannot be reached, and, therefore, that are self-defeating, is a recipe for failure. This is the time for "expert advice" and counsel. Talk knowledgeably about goals, expectations, and the process. Allow the client to make his or her own decisions about when to start, when they "feel" ready, and when he or she will initiate those first steps. Your input is valuable in helping him or her set goals and for providing specific advice about the initial steps of the program. Try to individualize the information or process, so that it fits your client and his or her situation. A "shotgun" approach rarely works.

Many clients who seek out an Exercise Professional are likely to be in preparation or action stages, though some may be in contemplation. Regardless, the strategies for those clients include setting very specific (and quantifiable) goals, identifying good support systems, and setting up some kind of reinforcement and reward system.

DIGGING DEEPER

The Coaching Process

Coaching is a relatively new concept in its application to behavior change. It started as a hybrid of "motivational interviewing" and other psychological models of behavior change, including TTM and SCT as discussed previously (3,16,22). Subsequently, there have been many papers and significant research published demonstrating that coaching is effective for people who are interested in "life change" (5,9,10). In fact, "life coaches" abound, and they are expanding their skills into a variety of interesting and important areas, including wellness. Margaret Moore, the founder of Wellcoaches, Inc., and her colleague have written a "white paper" about coaching that is comprehensive and explanatory. This paper is part of the recommended reading for this chapter. "INTERxVENT USA (www.interventusa.com) is another well-researched and user-friendly approach to lifestyle management and disease prevention coaching (10). We recommend that your exploration of coaching start with these examples. Stages of change and TTM are integral parts of the coaching process (as are other psychological models of behavior change). Assessment of SOC and then tailoring interventions using the appropriate process or strategy are integral to the coaching process.

(continued)

Wellness coaching also walks a line that "experts" often find difficult to navigate (16). Experts are expected to give advice and then structure interventions (in many specialties, especially medicine and health) to assist clients in achieving specific outcomes often aimed at disease management. These goals and outcomes are commonly set with little input from the individual. The standards for blood lipids and the recommendations for exercise are well known and established. Medical and Exercise Professionals often give this expert advice in a directive way: "Your cholesterol needs to be less than 200 and you need to exercise and eat a low-fat diet." In many cases, clients have little choice regarding specific health behaviors (i.e., medicine or physical therapy), expected outcomes, or how they will achieve them because of evidence-based recommendations.

The challenge for Exercise Professionals is to balance the established standards for health outcomes (e.g., lipids, blood pressure, and weight and body composition) with the methods and lifestyle behaviors that are required to achieve them. Using an optimal dietary pattern (Dietary Approaches to Stop Hypertension or Indo-Mediterranean) to achieve these goals is the lifestyle required. A goal such as lowering cholesterol or achieving an ideal body weight qualifies as a disease-preventing outcome. These are established *standards, not goals*. Exercise Professionals (functioning as "experts") should provide these established standards and outcomes to clients, then (as coaches) help them seek methods and means to reach those outcomes through lifestyle change.

The more traditional approach to health behavior change is usually stimulated by a serious health problem that limits the patient's role in the process. An expert (perhaps the doctor or the nurse) generally determines goals and outcomes guided by evidence-based standards and guidelines. We know that this traditional method of "prescribing" lifestyle change is not effective. The clinical literature is filled with studies using "usual care" groups who do not change with respect to achieving those evidence-based guidelines. In fact, relapse to previous health behaviors is the rule rather than the exception in many cases of combined medical therapy and lifestyle behavior change. This approach says, "You are not in charge, I am" (16). The traditional path does not assist clients to seek or find their own road to health behavior change.

Rather than give one-way expert advice, the aim of coaching is to let clients develop their own personal pathway to these behaviors. The client is at the center of the coaching process, not the receptacle. Coaches help clients set goals that are specific to their own needs and, more importantly, specific to their strengths and abilities. Coaches can offer expert advice, but they should do so in the context of questions that direct the individual to formulate his or her own program and his or her own pathway to successful change. Coaches focus on positive energy and forward progress in the effort to make the behavior change something that the "client owns," not that is forced on the client.

The behavior change research clearly shows that long-term change does not necessarily depend on will-power, or on external motivation, but rather on the individual's own value system for the best chance of success (see "Processes and Strategies", as well as Table 10.2). The individual must be guided to making choices that bring about those goals, that is, optimal health behaviors. The new behavior must be internalized by the person making the change for it to become permanent. For a change to become permanent, it cannot be imposed (12,23).

Coaching also fosters and nurtures self-efficacy (see above discussion). As we stated earlier, self-efficacy is critical to success and in fact, must be part and parcel of the behavior change process. This process is central to the coaching effort and to the models that coaches use to elicit the information and values that clients must express and clarify to find a personal pathway to successful change.

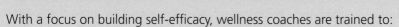

DID YOU KNOW?

Building Self-Efficacy in Coaching

With a focus on building self-efficacy, wellness coaches are trained to:

- accept and meet us where we are today;
- ask us to take charge;
- guide us in doing the mindful thinking and doing work that builds confidence;
- help us define a higher purpose for wellness and uncover our natural impulse to be well;
- help us tap into our innate fighting spirit;
- address mental and physical health together;
- help us draw a personal wellness blueprint;
- help us set realistic goals; small victories lay the foundation for self-efficacy;
- harness the strengths we need to overcome our obstacles;
- help us view obstacles as opportunities to learn and grow;
- help us build a support team; and
- inspire and challenge us to go beyond what we would do alone.

Altered with permission. Margaret Moore, CEO, Wellcoaches, Inc. (16).

Coaches help individuals develop the self-efficacy necessary for success, and they help them create individualized plans and pathways to successful behavior change. Coaches are also expected, in appropriate situations, and at appropriate "coaching moments," to be the expert. They can and do offer the expert advice that health and Exercise Professionals have been offering for years. The key in coaching is to offer that advice at the right time, in the right context, and when the client is ready (SOC and TTM are crucial to the whole coaching process).

Significant RESEARCH

Two articles are highly recommended in this chapter. The first is a comprehensive chapter about behavior change that summarizes much of this information, but in more detail. Dr. Melissa Napolitano has summarized basic information, principles, and background theory into a single book chapter that is easy to read, informative, and complete. The second is a "white paper" by Margaret Moore and her colleague, Dr. Lori Boothroyd, a clinical psychologist. This is a comprehensive discussion of coaching and how it might relate to the obesity epidemic. Both of these articles are well worth the effort.

Health Behavior Change

Napolitano MA, Lewis BA, Whiteley JA, et al. Principles of health behavior change. In: Ehrman JK, et al., eds. ACSM's Resource Manual for Guidelines for Exercise Testing and Prescription. 6th Ed. Baltimore, MD: Lippincott Williams & Wilkins Publishing, 2009, pp. 710–723.

(continued)

This is a comprehensive chapter about behavior change that covers most of the prominent and important theories about how people change their behavior. Dr. Napolitano divides the chapter into sections that address each of the major theories, including stages of change, Decision-Making theory, Social Cognitive theory, the theory of Reasoned Action, the theory of Planned Behavior, and Relapse Prevention theory. Each of these is further subdivided into specific sections that explain the theory, discuss research, and give practice implications. The chapter is easy to read, provides practical tips, and is highly recommended for Exercise Professionals who will have to deal with behavior change in their client population.

Coaching and the Obesity Epidemic

Moore M, Boothroyd L. A Whitepaper: The Obesity Epidemic: A Confidence Crisis Calling for Professional Coaches. Wellcoaches, Inc. Wellesley, MA. Available at http://www.wellcoaches.com/images/whitepaper.pdf.

Moore and Boothroyd have written an excellent paper that describes the unique qualities and characteristics of "wellness coaching." Coaching, sometimes called "motivational interviewing" in the literature, seems to be the wave of the future with respect to behavior change. "We" (Exercise Professionals) cannot make or even really "motivate" our clients to change health behaviors. Exercise, Physical Activity and dietary pattern are habits formed over the course of a lifetime. Implementing changes in these, perhaps the most important of health behaviors, can be challenging and difficult.

Moore lays out the foundations of coaching in behavioral, cognitive, and positive psychology. She discusses qualities that coaches posses along with the difference between coaching and therapy. Finally, she lays out the future in behavior change quite nicely. She speculates that the potential for partnership between health care providers and coaches has the potential to change how we act, live, and behave. This is an excellent article from which the Exercise Professional can glean much valuable information, not only about coaching but about behavior change as well.

REFERENCES

1. American College of Sports Medicine. ACSM's Guidelines for Exercise Testing and Prescription. 8th Ed. Baltimore, MD: Lippincott Williams & Wilkins, 2009.
2. Anderson JV, Mavis BE, Robinson JI, et al. A worksite weight management program to reinforce behavior. J Occup Med. 1993;35:800–804.
3. Bandura A. Self-Efficacy: The Exercise of Control. New York: W.H. Freeman, 1997.
4. Bovend'Eerdt TJH, Botell RE, Wade DT. Writing SMART rehabilitation goals and achieving goal attainment scaling: a practical guide. Clin Rehabil. 2009;23:352–361.
5. Burke BL, Arkowitz H, Menchola M. The efficacy of motivational interviewing: a meta-analysis of controlled clinical trials. J Counsult Clin Psychol. 2003;71(5):843–861.
6. Chambliss HO, King AC. Behavioral strategies to enhance physical activity participation. In: Ehrman JK, et al. eds. ACSM's Resource Manual for Guidelines for Exercise Testing and Prescription. 6th Ed. Baltimore, MD: Lippincott Williams & Wilkins Publishing, 2010, pp. 710–723.
7. Fry JP, Neff RA. Periodic prompts and reminders in health promotion and health behavior interventions: systematic review. J Med Internet Res. 2009;11(2):e16.
8. Garber CE, Alisworth JE, Marcus BH, et al. Correlates of change for physical activity in a population survey. Am J Public Health. 2008;98:897–904.
9. Gordon NF. Innovative approaches to CVD risk reduction: focus on therapeutic lifestyle changes. Lipid Spin. 2005;3:7–9.
10. Gordon NF, English CD, Contractor AS, et al. Effectiveness of three models for comprehensive cardiovascular disease risk reduction. Am J Cardiol. 2002;89:1263–1268.
11. Macauley E, Morris KS, Motl RW, et al. Long-term follow-up of physical activity behavior in older adults. Health Psychol. 2007;26(3):375–380.

12. Marcus BH, Forsyth LH. Motivating People to be Physically Active. 2nd Ed. Champaign, IL: Human Kinetics Publishers, 2009.

13. Marcus BH, Rossi SJ, Selby VC, et al. The stages and processes of exercise adoption and maintenance in a worksite sample. Health Psychol. 1992;11(6): 386–395.

14. Marshall SJ, Biddle JH. The transtheoretical model of behavior change: a meta-analysis of applications to physical activity and exercise. Ann Behav Med. 2001;23(4):229–246.

15. Michie S, Abraham C, Whittington C, et al. Effective techniques in healthy eating and physical activity interventions: a meta-regression. Health Psychol. 2009;28(6):690–701.

16. Moore M, Boothroyd L. A Whitepaper: The Obesity Epidemic: A Confidence Crisis Calling for Professional Coaches. Wellcoaches, Inc. Wellesley, MA. Available at: http://www.wellcoaches.com/images/whitepaper.pdf accessed on 3/13/2009.

17. Napolitano MA, Lewis BA, Whiteley JA, et al. Principles of health behavior change. In: Ehrman JK, et al. eds. ACSM's Resource Manual for Guidelines for Exercise Testing and Prescription. 6th Ed. Baltimore, MD: Lippincott Williams & Wilkins Publishing, 2010, pp. 710–723.

18. Noar SM, Benac CN, Harris MS. Does tailoring matter? Meta-analytic review of tailored print health behavior change interventions. Psychol Bull. 2007;133(4):673–693.

19. Okun MA, Karoly P. Perceived goal ownership, regulatory goal cognition and health behavior change. Am J Health Behav. 2007;31(1): 98–109.

20. Perri MG, Nezu AM, McKelvey WF, et al. Relapse prevention training and problem-solving therapy in the long-term management of obesity. J Consult Clin Psychol. 2001;69(4):722–726.

21. Prochaska JO. Decision making in the transtheoretical model of behavior change. Med Decis Making. 2008;28:845–849.

22. Prochaska JO, DiClemente CC. Stages and processes of self-change in smoking: towards an integrative model of change. J Consult Clin Psychol. 1983;51(3): 390–395.

23. Prochaska JO, Norcross JC, Diclemente CC. Changing for Good: A Revolutionary Six-Stage Program for Overcoming Bad Habits and Moving Your Life Forward. New York, NY: Avon Books, 1994, pp. 222–236.

24. Trost SG, Owen N, Bauman AE, et al. Correlates of adults' participation in physical activity: review and update. Med Sci Sports Exerc. 2002;34(12):1996–2001.

25. Williams DM, Matthews CE, Rutt C, et al. Interventions to increase walking behavior. Med Sci Sports Exerc. 2008;40(7, Suppl):567–573.

26. Yap TL, Davis LS. Process of behavioral change as it relates to intentional physical activity. AAOHN J. 2007;55(9):372–378.

The Optimal Program for Prevention of Chronic Disease

ABBREVIATIONS

CAD	Coronary artery disease	PA	Physical activity
CREF	cardiorespiratory endurance fitness	PF	Physical fitness
DASH	Dietary Approach to Stop Hypertension	PPL	Postprandial lipemia
		RAAS	Renin-angiotensin aldosterone system
HDL	High-density lipoprotein		
OVD	Occlusive vascular disease	RT	Resistance training

The goal of this final chapter is to consolidate the information in this book on prevention of chronic disease for Exercise Professionals. A basic, functional understanding of exercise and diet and their complimentary roles in preventing chronic disease is essential for achieving optimal outcomes when working with clients who have risk factors or who have controlled chronic disease.

What is the most effective exercise program for preventing heart disease or hypertension? What is the optimal intensity and duration for weight loss and prevention of weight regain? What is the ideal frequency of exercise for people with type 2 diabetes? These and other questions will be answered clearly and concisely in this chapter.

Information from previous chapters will be briefly reviewed, including pathophysiology, exercise, chronic disease, and behavior change. The "optimal" exercise prescription, as well as the "optimal" dietary pattern for preventing chronic disease, will be presented. This chapter is intended to be a summary that the Exercise Professional can utilize quickly and easily with clients and patients who present with a chronic disease or who have risk factors for chronic disease.

Exercise Professionals must be informed and knowledgeable about the physiology and pathophysiology of chronic disease processes as well as optimal programs to prevent them. It is clear that they will encounter clients on a daily basis, with either risk factors or overt chronic disease. Unquestionably, more and more people have diseases that stem from a sedentary lifestyle and an unhealthy (Western) dietary pattern. Together with smoking, poor stress management, and excess alcohol consumption, these modifiable lifestyle risk factors play a significant role in up to 70% to 90% of all chronic diseases (34,35). These diseases can be prevented; in fact, they can be largely alleviated. The pathophysiology of the disease can be controlled and/or largely eliminated, but unhealthy behaviors always have the potential to affect the expression of pathophysiology discussed in this book.

COMMON PATHOPHYSIOLOGY

The following pathophysiologies are common to all of the chronic diseases that we have discussed in this book:

- Low-grade systemic inflammation
- Vascular endothelial dysfunction
- Insulin resistance
- Hormonal dysfunction

Figure 11.1 illustrates these conditions common to many chronic diseases.

LOW-GRADE SYSTEMIC INFLAMMATION

The inflammation that is present in many chronic diseases is systemic and low level. It is not similar to the frank inflammation present in an infected wound but, rather, is detectable only by the presence of low levels of inflammatory markers in the blood, such as high-sensitivity c-reactive protein. It is directly associated with abnormal physiology and usually does not cause overt symptoms. In fact, in the absence of clinical disease and/or symptoms, this low-level systemic inflammation is rarely detected. As stated earlier, the inflammation does cause physiological dysfunction (pathophysiology). Moderate exercise has been demonstrated to be anti-inflammatory.

Pathophysiology common to chronic disease

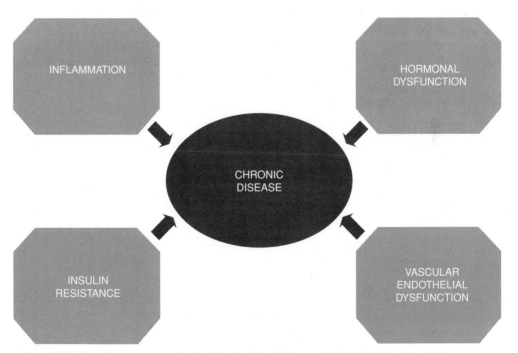

FIGURE 11.1 A set of common pathophysiological conditions underlie all of the chronic diseases discussed in this book.

The original source of this inflammation is unknown and controversial, but proinflammatory health behaviors are well-known, documented, and prevalent in the population. This systemic, low-level inflammation is present in very young people with risk factors for chronic disease such as inactivity, obesity and high blood pressure, or who are exposed to second-hand smoke, for example (27,30). In addition, there are many health behaviors that are proinflammatory (7,27). They include smoking, Western dietary pattern, specific foods, stress, and some specific types of behavior (anger, for example), overweight and obesity, and sedentary lifestyle (20,38). Thus, there are many "suspect" characteristics and behaviors that may contribute to the initial inflammatory insult and subsequent ongoing systemic, low-level inflammatory state.

VASCULAR ENDOTHELIAL DYSFUNCTION

The endothelium is a single layer of cells that is present as the lining of blood vessels throughout the vascular system. Normal vascular function is, in large part, controlled by the endothelium, but other external controls, such as the nervous system and physiological sensors (e.g., chemoreceptors, baroreceptors), provide input about the state of such things as blood flow, oxygenation, and pH. The endothelium also has major control functions for blood flow (e.g., vasoconstriction and vasodilation) as well as influence over things such as coagulation and intracellular metabolism through substances that it produces and secretes.

Vascular dysfunction is usually called "endothelial dysfunction." One example of endothelial dysfunction is that small arteriolar vessels vasoconstrict (rather than dilate) in response to increased metabolic demand. The end effect of this paradoxical vasoconstriction is that blood flow is reduced rather than increased with increased metabolic demand. This dysfunction extends to abnormal blood clotting and even to the production and release of proinflammatory substances that further exacerbate the dysfunction and the inflammation. Therefore, one potential source of this vascular endothelial dysfunction is inflammation.

Exercise has been demonstrated to improve and normalize endothelial function (21). This, in turn, produces beneficial effects that help with prevention of vascular diseases as well as other chronic diseases that have these common pathophysiologies (36). Table 11.1

TABLE 11.1 Summary of Pathophysiology of Chronic Disease		
Disease	**Central Pathophysiology**	**Etiology or Origin**
Excess adipose tissue (overweight/obesity)	Inflammation Vascular dysfunction Insulin resistance	Adipokines (adipose tissue) Proinflammatory substances Hyperinsulinemia
Type 2 diabetes (metabolic syndrome)	Insulin resistance Hyperglycemia Hyper/hypoinsulinemia	Adipokines (adipose tissue) Hyper/hypoinsulinemia Beta cell dysfunction
Occlusive vascular disease	Endothelial dysfunction Inflammation	Nitric oxide system dysfunction Proinflammatory substances
Hypertension	Inflammation Hormonal dysfunction Vascular remodeling	

shows some of the pathophysiology central to chronic disease as well as the theoretical origins of that pathophysiology.

INSULIN RESISTANCE

Insulin receptors are specialized receptors located on the membranes of cells that utilize glucose. These receptors facilitate the entry of glucose into the cell and, thus, are important in regulating blood glucose and cellular metabolism.

Insulin resistance occurs when insulin receptors do not properly facilitate the uptake of glucose into cells. Muscle and brain tissue are the most significant organ systems that utilize glucose for metabolic purposes. Insulin resistance results in hyperglycemia, hyperinsulinemia, and ultimately hypoinsulinemia, as well as other associated physiological dysfunction.

In addition, insulin is involved in such physiological processes as vascular function, fat metabolism, and processes that promote the development and progression of vascular plaque that is present in atherosclerosis and coronary artery disease (CAD). The presence of normal quantities of insulin, as well as little to no insulin resistance, is required for normal cellular and vascular function (33).

Thus, the relationship between insulin resistance, inflammation, and cardiovascular disease is well established (33). Insulin resistance is associated with inflammation as well as vascular, metabolic, and insulin abnormalities. Determining the origin of the insulin resistance is problematic, at best. The presence of inflammation and associated inflammatory substances is one factor that causes this, but all of the factors that we've discussed previously influence the physiological dysfunction. Thus, it becomes difficult to assign responsibility to any single factor or to say which comes first.

Exercise normalizes insulin resistance within some limitations (9,25). Those limitations are the presence of those other risk factors, such as Western dietary pattern and excess adipose tissue. Thus, exercise can and does normalize insulin resistance, but if dietary pattern excess adipose tissue is present, or if the low-level inflammation is exacerbated by other risk factors, then exercise cannot, by itself, normalize insulin resistance (25).

HORMONAL DYSFUNCTION

We did not thoroughly discuss hormonal dysfunction in this book, but it is a fact that endocrine function is not normal in most chronic diseases. Insulin (above) is one obvious example. Another example is the dysfunction present in hypertension (see discussion of the renin-angiotensin aldosterone system [RAAS] in Chapter 8). There are hormonal and neurohormonal abnormalities that accompany high blood pressure. Those abnormalities make hypertension worse and, thus, are similar to inflammation or insulin resistance, in that they are self-propagating. That is, they not only negatively affect other physiology but also result in increased pathophysiology simply because they persist. Thus, insulin resistance, insulin abnormalities, and inflammation underlie all of the chronic diseases discussed in this book in some form. They contribute to, may cause, and are definitely associated with overweight/obesity, dyslipidemia, hypertension, cardiovascular disease, metabolic syndrome, and diabetes.

It has been shown that some of these hormonal abnormalities can be modified by exercise. One example is the RAAS (renin-angiotensin-aldosterone system) that is a major (hormonal) control system for blood pressure. Exercise has effects within this system on a multilevel basis. Contrast this with many antihypertensive drugs that have effects on only a single part of the system, for example, drugs called angiotensin II receptor blockers, which are used in treating hypertension. Their effects are isolated to a single part of the RAAS, whereas exercise has normalizing effects on the system at many control points (see Chapter 8) (14,52). Thus, exercise is the preferred and is a centrally effective therapeutic treatment for hypertension.

EFFECTS OF EXERCISE

PHYSICAL ACTIVITY AND PHYSICAL FITNESS

Moderate exercise is antiinflammatory, normalizes vascular function, improves insulin resistance, and has positive effects on hormonal function. ACSM defines "moderate" as 40%–59% HRR or VO_2R. Clearly the effects of exercise are varied and different according to the intensity, duration, and total energy expenditure of the exercise. We will attempt, as much as is possible, to summarize the information concerning the optimal amount of exercise for each of these effects and preventive purposes.

Physical activity (PA) and physical fitness (PF) are both important in the prevention of chronic disease. The discussion in Chapter 3 on exercise includes a relatively detailed discussion on PA versus PF with respect to prevention of chronic disease. It is safe to say that most researchers conclude that both are important but that PF is more important in protection from heart disease (no conclusions are possible with respect to the general category of "chronic disease") (44,71).

The connection between PA and PF is strong, and, though there is certainly a genetic element in PF, it is difficult to increase PF without increasing PA (exercise, to be exact). Thus, the primary principle for the Exercise Professional should initially be to get clients to increase daily PA levels and to engage in some kind of regular exercise that improves PF as much as possible within the context and limitations of any pathophysiology that may be present. The recent "movement" for people to get 10,000 steps per day seems reasonable for most people, though the actual level for protection and prevention may be higher for some. Increasing PF and PA is beneficial and contributes to preventing chronic disease.

The principles of prescribing exercise as well as PA are discussed in Chapter 3. Mixing intensity, duration, and frequency with different modes of exercise for exercise prescription is an art as well as a science. The prescription of both PA and PF are important for the most effective program in prevention of chronic disease. The literature supports that decreasing sedentary time and even breaks in sedentary time are additionally preventive even in the presence of increased PA and PF (23,50,69).

CARDIORESPIRATORY ENDURANCE FITNESS

In Chapter 3, we referred to the importance of cardiorespiratory endurance fitness (CREF) as the type of fitness that is instrumental in preventing chronic disease. CREF is, by definition, improved by cardiovascular endurance exercise. Resistance training (RT) without cardiovascular endurance exercise is less effective for prevention of chronic disease and for most risk factor modification than aerobic exercise; therefore, RT should be combined with aerobic exercise for best results.

The principles of exercise prescription for increasing CREF can be found in Table 11.2. These principles are basic, were established many years ago, and are relatively simple and

TABLE 11.2	Principles of Exercise Prescription for CREF*	
Variable	**Minimum Criteria for Increase**
Frequency	3–5 d/wk
Intensity	64%–93% Max HR
	40%–85% of HRR
	40%–85% of VO$_2$R
Duration	20–60 min/session

CREF, cardiorespiratory endurance fitness; HR, heart rate; HRR, heart rate reserve; VO$_2$R, maximal oxygen uptake reserve.

*Modified from ACSM's Guidelines for Exercise Testing and Prescription, 8th Ed. Lippincott, Williams & Wilkins, 2010. These are summary recommendations. For more a more complete table, please see Table 3.1.

straightforward (1). They are, however, only part of the equation with respect to prevention of chronic disease. As we stated earlier, it is important to increase PA and PF for prevention of chronic disease.

We also discussed the "subacute" effects of exercise in Chapter 3. These are temporary effects (lasting from a few to 24 or more hours) that accrue from a single exercise session. Obtaining specific subacute effects may depend on intensity and duration of exercise. We believe, and the research literature confirms, that these effects are preventive. The physiology affecting insulin resistance and endothelial function, for example, are subacute effects. They are stimulated by a single session of exercise and, for all practical purposes, disappear after several hours. Thus, daily exercise and activity are most appropriate for optimal prevention of chronic disease (12).

PRESCRIPTION OF PA

Prescribing increases in PA, as well as exercise for CREF is important to achieving optimal prevention of chronic disease. Sedentary time is the majority of almost everyone's day. With the exception of those few individuals who have very active occupations, most individuals spend too much time sitting or being totally sedentary (43). The optimal exercise prescription for weight loss and maintenance (see Table 11.3) also contains the general prescription for PA. We will not repeat this explanation in further tables, except to refer to the prescription of PA as a critical component of the optimal program.

OPTIMAL PROGRAMS FOR PREVENTING CHRONIC DISEASE

OVERWEIGHT AND OBESITY (EXCESS ADIPOSE TISSUE)

Obesity is, perhaps, the most widespread chronic disease with respect to prevalence in the population of the United States. Since it seems to be an "underlying" chronic disease, common to other highly prevalent chronic diseases such as heart disease and type 2 diabetes, we will summarize the optimal program for obesity and overweight first. Multiple standards have been used to define excess adiposity. Table 6.3 summarizes those standards.

The underlying pathophysiology that connects excess adiposity to other chronic disease seems to be systemic inflammation and insulin resistance. Though not all people with excess adiposity have both systemic inflammation and insulin resistance, adipose tissue produces and secretes substances (adipokines) that are proinflammatory and promote insulin resistance (3,20,38).

The optimal exercise program for weight loss as well as maintenance of weight loss is summarized in Table 11.3. A negative energy balance is critical for successful weight loss. Energy balance is defined as the sum of caloric expenditure (including basal metabolic rate) and caloric intake. A negative energy balance is easier to achieve if some form of exercise and

TABLE 11.3	Optimal Exercise Prescription for Weight Loss and Maintenance
Optimal exercise for excess adiposity	
Frequency	CREF: 7 days per week if tolerated; a minimum of 5 d/wk is recommended.
Intensity	Moderate: 40%–59% max HRR or VO$_2$R, RPE: 11–13 range (on a 6–20 scale).
Duration	CREF: 60 minutes per day—may be divided into shorter sessions but prefer not less than 15 minutes and at least one session longer than 30 minutes, 3 days per week. Duration should be emphasized in the early exercise prescriptions.
Type	Walking or other weight-bearing exercise is preferred; swimming or water aerobics may be substituted but because of buoyancy, may be less effective; RT may be used as an excellent adjunct, but should be in addition to the cardiovascular endurance exercise and is an excellent combined program for muscular and cardiovascular fitness.
Caloric expenditure	Caloric expenditure should be >2000 kcal/wk outside normal daily activities. Preventing weight regain may require >3000 cal/wk. LTPA should be added to the exercise program in amounts equaling the caloric expenditure during exercise. We also recommend a step counter to quantify daily activity with a goal of 8–10,000 steps per day outside the exercise activity. Total steps, including exercise and activity, should be approximately 11,000–14,000 in weight loss programs.
Physical activity prescription	
LTPA	Some PA > "light" (20%–39% HRR) every 2 hours. Recommend at least 3–5 minutes each for a total of 60 minutes per day.
Sedentary time	Decrease sitting and other sedentary time as much as possible. Preferably no more than 1 hour continuously throughout the day.

CREF, cardiorespiratory endurance fitness; RPE, ratings of perceived exertion; RT, resistance training; PA, physical activity; LTPA, leisure-time physical activity; HRR, heart rate reserve.

activity are prescribed as part of the weight loss program. Prescription of PA as well as "exercise" contributes significant numbers of calories to a negative energy balance. Research demonstrates that maintaining weight loss may require larger energy expenditure than the initial weight loss required. In addition, it appears that higher than usual levels of PA are required to prevent weight gain with aging (24,37). The reasons are complex, but loss of lean and fat mass as well as altered metabolic function seem to combine to contribute to this puzzling problem. Successful weight loss programs are characterized by reduced calorie intake and increased calorie expenditure. Calorie expenditures exceeding 2000 calories per week are required for weight loss, and weekly calorie expenditures of greater than 3000 calories per week are common to successful long-term maintenance of weight loss that exceeds 50 pounds (24,61).

The optimal nutritional program for weight loss and weight maintenance should aim at a negative caloric balance. Recent research shows that calories make a difference and that the dietary content of carbohydrates, fat, and protein may not be as important as total calorie intake (57). Some research has shown that reducing simple and refined carbohydrates may be as or more effective for weight loss programs than low-fat diets (18). At this time, a definitive answer is not known, but it is clear that calories do count! (See the box titled "Critical Nutritional Principles of Weight Loss Programs") summarizes important nutritional principles for weight loss programs.

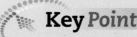

Key Point

The overall objective in prescribing PA should be a reduction of sedentary time. The use of step counters or other activity monitors, including personal logs, is encouraged. At the very least, the client should be encouraged to be physically active for brief periods (5 or more minutes) in every waking hour. Activities such as walking, stretching, activities of daily living, or similar active pursuits (but perhaps not "exercise" by definition) can contribute significantly to daily calorie expenditure.

DID YOU KNOW?
Critical Nutritional Principles of Weight Loss Programs

Caloric restriction should be moderate and should involve both carbohydrates and fats. Generally greater restriction in carbohydrates may lead to greater weight loss early in a program, but not necessarily in the long term.

Fat restriction centers on foods containing saturated and trans fat. A nutritional plan should include foods containing monounsaturated and polyunsaturated fat for their health benefits (see Chapters 4 and 6). Using these principles produces positive changes in nutritionally related risk factors, including blood lipids, glucose and fat metabolism, and inflammatory state.

Carbohydrate restriction should center on simple sugars and refined carbohydrates. Restricting these requires, by default, consuming mostly complex and high-fiber carbohydrates. This is a healthier dietary pattern and one that decreases hunger and enhances satiety.

Very low–calorie diets should not be used without the ongoing supervision of a physician. Extreme caloric restriction is inappropriate for all but the most obese.

Any diet should limit the consumption of high-caloric-density foods because they are often high in fat or simple carbohydrates and because high-caloric-density foods are usually low-volume foods with little nutritional value. Thus, hunger can be a constant problem with these foods in the dietary pattern.

DID YOU KNOW?
Principles of Energy Balance (24)

Traditional methods of producing a negative energy balance for intake and expenditure with food and exercise may be ineffective for those with a significant genetic component to obesity.

Energy flux is important to the effectiveness of weight loss when altering energy balance. A greater energy flux may ensure more success than a smaller energy flux. Significantly increased levels of PA may allow people to regulate energy intake more effectively. Lower energy flux may not allow sufficient calorie restriction for weight loss or maintenance of weight loss.

Diet composition may variably affect weight loss depending on whether a person is in negative, positive, or in energy balance (intake = expenditure). When total caloric restriction is equal between diets and a negative energy balance is present, there is little difference in weight loss associated with diet composition.

Small increases in PA may help prevent weight gain, but relatively large increases in PA are necessary to prevent weight gain after weight loss.

Maintaining weight loss is more difficult because losing weight causes decreased energy requirements both at rest and during exercise. After a weight loss, maintaining that loss may require even greater increases in energy expenditure.

Systematic changes in both the "food" environment and the PA/exercise environments are critical to losing and maintaining weight loss.

See Chapter 6 for a more detailed explanation of the principles of energy balance.

HEART AND VASCULAR DISEASE (ATHEROSCLEROSIS)

For this discussion, we will refer to these diseases collectively as occlusive vascular disease (OVD). Though cerebral vascular disease and peripheral vascular disease are found in different anatomical locations, they are all the same disease. CAD has the common underlying pathophysiology that we have described earlier. The hallmark of the disease is accumulation of plaque (forming a blockage) under the endothelium. These blockages are deposits of fat, cholesterol, white blood cells, smooth muscle, and other substances. Figure 2.3 illustrates atherosclerotic plaque. The plaque, coupled with endothelial dysfunction and inflammation, leads to coagulation abnormalities as well as more physiological and vascular dysfunction. Under some circumstances, this plaque becomes increasingly prone to rupture. Plaque rupture is the primary event associated with myocardial infarction and stroke as well as much of the incidence of unstable angina, transient ischemic attacks, and other complications associated with OVD (40). The optimal exercise program for OVD is shown in Table 11.4.

Exercise and diet have long been shown to be associated with lower prevalence and incidence of and mortality from CAD. Increased PF and PA are each protective. Dietary patterns with increased amounts of monounsaturated fatty acids, polyunsaturated fatty acids, fiber, and lower amounts of saturated and trans-fats, red meat, and refined grains are also associated with lower rates of and death rates from OVD (8).

The optimal program for preventing atherosclerosis includes the exercise prescription (see Table 11.4) along with an optimal dietary pattern perhaps best described as "Indo-

TABLE 11.4	**Optimal Exercise Prescription for Prevention of Atherosclerosis**
Frequency	CREx exercise: 3–4 d/wk. Resistance exercise: 2–3 d/wk. LMEx: 3–4 d/wk (opposite CREF exercise). Total: exercise 7 d/wk.
Intensity	CREx: 60%–85% VO_2R. LMEx: 30%–60% VO_2.
Duration	CREx: 30 minutes or more of continuous exercise. LMEx: 15–30 minutes (continuous or intermittent).
Type	CREx: repetitive, large muscle group exercise, for example, walking, jogging, swimming, and so on. LMEx: Any other activities, including team sports, recreational activities, job-related or household activities, are included in this category
Physical Activity	See Table 11.3 for PA prescription.

CREx, cardiorespiratory endurance exercise; LMEx, low- to moderate-intensity exercise (including LTPA); PA, physical activity.

Mediterranean" is presented in the following Did You Know? box. That optimal dietary pattern is described in Chapter 4 on nutrition and presented in Table 4.14. The Indo-Mediterranean dietary pattern discussed in the following box is similar to the optimal nutritional pattern described in Table 4.14.

Please note that these recommendations are specific to OVD and that the summary recommendations for the optimal nutritional plan found in Table 4.14 are consistent with

DID YOU KNOW?
Characteristics of a Mediterranean-type Diet

- Four or more servings of vegetable per day—½ cup raw or cooked, 1 cup leafy raw greens, or ½ cup of vegetable juice
- Four or more servings of fruit per day—½ cup of fresh, frozen, or canned fruit, ¼ cup of dried fruit, one medium-sized fruit, or ½ cup of fruit juice
- Six or more servings of whole grains per day—a serving is 1 cup of dry breakfast cereal, ½ cup of cooked cereal, whole-grain rice or pasta, or one slice of whole-grain bread
- Olive oil is the primary oil used in dressings and cooking
- Two or more servings of fish per week—a serving is 4 ounces
- One serving of yogurt or cheese per day—8 ounces of yogurt or 2 ounces of cheese
- One serving of beans or nuts per day—for cooked beans, ½ cup is a serving; for nuts, 1.5 ounces or a "handful" is a serving
- Limit alcohol to 1 drink for women and 2 for men—one drink is 5 ounces of wine, 12 ounces of beer, or 1.5 ounces of liquor

these recommendations. A more structured program is the most recent version of the Dietary Approach to Stop Hypertension (DASH) diet that has been demonstrated to be effective in preventing OVD, hypertension, and other chronic diseases. DASH is an excellent alternative and has sufficient structure if clients require more than just the recommendations found in Table 4.4 along with a detailed discussion of these dietary patterns.

TYPE 2 DIABETES AND METABOLIC SYNDROME

The incidence of MetS and type 2 diabetes are increasing in the United States and in most industrialized countries around the world (46). The incidence of both is directly proportional to the increasing incidence and prevalence of overweight and obesity. MetS is defined (clinically) by the presence of 3 out of 5 risk factors. Those risk factors include abdominal obesity, high triglycerides, low high-density lipoprotein (HDL) cholesterol, elevated blood pressure, and hyperglycemia. Thus, when these risk factors "cluster" (are found together in individuals), the risk for both type 2 diabetes and CAD increase by 5-fold and 2-fold, respectively (13).

MetS and type 2 diabetes have two major, common, pathophysiological characteristics—insulin resistance and systemic inflammation. MetS and type 2 diabetes are commonly accompanied by obesity (or overweight) and sedentary lifestyle. Though most people with MetS or type 2 diabetes are obese and have lipid abnormalities, these are not necessarily consistent with everyone. Most researchers believe that the etiology of MetS and type 2 diabetes originates with the combination of excess adiposity and a sedentary lifestyle (19). Finally, the influence and actions of adipokines (see Chapter 6 for a detailed discussion) is thought to be operative in initiating and potentiating the pathophysiology associated with these diseases (20,38,56).

The optimal program for prevention of MetS and type 2 diabetes, utilizing both exercise and diet, has been shown to be effective in both prevention and moderation of these diseases (6,47). Weight loss and caloric restriction have been shown to be preventive (15,65). Dietary patterns similar to the DASH or Omni-Heart diet—low in saturated and trans-fats, high in fiber, and complex carbohydrates—are preventive (26). More importantly, the change in insulin resistance that is attributed to exercise is a subacute effect that is short-lived. Thus, the exercise prescription for MetS and type 2 diabetes is a daily (or almost daily) routine of exercise and PA (6,47). The optimal exercise program for type 2 diabetes and MetS can be seen in Table 11.5.

HYPERTENSION

Aside from excess adipose tissue, hypertension is the most prevalent chronic disease in the United States. More than 70 million people have hypertension, but only about 70% of those with hypertension are aware of it. Less than 35% of people with hypertension are being effectively treated (45). Hypertension is more prevalent in some ethnic groups (non-Hispanic black men, for example) and death rates in these groups are also higher (29).

National Guidelines for Prevention and Treatment of Hypertension state that normal blood pressure is <120 mm Hg (systolic) and <80 mm Hg (diastolic) but also state that CVD risk increases beginning at blood pressures of 115/75 mm Hg (29). They also specify

TABLE 11.5	Optimal Exercise Program for Preventing Type 2 Diabetes and Metabolic Syndrome
Optimal exercise for preventing type 2 diabetes and metabolic syndrome	
Frequency	CREF: 7 days per week if tolerated, or work toward 6–7 days per week.
Intensity	Moderate: 40%–59% HRR. RPE: 11–13 range (on a 6–20 scale).
Duration	60 minutes per day—may be divided into shorter sessions but not less than 15 minutes and preferably at least one session longer than 30 minutes 3 days per week.
Type	CREF exercise is preferred and most effective. Walking can be effective if performed according to guidelines above with respect to intensity and duration; RT is an excellent adjunct, but should be performed in addition to the CREF.
Caloric expenditure	Caloric expenditure should equal >2000 kcal/wk in addition to normal daily activities.
Physical activity	See Table 11.3 for PA prescription.

CREF, cardiorespiratory endurance fitness; HRR, heart rate reserve; RPE, ratings of perceived exertion; RT, resistance training; PA, physical activity.

that people with systolic blood pressure of 120 to 129 or diastolic blood pressure of 80 to 90 have "prehypertension" and thus should be followed by a physician and treated with lifestyle changes.

Hypertension is considered to be a primary risk factor for OVD, but it also multiplies the risk of chronic disease in the presence of other risk factors (29). Thus, hypertension is not only a chronic disease that requires treatment but also a risk factor (not unlike excess adipose tissue) that interacts with other risk factors to further increase risk of disease. Systemic inflammation is associated with hypertension, but the etiology is controversial since the presence of other risk factors and a proinflammatory dietary pattern is common. A low-level, systemic inflammation is present in the earliest phases of hypertension (11). Vascular stiffening, which is a coincident with vascular remodeling due to the chronically increased pressure in arteries, is present in longer-standing hypertension. This stiffening results in further increases in blood pressure that come from the vascular remodeling and from the increased stiffness itself—this is an example of a positive feedback loop (2,14,68,74).

Though the Seventh Edition of the National Guidelines for Prevention and Treatment of Hypertension guidelines emphasize lifestyle in the prevention and control of hypertension, it is only a small part of the text and relatively few recommendations are in the document (29). Our recommendation is that lifestyle should be *the* primary mode of treatment. Specifically, exercise and diet must be central to any effort to reduce and prevent hypertension and should be used in all persons who are medicated for hypertension. The optimal exercise and activity prescription for preventing and treating hypertension is found in the Table 11.6.

Dietary pattern has been demonstrated to be inextricably linked to the presence of hypertension and is critical to prevention and control. High sodium, low potassium, and

TABLE 11.6	Optimal Exercise and Physical Activity Program for Hypertension
Frequency	CREF: 3–4 d/wk. RT: 2–3 d/wk. LMEx: 3–4 d/wk (opposite CREF exercise). Total: exercise 7 d/wk.
Intensity	CREF: 60%–85% VO_2R. LMEx: 50%–70% VO_2.
Duration	CREF: 30 minutes or more of continuous exercise per day. LMEx: 15–30 minutes.
Type	CREF: Repetitive, large muscle group exercise, for example, walking, jogging, swimming, cycling, etc. LMEx: Any other activities, including team sports, recreational activities, job-related or household activities, are in this category
PA	See Table 11.3 for PA prescription.

CREF, cardiorespiratory endurance fitness; LMEx, low- to moderate-intensity exercise; PA, physical activity; VO_2 and VO_2R, maximal oxygen uptake and maximal oxygen uptake reserve.

excessive alcohol intake are related to hypertension. The DASH dietary pattern (Table 4.6) has been demonstrated to be effective in reducing elevated blood pressure (57).

DYSLIPIDEMIA

Dyslipidemia is a widespread chronic disease in the United States. Somewhere between 30% and 50% of the adult population have some form of dyslipidemia (16). The plaque that forms blockages in arteries is primarily composed of lipid-filled "foam" cells, along with many other types of cell and cellular debris (40). Lipids are transported in blood by proteins; thus, "specific lipoproteins," for example LDL or triglycerides, may contribute to the development and progression of plaque by depositing fat into the plaque. On the other hand, some lipids are protective and actually remove fat from plaque, for example, HDL. Postprandial lipemia (PPL) is the increase in lipoproteins (particularly triglycerides) that occurs shortly after a meal. High-fat meals cause a large influx of lipoproteins and triglycerides into the blood; thus, a significant degree of PPL is apparent after high-fat meals. Abnormally high levels of PPL are a risk factor for atherosclerosis (62).

Exercise, dietary pattern (and macronutrients), and weight loss are primary tools for prevention and moderation of dyslipidemia. Positive changes in HDL, triglycerides, and low-density lipoprotein particle size have been shown to be associated with exercise, diet, and weight loss (31,32,58,60,71,72). The effects of RT are less well defined, but some studies suggest that there is a positive effect, especially in combination with other aerobic exercise training (31,32). Exercise has also been shown to have positive effects on moderating PPL, but the exercise must be performed 8 to 12 hours before ingestion of that meal (4,62,63).

The optimal exercise prescription for dyslipidemia is a bit different from the other programs. Some of the research demonstrates that intermittent exercise sessions, as few as

TABLE 11.7	Optimal Program for Exercise Management of Dyslipidemia
Optimal exercise for preventing type 2 diabetes and metabolic syndrome	
Frequency	CREF: 4–7 d/wk. RT: 2–3 d/wk.
Intensity	CREF: 40%–85% HRR. RPE: 12–16 RPE range (on a 6–20 scale). RT: 50%–80% 1 RM. Discontinue repetitions before volitional fatigue.
Duration	CREF: 30–60 minutes per session. RT: 30–45 minutes per session; 2–3 sets, 8–15 repetitions.
Type	8–12 large muscle exercises preferable.
Caloric expenditure	Caloric expenditure should equal ≥2000 kcal/wk in addition to normal daily activities.
Physical activity	See Table 11.3 for PA prescription.

CREF, cardiorespiratory endurance fitness; RT, resistance training; RPE, ratings of perceived exertion; 1 RM, one repetition-maximum; LMEx, low- to moderate-intensity exercise; PA, physical activity.

three 10-minute sessions, can result in significant changes in lipoproteins but the research remains inconclusive (4). Other than that, the exercise prescription calls for a dose of exercise that is similar but not identical to other optimal programs for chronic diseases. Table 11.7 shows the optimal exercise program for dyslipidemia.

OPTIMAL NUTRITION

The predominant dietary pattern in the United States is the "Western Dietary Pattern" (5,17). Recently, much of the nutritional research literature that addresses health and nutrition has centered on dietary pattern, as opposed to specific nutrients or macronutrients (e.g., fat or carbohydrates). Dietary patterns such as the Mediterranean, the Indo-Mediterranean, and the "prudent" dietary pattern have been demonstrated to be effective in preventing and ameliorating several chronic diseases. (See the box titled "Characteristics of the 'Prudent' and the 'Western Diet'" compares the Western dietary pattern with the prudent dietary pattern (5,10,17).

Several key nutritional studies investigated the Western and the prudent dietary pattern with respect to incidence of heart and other chronic disease. Others, for example, INTER-HEART (73) and Van Dam (67), studied chronic disease and lifestyle behavior. INTERHEART identified nine risk factors that were present in 94% of all cases of myocardial infarction; six of the nine risk factors are diet related (73). Van Dam (67) identified five behaviors that were preventive. Those included no history of smoking, regular PA, a healthy diet, body mass index <25.0, and light or moderate alcohol consumption (three risk factors are diet related).

Whole food–based diets, including Dietary Approach to Stop Hypertension (DASH), Portfolio, Ornish, Pritikin, and the Indo-Mediterranean, have been shown to be preventive (28,49,50,57,59). The characteristics of these and other dietary patterns are shown throughout Chapter 4. These are based on the research noted earlier and have been demonstrated to be effective for preventing chronic disease.

DID YOU KNOW?

Characteristics of the "Prudent" and the "Western Diet"

Western	Prudent
High intake of simple carbohydrates such as French fries and simple sugar	High intake of complex carbohydrates
	Few sweetened products
Simple sugar sweetened products	
High intake of refined grains; few whole grains, nuts, and legumes	Little if any refined grains
	Whole grains, nuts, and legumes
Low fiber	High Fiber
Few fruits and vegetables	Fruits and vegetables
High sodium and fat	Low fat, lower sodium
High intake of red meat	Limited intake of red meats (unsaturated plant sources); little if any processed, meats
Frequent intake of processed meats	
Frequent intake of fast foods	
High- or moderate-fat dairy	High intake of mono- and polyunsaturated fats from plant sources
	Low-fat dairy
	Omega-3 fatty acids from fish
	Infrequent consumption of fast foods

Food pyramids can be useful visual tools to guide dietary pattern. Three of them may be particularly helpful. The Healing Foods Pyramid (University of Michigan) emphasizes "functional foods" that have been shown to promote healthy physiology (66). Examples are whole grains, legumes, healthy fats, and the emphasis on eating many different colors of food. The Healthy Eating Pyramid developed by the Harvard Public Health researchers (22) emphasizes exercise and weight control at the base of the pyramid as part of a healthy lifestyle. Fruits, vegetables, whole grains, and healthy fats are emphasized, as in other healthy nutritional patterns. Finally, the Ornish Pyramid emphasizes vegetables, whole grains, fruits, and legumes at the base, with nuts and plant oils for healthy fats (49). All of these food pyramids can be found in Chapter 4.

We have used those pyramids as well as the key nutrition and chronic disease studies to formulate recommendations for our optimal dietary pattern shown on Table 4.14. A wide variety of foods is recommended and available with this pattern. Functional foods are available, and attention to low sodium and high fiber are central to the pattern.

OPTIMAL BEHAVIOR CHANGE

For individuals who do not practice these optimal lifestyle behaviors, none of these programs can be actualized unless behavior change is initiated and accomplished. Changing a lifelong habit such as dietary pattern or activity level can be extremely difficult and challenging even to the most motivated and diligent person. Practicing a new habit for 6 to 12 months or more is necessary for it to be considered permanent; even then the risk of lapse and relapse continues at some level (42).

The critical pieces for the Exercise Professional to understand include the Transtheoretical Model of behavior change and self-efficacy. Providing ongoing support is something that most people require to maintain a new behavior. "Enabling" and "codependency" can take many forms, but reminding and being present for clients as well as being someone for clients to be accountable to, while reinforcing appropriate behaviors, are all part of the Exercise Professional's tool kit for facilitating change in clients. Assessing stage of change is quick and easy and should be a part of the Exercise Professionals assessment package for any client who has not initiated or reached maintenance stage of the desired health behavior. Figure 10.5 and the accompanying box in Chapter 10 provides a brief questionnaire that can help assess a person's stage of change.

The Transtheoretical Model is a model that was originally conceived to explain and understand behavior change. It includes (55)

- stages of change
- processes of change
- decisional balance and
- self-efficacy.

Although people who are attempting to habituate a new behavior progress through stages of change in order, it does not necessarily happen in a linear and chronological fashion. In fact, progression usually involves cycling back and forth between stages. For example, it is not uncommon for someone to progress from the preparation stage to the action stage and then drift back to the preparation stage during the process. Likewise, individuals take varying amounts of time to progress through the stages to maintenance.

Some strategies seem to be more effective when they are utilized during specific stages (17,48). Informing the client about pros and cons of the change is useful, but it has been demonstrated that the pros are more important than the cons and that they (the pros) become progressively more important as an individual progresses through the stages (48,54). In addition, strategies such as reminders and support systems are important throughout the change process. However, some individuals may require differing amounts of support, so the Exercise Professional must be aware of these individual differences and act to support and reinforce appropriately.

DID YOU KNOW?

Best-Practice Behavior Change Techniques

- Assess stage of change (see Table 10.5).
- Set specific behavioral goals, outcomes, and time frames that can be objectively monitored.
- Formulate a system that rewards behavior as it occurs (not at the end) and that does not defeat the purpose of the behavior change.
- Specify support systems.
- Attempt to foresee barriers and obstacles in formulating a lapse/relapse plan. Always develop a plan to "restart" lapsed behavior.
- Assure that behavior change processes fit the stage of readiness.
- Model and provide models for the appropriate behavior.
- Always reinforce correct behavior and success!

Self-efficacy is the extent to which an individual believes that they can succeed in the behavior change process. Individuals differ in the belief about their ability to change and to achieve the goal behavior. In the case of PA, for example, it has been stated the self-efficacy is the single "most consistent correlate of physical activity behavior" (64). Exercise Professionals can encourage, reinforce, and model (or provide models for) appropriate kinds of PA behavior; thus, they can (and should) positively influence and reinforce self-efficacy.

Perhaps one of the most important parts of the behavior change process with respect to an Exercise Professional's involvement is preparing and anticipating lapse and relapse behavior in the change process. Lapse is inevitable. Individuals not only need to be aware of it but also need to be prepared for lapses and relapses. Foreseeing obstacles and events that may provoke lapse is one way to prepare. Planning what to do in case of lapse is another. The Exercise Professional must assist clients to overcome these slips in behavior and get back on track in the behavior change process.

REFERENCES

1. ACSM's Guidelines for Exercise Testing and Prescription (ed. Thompson WR). 8th ed. Baltimore, MD: Lippincott Williams & Wilkins, 2010.
2. Adams V, Linke A, Krankel N, et al. Impact of regular physical activity on NAD(P)H oxidase and angiotensin receptor system in patients with coronary artery disease. Circulation. 2005;111:555–562.
3. Aggoun Y. Obesity, metabolic syndrome, and cardiovascular disease. Pediatr Res. 2007;61(6):653–659.
4. Altena TS, Michaelson JL, Ball SD, et al. Single sessions of intermittent and continuous exercise and postprandial lipemia. Med Sci Sports Exerc. 2004;36:1364–1371.
5. Bassuk SS, Manson JE. Lifestyle and risk of cardiovascular disease and type 2 diabetes in women: a review of epidemiologic findings. Am J Lifestyle Med. 2008;2:191–213.
6. Bazzano LA, Serdula M, Liu S. Prevention of type 2 diabetes by diet and lifestyle modification. J Am Coll Nutr. 2005;24(5):310–319.
7. Berenson GS, Wattigney WA, Tracy RE, et al. Atherosclerosis of the aorta and coronary arteries and cardiovascular risk factors in persons aged 6 to 30 years and studied at necropsy (The Bogalusa Heart Study). Am J Cardiol. 1992;70:851–858.
8. Blair SN, Horton E, Leon AS, et al. Physical activity, nutrition, and chronic disease. Med Sci Sports Exerc. 1996;28(3):335–349.
9. Borghouts LB, Keizer HA. Exercise and insulin sensitivity: a review. Int J Sports Med. 2000;21:1–12.
10. Carlson JJ, Monti V. The role of inclusive dietary patterns for achieving secondary prevention cardiovascular nutrition guidelines and optimal cardiovascular health. J Cardiopulm Rehabil. 2003;23:322–333.
11. Chae CU, Lee RT, Rifai N, et al. Blood pressure and inflammation in apparently healthy men. Hypertension. 2001;38:399–403.
12. da Nobrega ACL. The subacute effects of exercise: concept, characteristics and clinical implications. Exerc Sports Sci Rev. 2005;33(2):84–87.
13. Dandona P, Aljada A, Chaudhuri A, et al. Metabolic syndrome: a comprehensive perspective based on interactions between obesity, diabetes, and inflammation. Circulation. 2005;111(11):1448–1454.
14. Fagard RH, Cornelissen VA. Effect of exercise on blood pressure control in hypertensive patients. Eur J Cardiovasc Prev Rehabil. 2007;14:12–17.
15. Fontana LA. Calorie restriction and cardiometabolic health. Eur J Cardiovasc Prev Rehabil. 2008;15(1):3–9.
16. Ford ES, Chaoyang L, Zhao G, et al. Hypertriglyceridemia and its pharmacologic treatment among US adults. Arch Intern Med. 2009;169:572–578.
17. Garber CE, Alisworth JE, Marcus BH, et al. Correlates of change for physical activity in a population survey. Am J Public Health. 2008;98:897–904.
18. Gardner CD, Kiazand A, Alhassan S, et al. Comparison of the Atkins, Zone, Ornish, and LEARN diets for change in weight and related risk factors among overweight premenopausal women: the A TO Z Weight Loss Study: a randomized trial. JAMA. 2007;297:969–977.
19. Grundy SM. Metabolic syndrome pandemic. Arterioscler Thromb Vasc Biol. 2008;28:629–636.
20. Gustafson B, Hammarstedt A, Andersson CX, et al. Inflamed adipose tissue: a culprit underlying the metabolic syndrome and atherosclerosis. Arterioscler Thromb Vasc Biol. 2007;27(11):2276–2283.
21. Hamer M. Exercise and psychobiological processes: implications for the primary prevention of coronary heart disease. Sports Med. 2006;36(10):829–838.
22. Harvard School of Public Health. Nutrition Source: Healthy Eating Pyramid: The Bottom Line. Cambridge, MA. Available at: http://www.hsph.harvard.edu/nutritionsource/what-should-you-eat/pyramid/.

23. Healy GN, Dunstan DW, Salmon J, et al. Breaks in sedentary time: beneficial associations with metabolic risk. Diabetes Care. 2008;31(4):661–666.

24. Hill JO. Understanding and addressing the epidemic of obesity: an energy balance perspective. Endocr Rev. 2006;27:750–761.

25. Houmard JA, Tanner CJ, Slentz CA, et al. Effect of the volume and intensity of exercise training on insulin sensitivity. J Appl Physiol. 2004;96(1):101–106.

26. Hu FB. Dietary pattern analysis: a new direction in nutritional epidemiology. Curr Opin Lipidol. 2002; 13(1):3–9.

27. Jarvisalo MJ, Harmoinen A, Hakanen M, et al. Elevated serum c-reactive protein levels and early arterial changes in healthy children. Arterioscler Thromb Vasc Biol. 2002;22:1323–1328.

28. Jenkins DJA, Josse AR, Wong JMW, et al. The Portfolio Diet for cardiovascular risk reduction. Curr Atheroscler Rep. 2007;9:501–507.

29. Joint National Committee on Prevention, Detection, Evaluation, and Treatment of High Blood Pressure. National High Blood Pressure Education Program. The sixth report of the Joint National Committee on Prevention, Detection, Evaluation, and Treatment of High Blood Pressure. Hypertension. 2003;42:1206–1252.

30. Kapiotis S, Holzer G, Schaller G, et al. A proinflammatory state is detectable in obese children and is accompanied by functional and morphological vascular changes. Arterioscler Thromb Vasc Biol. 2006; 26:2541–2546.

31. Kelley GA, Kelley KS. Aerobic exercise and lipids and lipoproteins in men: a meta-analysis of randomized controlled trials. J Mens Health Gend. 2006;3:61–70.

32. Kelley GA, Kelley KS, Tran ZV. Exercise, lipids, and lipoproteins in older adults: a meta-analysis. Prev Cardiol. 2005;8:206–214.

33. Kim J, Monagnani M, Kwand KK, et al. Reciprocal relationships between insulin resistance and endothelial dysfunction: molecular and pathophysiological mechanisms. Circulation. 2006;113: 1888–1904.

34. King DE, Mainous AG, Carnemolla M, et al. Adherence to healthy lifestyle habits in U.S. adults, 1988–2006. Am J Med. 2009;122:528–534.

35. Kvaavik E, Batty GD, Ursin G, et al. Influence of individual and combined health behaviors on total and cause-specific mortality in men and women: the United Kingdom health and lifestyle survey. Arch Intern Med. 2010;170(8):711–718.

36. Laughlin HM. Physical activity in prevention and treatment of coronary disease: the battle line is in exercise vascular cell biology. Med Sci Sports Exerc. 2004;36(3):352–362.

37. Lee IM, Djoussé L, Sesso SD, et al. Physical activity and weight gain prevention. JAMA. 2010;303:1173–1179.

38. Lee YH, Pratley RE. Abdominal obesity and cardiovascular disease risk: the emerging role of the adipocyte. J Cardiopulm Rehabil Prev. 2007;27(1):2–10.

39. Lee CD, Sui X, Blair SN. Combined effects of cardiorespiratory fitness, not smoking and normal waist girth on morbidity and mortality in men. Arch Intern Med. 2009;169(22):2096–2101.

40. Libby P. Atherosclerosis: the new view. Sci Am. 2002;286:47–53.

41. Lusis AJ, Attie AD, Reue K. Metabolic syndrome: from epidemiology to systems biology. Nat Rev Genet. 2008;9(11):819–830.

42. Marshall SJ, Biddle SJH. The transtheoretical model of behavior change: a meta-analysis of applications to physical activity and exercise. Ann Behav Med. 2001;23(4):229–246.

43. Matthews CE, Jurj AL, Shu X, et al. Respond to "A Challenge for Physical Activity Epidemiology." Am J Epidemiol. 2007;165(12):1354–1355.

44. Myers J, Kaykha A, George S, et al. Fitness versus physical activity patterns in predicting mortality in men. Am J Med. 2004;117:912–918.

45. Centers for Disease Control and Prevention. National Health and Nutrition Examination Survey. Available at: http://www.cdc.gov/nchs/nhanes.htm.

46. National Institutes of Health. Available at: http:// www.nhlbi.nih.gov/health/dci/Diseases/ms/ms_ whatis.html.

47. Nicklas BJ, You T, Pahor M. Behavioural treatments for chronic systemic inflammation: effects of dietary weight loss and exercise training. Can Med Assoc J. 2005;172(9):1199–1209.

48. Noar SM, Benac CN, Harris MS. Does tailoring matter? Meta-analytic review of tailored print health behavior change interventions. Psychol Bull. 2007; 133(4):673–693.

49. Ornish D, Scherwitz LW, Billings JW, et al. Intensive lifestyle changes for reversal of coronary heart disease. JAMA. 1998;280:2001–2007.

50. Owen N, Healy GN, Matthews CE, et al. Too much sitting: the population health science of sedentary behavior. Exerc Sport Sci Rev. 2010;18(3):105–113.

51. Pangiota NM, Kipnis V, Thiebaut ACM, et al. Mediterranean dietary pattern and prediction of all cause mortality in a US population. Arch Intern Med. 2007;167:2461–2468.

52. Pescatello LS, Franklin BA, Fagard R, et al. American College of Sports Medicine position stand: exercise and hypertension. Med Sci Sports Exerc. 2004;36(3):533–553.

53. Preventive Medicine Research Institute. Available at: http://www.pmri.org.

54. Prochaska JO. Decision making in the transtheoretical model of behavior change. Med Decis Making. 2008;28:845–849.

55. Prochaska JO, DiClemente CC. Stages and processes of self-change in smoking: towards an integrative model of change. J Consult Clin Psychol. 1983;51(3): 390–395.

56. Rizvi AA. Type 2 diabetes: epidemiologic trends, evolving pathogenic concepts, and recent changes in therapeutic approach. South Med J. 2004;97(11): 1079–1087.

57. Sacks FM, Bray GA, Carey VJ, et al. Comparison of weight-loss diets with different compositions of fat, protein, and carbohydrates. N Engl J Med. 2009;360: 859–873.

58. Shai I, Schwarzfuchs D, Henkin Y, et al. Weight loss with a low carbohydrate, Mediterranean, or low fat diet. N Engl J Med. 2008;359:229–241.

59. Singh RB, Dubnov G, Niaz MA. Effect of an Indo-Mediterranean diet on progression of coronary artery disease in high-risk patients: a randomized single-blind trial. Lancet. 2002;360:1455–1461.

60. Sorace P, LaFontaine TP, Thomas TR. Know the risks: lifestyle management of dyslipidemia. Health Fit J. 2006;10:18–25.

61. Tate DF, Jeffery RW, Sherwood NE, et al. Long-term weight losses associated with prescription of higher physical activity goals. Are higher levels of physical activity protective against weight regain? Am J Clin Nutr. 2007;85(4):954–959.

62. Thomas TR, LaFontaine TP. Exercise, nutritional strategies, and lipoproteins. In: Roitman J, ed. Resource Manual for Guidelines for Exercise Testing and Prescription. Baltimore, MD: Lippincott Williams & Wilkins, 2001, pp. 294–301.

63. Thomas TR, Liu Y, Linden MA, et al. Interaction of exercise training and n-3 fatty acid supplementation on postprandial lipemia. Appl Physiol Nutr Metab. 2007;32:473–480.

64. Trost SG, Owen N, Bauman AE, et al. Correlates of adults' participation in physical activity: review and update. Med Sci Sports Exerc. 2002;34(12):1996–2001.

65. Ungvari Z, Parrado-Fernandez C, Csiszar A, et al. Mechanisms underlying caloric restriction and lifespan regulation: implications for vascular aging. Circ Res. 2008;102(5):519–528.

66. University of Michigan Integrative Medicine. Healing Foods Pyramid 2010. Available at: http://med.umich.edu/umim/food-pyramid/index.htm.

67. van Dam RM, Li T, Spiegelman D, et al. Combined impact of lifestyle factors on mortality: prospective cohort study in the US women. BMJ. 2008;337:1440–1447.

68. Wan WH, Powers As, Li J, et al. Effect of post-myocardial infarction exercise training on the renin-angiotensin-aldosterone system and cardiac function. Am J Med Sci. 2007;334:265–273.

69. Warren TY, Vaughn B, Hooker SP, et al. Sedentary behaviors increase risk of cardiovascular disease mortality in men. Med Sci Sports Exerc. 2010; 42(5):879–885.

70. Williams PT. Physical fitness and activity as separate heart disease risk factors; a meta-analysis. Med Sci Sports Exerc. 2001;33(5):754–761.

71. Williams PT, Stefanick ML, Vranizan KM, et al. The effects of weight loss by exercise or dieting on high-density lipoprotein (HDL) levels in men with low, intermediate, and normal-to-high HDL at baseline. Metabolism. 1994;43:917–924.

72. Wood PD, Stefanick ML, Williams PT, et al. The effects on plasma lipoproteins of a prudent weight-reducing diet, with or without exercise, in overweight men and women. N Engl J Med. 1991;325:461–466.

73. Yusuf S, Hawken S, Qunpuu S, et al. Effect of potentially modifiable risk factors associated with myocardial infarction in 52 countries (The INTERHEART Study and Control Study). Lancet. 2004;364:937–952.

74. Zieman SJ, Melenovsky V, Kass DA. Mechanisms, pathophysiology and therapy of arterial stiffness. Arterioslcler Thromb Vasc Biol. 2005;25:932–943.

General Guidelines for Resistance Exercise Training

Resistance training (RT) is a critical component of an evidence-based comprehensive exercise program for the prevention and management of chronic diseases. Resistance training is recognized as the primary means of increasing muscular hypertrophy, strength, power, and endurance. During the last two to three decades, a large body of literature has accumulated that supports the use of RT in virtually all populations including youth, healthy adults, elderly, and numerous clinical populations. Table A1 presents a summary of the documented benefits of RT.

TABLE A1	Evidence-based Effects of Resistance Training on Health and Fitness Variables

Variable	Magnitude of Effects
Muscle strength	+++*
Muscle size (hypertrophy)/lean body mass	+++
Percent body fat	++†
Bone mineral density	++
Insulin sensitivity	++
LDL-cholesterol	+‡
HDL-cholesterol	+
Triglycerides	+
Resting and exercise blood pressure	+
Physical working capacity	++
Maximal oxygen uptake	+
Submaximal endurance	++
Maximal endurance capacity	+
Basal metabolic rate	+
Health-related quality of life	++
Muscle power	+++
Sarcopenia	+++
Resting and exercise rate pressure product (HR × systolic BP/100)	+

LDL, Low-density lipoprotein; HDL, high-density lipoprotein; HR, heart rate; BP, blood pressure.

*Well-documented and observed outcome.

†Considerable evidence supports outcome.

‡Limited scientific evidence supports improvement in this variable as a consistent outcome.

Resistance training is now recommended by essentially all major exercise, health, and sports medicine organizations. A summary of the guidelines for RT from a representative sample of association adult guidelines for physical activity, exercise, and health is provided in Table A2.

TABLE A2 Guidelines for Resistance Training						
Association	Exercises (n)	Reps	Sets	Load	Frequency	Comment
AHA Cardiovascular Disease (12)	8–10	8–12 for <50–60 years of age and 10–15 for >50–60 years of age	1	30%–80%	2–3	30%–40% for upper body initially, 50%–60% for lower body. States that most studies used loads of 30%–80%
AHA Type 2 diabetes mellitus (6)	Not specified	8–10	2–4	Moderate to high	3	States that large group multijoint exercises preferred and using weight that cannot be lifted >8–10 reps.
ACSM Hypertension (7)	Not specified	NA	NA	NA	NA	RT should supplement endurance physical activity
ACSM Diabetes (1)	8–10	10–15	1	NA	2	Increased intensity of exercise, additional sets, or combinations of volume and intensity may produce more benefits and may be appropriate for some individuals
ACSM Bone health (3)	NA	NA	NA	Moderate to high in terms of bone loading	2–3	Intensity should be <60% for safety reason—but some higher intensity loading may be appropriate

TABLE

Guidelines for Resistance Training (continued)

Association	Exercises (n)	Reps	Sets	Load	Frequency	Comment
AHA/ACSM Healthy older adults (5)	8–10	8–12	1	Moderate to high	2+	Recommended two or more nonconsecutive days. Sets to volitional or substantial fatigue recommended
AACVPR Cardiac Patients (2)	8–10	12–15	1	30%–50% 1RM	2–3	Suggests using 11–13 RPE and states also that stable patients can be progressed toward higher intensity
DHHS Healthy Adults (11)	All major muscle groups	8–12	2–3	Moderate to high	2	Muscle-strengthening exercises should be performed to the point at which it would be difficult to do another repetition without help
AGS Older adults (4)	Not specified	10–15	NA	40-60% 1 RM > 60% as tolerated	2–3	Also recommended stretching 3–5 d/wk, three to five stretches per key muscle group, 20–30 seconds
ADA Diabetes (9)	All major muscle groups	8–10	3	8–10 reps maximum	3	Statement recommends progressing gradually to three sets

NA, not available; AHA, American Heart Association; ACSM, American College of Sports Medicine; AACVPR, American Association of Cardiovascular and Pulmonary Rehabilitation; DHHS, Department of Health and Human Services; AGS, American Geriatric Society; ADA, American Diabetes Association; RT, resistance training; 1RM, one repetition maximum; RPE, rating of perceived exertion; Reps, repetitions.

Resistance training involves the careful manipulation of many variables to optimize desired outcomes and health benefits. Two recent documents referenced below provide excellent information on planning and implementing a safe and effective RT program (8,10). Ratamess discusses the key variables that need to be manipulated systematically to develop an optimal RT program (8). This position statement of the American College of Sports Medicine discusses topics such as periodization, intensity or loading, volume, sets, repetitions, order of exercises, rest periods, and so forth, and how they need to be manipulated in order to optimize characteristics such as muscle hypertrophy, strength, and muscle endurance. The second reference is a recent textbook devoted specifically to the utilization of RT for special populations (10). It includes a compact disc that provides example plans and guidelines for developing an RT program for persons with numerous chronic diseases including types 1 and 2 diabetes, coronary heart disease, and obesity.

REFERENCES

1. Albright A, Franz M, Hornsby G, et al. Exercise and type 2 diabetes mellitus. Med Sci Sports Exerc. 2000;32:L1345–L1360.
2. American Association for Cardiovascular and Pulmonary Rehabilitation. Guidelines for Cardiac Rehabilitation and Secondary Prevention Programs. 4th Ed. Champaign, IL: Human Kinetics, 2004.
3. American College of Sports Medicine. Position stand. Physical activity and bone health. Med Sci Sports Exerc. 2004;36:1985–1996.
4. American Geriatrics Society Panel on Exercise and Osteoarthritis. Exercise prescription for older adults with osteoarthritis pain: consensus practice recommendations: a supplement to the AGS Clinical Practice Guidelines on the management of chronic pain in older adults. J Am Geriatr Soc. 2001;49:808–823.
5. Haskell WL, Lee IM, Pate RR, et al. Physical activity and public health. Circulation. 2007;116:1081–1093.
6. Marwick TR, Hordern MD, Miller T, et al. Exercise training for type 2 diabetes mellitus impact on cardiovascular risk. Circulation. 2009;119:3244–3262.
7. Pescatello LS, Franklin BA, Fagard R, et al. Exercise and hypertension. Med Sci Sports Exerc. 2004;36:533–553.
8. Ratamess NA, Alvar BA, Evetoch TK, et al. Progression models in resistance training for healthy adults. Med Sci Sports Exerc. 2009;41(3):687–708.
9. Sigal RJ, Wasserman DH, Kenny GP, et al. Physical activity/exercise and type 2 diabetes. Diabetes Care. 2004;27:2518–2539.
10. Swank AM, Hagerman P, eds. Resistance Training for Special Populations. Clifton Park, NY: Delmar Cengage Learning, 2010.
11. United States Department of Health and Human Services. 2008 Physical Activity Guidelines for Americans. Available at: 6-20-2010. http://www.health.gov/PAGuidelines/.
12. Williams MA, Haskell WL, Ades PA, et al. Resistance exercise in individuals with and without cardiovascular disease: 2007 update. Circulation. 2007;116:572–584.

Note: Page numbers followed by *f* indicates figure and those followed by *t* indicates table.